Emotions and Surgery in Britain, 1793–1912

•

In this innovative analytical account of the place of emotion and embodiment in nineteenth-century British surgery, Michael Brown examines the changing emotional dynamics of surgical culture for both surgeons and patients from the pre-anaesthetic era through the introduction of anaesthesia and antisepsis techniques. Drawing on diverse archival and published sources, Brown explores how an emotional regime of Romantic sensibility, in which emotions played a central role in the practice and experience of surgery, was superseded by one of scientific modernity, in which the emotions of both patient and practitioner were increasingly marginalised. Demonstrating that the cultures of contemporary surgery and the emotional identities of its practitioners have their origins in the cultural and conceptual upheavals of the later nineteenth century, this book challenges us to question our perception of the pre-anaesthetic period as an era of bloody brutality and casual cruelty. This title is also available as open access.

MICHAEL BROWN is a historian at Lancaster University. He is co-editor of *Martial Masculinities: Experiencing and Imagining the Military in the Long Nineteenth Century* (2019) and author of *Performing Medicine: Medical Culture and Identity in Provincial England, c.1760–1850* (2011), as well as numerous articles on the history of medicine, war, gender, and emotion. Between 2016 and 2021 he was the Principal Investigator on the Wellcome Trust Investigator Award project Surgery & Emotion (108667/Z/15/Z).

Emotions and Surgery in Britain, 1793–1912

Michael Brown

Lancaster University

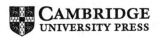
CAMBRIDGE
UNIVERSITY PRESS

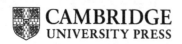

Shaftesbury Road, Cambridge CB2 8EA, United Kingdom

One Liberty Plaza, 20th Floor, New York, NY 10006, USA

477 Williamstown Road, Port Melbourne, VIC 3207, Australia

314–321, 3rd Floor, Plot 3, Splendor Forum, Jasola District Centre, New Delhi – 110025, India

103 Penang Road, #05–06/07, Visioncrest Commercial, Singapore 238467

Cambridge University Press is part of Cambridge University Press & Assessment, a department of the University of Cambridge.

We share the University's mission to contribute to society through the pursuit of education, learning and research at the highest international levels of excellence.

www.cambridge.org
Information on this title: www.cambridge.org/9781108792233

DOI: 10.1017/9781108877237

First published 2023
First paperback edition 2025

A catalogue record for this publication is available from the British Library

Library of Congress Cataloging-in-Publication data
Names: Brown, Michael, 1977– author.
Title: Emotions and surgery in Britain, 1793–1912 / Michael Brown.
Description: Cambridge, United Kingdom ; New York, NY :
Cambridge University Press, 2022. | Includes bibliographical references and index.
Identifiers: LCCN 2022023388 | ISBN 9781108834841 (hardback) |
ISBN 9781108877237 (ebook)
Subjects: MESH: General Surgery – history | Emotions | Surgeons – psychology |
History, 18th Century | History, 19th Century | History, 20th Century | United Kingdom |
BISAC: MEDICAL / History
Classification: LCC RD27.3.G5 | NLM WO 11 FA1 | DDC 617.0941–dc23/eng/20220819
LC record available at https://lccn.loc.gov/2022023388

ISBN   978-1-108-83484-1   Hardback
ISBN   978-1-108-79223-3   Paperback

Cambridge University Press & Assessment has no responsibility for the persistence or accuracy of URLs for external or third-party internet websites referred to in this publication and does not guarantee that any content on such websites is, or will remain, accurate or appropriate.

For Joanne, my love and my life

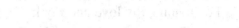

Contents

Figures

Acknowledgements

This book has come into being in what might fairly be described as 'interesting times'. I began work on it shortly after meeting someone who would very soon become my wife. We moved in together, and now share everything in our lives, including our research. This blessing has made the experience of researching and writing *Emotions and Surgery* all the more joyous. But there have been challenges too. Somewhat ironically, the writing of Chapter 5 coincided with my first ever experience of surgery under general anaesthetic. While this is not something I would care to repeat, I would like to thank the staff at Stoke Mandeville Hospital, particularly my surgeon, Aman Sethi, and my anaesthetist, Rich Kaye, for facilitating this enlightening perspective on surgery and emotion without my having to endure the pain, suffering, and anxiety that so many of those whose stories are featured in this book sadly did. To add to this, a not inconsiderable proportion of *Emotions and Surgery* has been written during the COVID-19 pandemic. Even as I type this, things are by no means over, and we face continued uncertainty about the duration and future severity of the pandemic. It might seem insensitive to even mention the relatively minor personal inconveniences caused by COVID-19 when so many people have lost their lives. In any case, my research was not as badly impacted as it might have been, largely because much of the relevant archival material had been compiled and processed before March 2020. Nonetheless, the anxieties produced by the pandemic, and the limitations it imposed, are baked into this book, albeit in ways so subtle and inconsequential that I hope no one will notice. Indeed, if anything, *Emotions and Surgery* and my research more generally have provided a valuable emotional and intellectual refuge from the frequently depressing world of politics and global affairs over the last five or so years.

As regards the genesis of this book, my first, and deepest, debt of gratitude is to the Wellcome Trust, which funded my Investigator Award project, Surgery & Emotion (108667/Z/15/Z). I am honoured that the Trust thought highly enough of my research plans to fund me, initially for four years, subsequently for five. Its support has provided me with an invaluable opportunity to undertake the research that I wanted to pursue and, ultimately, to write this book. Its incredibly generous Open Access funding scheme also means that *Emotions and Surgery*, and all the other research outputs from the project, are available for anyone to read, free of charge; this is an incalculable privilege. But the Trust did not just fund me. One of the joys of being Principal Investigator on the Surgery & Emotion project has been working with an incredibly talented and personable team on a range of activities, from policy and publications to public engagement. I would like to thank Agnes Arnold-Forster, James Kennaway, Alison Moulds, David Saunders, and Lauren Ryall-Waite for all their hard work on the project and for making the last few years as enjoyable as they have been. It has been a pleasure to work with you all, and wonderful to see you go on to such great things.

For the last decade and more, I have had the great privilege of being based in what is currently the School of Humanities and Social Sciences at the University of Roehampton. Roehampton has been my academic home since before my first book was published and it is a pleasure to reflect on how much I have flourished there. While I was undertaking the initial research for the Surgery & Emotion project, I was less involved in the day-to-day activities of the School than before. Nonetheless, I always felt deeply connected to the School and proud to fly the flag for Roehampton at the various events I organised and participated in. I have come to resume my teaching and leadership duties at a difficult time for the sector in general, and the School in particular. However, I believe that there is no finer place in the country to teach and learn history, nor do I believe that anyone could be as blessed as I am with such friendly, supportive, capable, and committed colleagues, or such curious, engaged, and resourceful students.

A book like *Emotions and Surgery*, which draws heavily upon archival sources, would not have been possible were it not for the tireless work of librarians and archivists in accessioning, maintaining, and making accessible the requisite research materials. I am therefore hugely grateful to staff at a number of different libraries and archives, including the University of Roehampton Library, the British Library, the National Archives, the Wellcome Library, the National Library of Scotland, and the Library and Archive of the Royal College of Surgeons of Edinburgh. However, my greatest single vote of thanks must go to the staff of the Library of the Royal College of Surgeons of England, who, for several months in a row, handled my incessant requests for material with unceasing professionalism, efficiency, and good grace. I hope this book has done justice to the materials you work so hard to preserve for posterity.

I enjoy the great fortune of being part of a wider historical research community, and to count among my friends and colleagues those whose opinions and insights I value highly. Due to the pressures of the COVID-19 pandemic on everyone's workloads, I have been less inclined to pass my work to already overburdened colleagues than might otherwise have been the case. However,

I would like to thank those who have been kind enough to read all, or parts, of *Emotions and Surgery* before publication. These include Joanne Begiato, Ian Burney, John Collins, James Kennaway, Allister Neher, and Matthew Roberts. I would also like to thank the two anonymous reviewers of the initial proposal, and the sole reviewer of the final manuscript, for the remarkable speed, depth, and generosity of their readings. Beyond those who have read the manuscript, I would like to thank those colleagues and friends with whom I have discussed the project over the years, and who attended the various seminars and lectures I have given about my research. Your questions, comments, and reflections have helped to shape my thinking in profound ways. There are too many of you to name and it would be futile of me to try and recall the myriad influences on my work. However, I am especially grateful for the many stimulating and provocative conversations I have had with Chris Lawrence, my mentor from my days as a master's student and, in more recent years, a dear friend. My thoughts are with you and Jan in difficult times.

I am so glad that *Emotions and Surgery* has found its home at Cambridge University Press, and special thanks must go to the senior commissioning editor for the history of science and medicine, Lucy Rhymer. Lucy has been incredibly supportive of this book ever since I first pitched the idea for it at the Society for the Social History of Medicine annual conference at Liverpool in 2018. Together with Emily Plater and Natasha Whelan, she has eased its journey to production with consummate professionalism.

Writing a book, as anyone who has done it knows, requires emotional as much as academic resources. In this sense I am enormously fortunate to enjoy the love, support, and encouragement of my family. Thanks go to my brother, Andrew, and his family, and to my parents, Monika and Stephen. They have been my inspiration throughout life: intelligent, perceptive, generous, and unstintingly kind. They have supported me with unwavering enthusiasm throughout my career in academia, consoling me in difficult times and celebrating my achievements with love and pride. I only hope I can live up to their example.

Finally, I must acknowledge the incalculable emotional debt that I owe to my wife, Joanne, and my stepson, Gabriel. It was in 2015, when I was awarded the grant that led to this book, that I first met Joanne. I have many cherished memories of those early months, not the least of which involves the two of us, after my funding interview with the Wellcome Trust, sitting in the sunshine outside the Jeremy Bentham pub, little knowing what would follow or where it would lead. It is astonishing to me that so much life can be crammed into the time it takes to write a book. But so it has been. In those six years, Gabriel has grown from a boy into a man, and our life as a family has blossomed. Joanne is not only my friend, my lover, and my confidante, but also my editor, my critic, and my intellectual guide to the history of emotions. Anyone who has read our respective works will be able to trace the story of our relationship through our acknowledgements. I can only beg their indulgence on this occasion and promise that the next book we write will be together and, as such, we will have to think of someone else to dedicate it to. Until that time, this book, as with everything else I have, is for her.

Note on the Text

Emotions and Surgery refers to a number of individuals who, like Charles Bell, Benjamin Brodie, or Astley Cooper, received knighthoods or baronetcies, or who, in the case of Joseph Lister, were made peers of the realm. However, for the sake of consistency and clarity, I have decided not to use the titles 'Sir' or 'Lord' in the text, given that this book covers the period both before and after these titles were bestowed.

For ease of identification, life dates are provided for named individuals at · the first mention in the body text. I have tried to do this for as many people as possible, but clear identities, let alone life dates, have not been possible to establish for everyone mentioned.

This book makes extensive use of manuscript sources, such as letters, diaries, and casebooks, in which spelling and punctuation do not necessarily conform to modern standard practice. These are presented unaltered, and clarification is provided only in cases where confusion might otherwise result.

Abbreviations

CAS-C	Cumbria Archives Service, Carlisle
NA	National Archives, London
NLS	National Library of Scotland, Edinburgh
ODNB	*Oxford Dictionary of National Biography*
RCSE	Royal College of Surgeons of England, London
RCSEd	Royal College of Surgeons of Edinburgh
WL	Wellcome Library, London

Introduction

A 'Black Whirlwind of Emotion': George Wilson's Surgery

In 1856, George Wilson (1818–59), then Professor of Technology at the University of Edinburgh, wrote a letter to the physician James Young Simpson (1811–70) in which he described the amputation of his foot by the surgeon James Syme (1799–1870) in 1842. Wilson composed this letter some ten years after the introduction of surgical anaesthesia about a procedure that had taken place four years prior to it. For Simpson, it therefore provided incontrovertible evidence for the value of anaesthesia 'from the patient's point of view', by describing, in highly eloquent and evocative terms, the experiential terrors of the recent past.[1] In his letter, Wilson recalled that, having been informed of the need for amputation:

I at once agreed to submit to the operation, but asked a week to prepare for it, not with the slightest expectation that the disease would take a favourable turn in the interval, or that the anticipated horrors of the operation would become less appalling by reflection upon them, but simply because it was so probable that the operation would be followed by a fatal issue, that I wished to prepare for death and what lies beyond it, whilst my faculties were clear and my emotions were comparatively undisturbed.[2]

'Before the days of anaesthetics', he wrote, 'a patient preparing for an amputation was like a condemned criminal preparing for execution'. He 'counted the days' and 'the hours' until the appointed moment arrived. He anxiously awaited the arrival of the surgeon, listening for the 'pull at the door bell', his 'foot on the stair', and 'his step in the room'. He watched in agonised anticipation at the 'production of his dreaded instruments', and attended the surgeon's 'few grave words', before he 'helplessly gave himself up to the cruel knife'.[3] As to the amputation itself:

---

[1] James Young Simpson, *Acupressure: A New Method of Arresting Surgical Haemorrhage* (Edinburgh: Adam and Charles Black, 1864), p. 566.

[2] Simpson, *Acupressure*, pp. 556–7.

[3] Simpson, *Acupressure*, p. 557.

Of the agony it occasioned I will say nothing. Suffering so great as I underwent cannot be expressed in words, and thus fortunately cannot be recalled. The particular pangs are now forgotten; but the black whirlwind of emotion, the horror of great darkness, and the sense of desertion by God and man, bordering close upon despair, which swept through my mind and overwhelmed my heart, I can never forget, however gladly I would do so.[4]

Wilson's account of his operation was conditioned by the intervening introduction of anaesthesia, and by the relative painlessness of contemporary operative surgery. Indeed, this was the very point of his letter, the reason that Simpson, who had identified the anaesthetic properties of chloroform in 1847, had solicited it in the first place. Perhaps because of this, Wilson expressed concern that Simpson might think his 'confessions exaggerated'. He assured him that they were not. These were 'not pleasant remembrances', he maintained, and 'For a long time they haunted me'. While they 'cannot bring back the suffering attending the events [...], they can occasion a suffering of their own, and be the cause of a disquiet which favours neither bodily nor mental health'. 'From memories of this kind', Wilson observed, 'those subjects of operations who receive chloroform are of course free', and he confessed that if there were 'some Lethean draught' to 'erase the memories I speak of, I would drink it, for they are easily brought back and they are never welcome'.[5]

Rare though such first-hand accounts might be, Wilson's letter can be taken as fairly representative of the experience of pre-anaesthetic surgery from the patient's perspective. After all, while clearly of deep personal significance, his operation, an amputation of the foot at the ankle, was neither the most technically demanding nor the most daunting of early nineteenth-century surgical procedures. In this regard, what is most remarkable about Wilson's letter is its relative lack of emphasis on the pain of the operation when compared to his vivid description of the emotional distress and mental turmoil that it had caused and, indeed, continued to cause. If the physical agonies of the procedure remained ineffable and unrecoverable, then the 'black whirlwind of emotion' that 'swept through' his mind and 'overwhelmed' his heart was, by contrast, indelible.[6]

In many ways, Wilson's recollections of his operation work contrary to our own cultural memory of the pre-anaesthetic era. If for him the emotions of the experience were far more enduring than the pain itself, for us it is the physical agonies of pre-anaesthetic surgery, rather than its emotional dynamics, that haunt our collective memory. This is not to say that the emotional sufferings of the pre-anaesthetic patient are entirely absent from popular consciousness. But, to modern minds habitually accustomed to analgesics, it is that most

[4] Simpson, *Acupressure*, p. 568.
[5] Simpson, *Acupressure*, pp. 568–9.
[6] For more discussion of the historical recollection of pain, see Chapter 3.

inconceivable of sensations, the pain of being sliced open and sawn apart while conscious, that captures the imagination most forcibly.

This book reorientates our cultural, intellectual, and imaginative perspective by putting emotions back at the heart of the history of surgery. It maps the emotional landscape of British surgery from the later eighteenth to the early twentieth centuries, analysing the changing place of emotions within surgical culture, practice, and experience. Although largely concerned with the professional identity and ideology of surgeons, it also seeks to comprehend the patient, not only in terms of experience and agency, but also as regards their shifting ontological status within surgical cosmology.[7] In short, it traces the elaboration of an 'emotional regime' of Romantic sensibility within British surgery, before charting its gradual eclipse, from around the middle of the nineteenth century, by a new emotional regime of scientific modernity.[8] It attributes this shift in emotional regimes to the rise of medical and surgical utilitarianism and the advent of anaesthesia, and locates its ultimate realisation in the aetiological reductionism and techno-scientific rationalism of Joseph Lister's (1827–1912) antisepsis. It demonstrates the profound impact that this shift in emotional regimes had on contemporary surgical culture, and explores the ways in which it reconfigured relations between surgeons and their patients, before ending with a consideration of its legacy for modern-day surgery.

Historiography and Context

Emotions and Surgery thus provides an analytical account of the history of emotions applied to British surgery in the long nineteenth century. During the last ten to fifteen years, the history of emotions has grown into one of the most flourishing and exciting fields of historical scholarship. The roots of this approach lie in the work of Carol and Peter Stearns in the 1980s, although they can probably be traced back even further to the abortive study of *mentalités* by the French *Annales* school, or to the historical sociology of Norbert Elias.[9] However, the history of emotions really came to fruition in the late 1990s and early 2000s when, building on the Stearns' model of 'emotionology', scholars such as William Reddy and Barbara Rosenwein fabricated a theoretical

---

[7] This word is chosen to suggest the parallels with Nicholas D. Jewson's landmark article 'The Disappearance of the Sick Man from Medical Cosmology, 1770–1870', *Sociology* 10 (1976), 225–44.

[8] William Reddy, *The Navigation of Feeling. A Framework for the History of the Emotions* (Cambridge, UK: Cambridge University Press, 2001), pp. 124–6.

[9] For example, see Carol Z. Stearns and Peter N. Stearns, *Anger: The Struggle for Emotional Control in America's History* (Chicago: Chicago University Press, 1986); Norbert Elias, *The Civilising Process: Sociogenetic and Psychogenetic Investigations* (Oxford: Blackwell, 1994 [1939]). For a historical account of the history of emotions, see Rob Boddice, *The History of Emotions* (Manchester: Manchester University Press, 2018), ch. 1.

framework for studying the affective cultures of the past with their respective concepts of emotional regimes and 'emotional communities'.[10] Since then, there has been a good deal of theoretical and terminological debate, as scholars have sought to nuance existing models, or develop new ones.[11] This is especially true of recent years, as the history of emotions has gained sufficient intellectual self-confidence to expand into new areas of study and to engage with other disciplines.[12] Meanwhile, beyond the theoretical debates, numerous scholars have sought to 'do' the history of emotions by applying these conceptual frameworks to the archival record, using feeling as an interpretive prism though which to rethink our understanding of past human relations.[13]

The histories of medicine and science have not, perhaps, been shaped by the emotions to the extent that other areas, such as histories of the family and domesticity, have been.[14] Indeed, in his 2009 introduction to a special section of the journal *Isis* on 'The Emotional Economy of Science', Paul White suggested that, far from following the 'emotional turn', historians of modern science were heading in the opposite direction, towards a study of objectivity.[15] White was one of the earliest historians of science and medicine to take the emotions seriously, as was his fellow contributor to this special issue, Fay Bound Alberti. In her article, Bound Alberti analyses the death of the Scottish

---

[10] Peter N. Stearns and Carol Z. Stearns, 'Emotionology: Clarifying the History of Emotions and Emotional Standards', *American Historical Review* 90:4 (1985), 813–36; Reddy, *Navigation*; Barbara H. Rosenwein, *Emotional Communities in the Early Middle Ages* (Ithaca, NY: Cornell University Press, 2006).

[11] For example, see Thomas Dixon, '"Emotion": The History of a Keyword in Crisis', *Emotion Review* 4:4 (2012), 338–44; Rob Boddice (ed.), *A History of Feelings* (London: Reaktion, 2019); Katie Barclay, *Caritas: Neighbourly Love and the Early Modern Self* (Oxford: Oxford University Press, 2021).

[12] For example, see Stephanie Downes, Sally Holloway, and Sarah Randles (eds), *Feeling Things: Objects and Emotions through History* (Oxford: Oxford University Press, 2018); Dolores Martín-Moruno and Beatriz Pichel (eds), *Emotional Bodies: The Historical Performativity of Emotions* (Urbana: University of Illinois Press, 2019); Mark Smith and Rob Boddice, *Emotions, Sense, Experience* (Cambridge, UK: Cambridge University Press, 2020).

[13] For example, see Nicole Eustace, *Passion Is the Gale: Emotion and the Coming of the American Revolution* (Chapel Hill: University of North Carolina Press, 2008); Joanne Bailey, *Parenting in England, 1760–1850: Emotion, Identity and Generation* (Oxford: Oxford University Press, 2012); Claire Langhamer, *The English in Love: The Intimate Story of an Emotional Revolution* (Oxford: Oxford University Press, 2013); Katie Barclay, *Men on Trial: Performing Emotion, Embodiment and Identity in Ireland, 1800–45* (Manchester: Manchester University Press, 2018); Sally Holloway, *The Game of Love in Georgian England: Courtship, Emotions and Material Culture* (Oxford: Oxford University Press, 2018); Joanne Begiato, *Manliness in Britain, 1760–1900: Bodies, Emotion, and Material Culture* (Manchester: Manchester University Press, 2020).

[14] For example, see Susan Broomhall (ed.), *Emotions in the Household, 1200–1900* (Basingstoke: Palgrave Macmillan, 2008).

[15] Paul White, 'Introduction: The Emotional Economy of Science', *Isis* 100:4 (2009), 792–7, p. 792. White refers here, among other things, to Lorraine Daston and Peter Galison, *Objectivity* (New York: Zone Books, 2007).

surgeon-anatomist John Hunter (1728–93), caused, according to his contemporaries, by heart failure induced by 'affections of the mind', to highlight the intimate relationship between mind and body in pre-modern medicine and to assert the powerful role that emotions played in shaping ideas about health, disease, and embodied experience.[16]

Bound Alberti's earlier collection, *Medicine, Emotion and Disease, 1700–1950* (2006), is often cited as a seminal text for the entwined histories of emotion, medicine, and the body.[17] It certainly serves as a snapshot in time, its list of contributors including scholars, such as Thomas Dixon, Rhodri Hayward, and Bound Alberti herself, who would soon be associated with the Centre for the History of Emotions at Queen Mary University of London. This was founded in 2008 as the first dedicated research centre for the historical study of the emotions in the United Kingdom. While this development certainly helped to drive interest in the history of emotions in this country, it has taken some time for historians of medicine as a whole to pay serious attention to the emotions. This is now beginning to change, and recent years have seen the publication of several important works, such as those by Mark Neuendorf on psychiatric reform or Rob Boddice on the emotional politics of vivisection.[18] Boddice's valuable research on the concept of sympathy within late nineteenth-century medicine and science resonates with some of the arguments developed later in this book, even if my understanding of the earlier period is somewhat at odds with his.[19] Furthermore, the somatic turn in the history of emotions provides ever greater opportunities for historians of medicine to make a significant contribution to the field, while historians from other specialities are increasingly bringing emotions, medicine, and the body together in productive ways.[20] *Emotions and Surgery* pushes this project forward, demonstrating the value of an emotions-orientated approach to the

[16] Fay Bound Alberti, 'Bodies, Hearts, and Minds: Why Emotions Matter to Historians of Science and Medicine', *Isis* 100:4 (2009), 798–810. See also Bound Alberti, *Matters of the Heart: History, Medicine and Emotion* (Oxford: Oxford University Press, 2010), ch. 2.

[17] Fay Bound Alberti (ed.), *Medicine, Emotion and Disease, 1700–1950* (Basingstoke: Palgrave Macmillan, 2006).

[18] Rob Boddice, *The Science of Sympathy: Morality, Evolution and Victorian Civilization* (Urbana: University of Illinois Press, 2016); Boddice, *The Humane Professions: The Defence of Experimental Medicine, 1876–1914* (Cambridge, UK: Cambridge University Press, 2020); Mark Neuendorf, *Emotions and the Making of Psychiatric Reform in Britain, c. 1770–1820* (London: Palgrave Macmillan, 2021).

[19] This is especially true of his characterisation of feeling and gender in the early nineteenth century: Boddice, *Sympathy*, pp. 44–5.

[20] Martín-Moruno and Pichel (eds), *Emotional Bodies*. The latter is particularly true of recent literature on the First World War, e.g. Ana Carden-Coyne, *The Politics of Wounds: Military Patients and Medical Power in the First World War* (Oxford: Oxford University Press, 2014); Jessica Meyer, *An Equal Burden: The Men of the Royal Army Medical Corps in the First World War* (Oxford: Oxford University Press, 2019).

history of surgery by showing how a sensitivity to the emotions enables us to reframe our perspective and question some of our most basic historical assumptions.

The history of pain might be regarded as a cognate of the history of emotions.[21] The intimate connection between the histories of surgery, pain, and the emotions is intuitively understood, especially because surgical treatment, both operative and therapeutic, has historically involved a considerable amount of pain, and because, as Wilson's testimony suggests, the 'conquest' of surgical pain in the form of anaesthesia had profound implications for surgery's emotional dynamics. *Emotions and Surgery* is not conceived as a surgical history of pain, per se. Nonetheless, pain features prominently in our discussion of pre-anaesthetic surgery, and comes into particularly sharp relief in the debates surrounding its prospective elimination. *Emotions and Surgery* also elaborates Joanna Bourke's suggestion that the traditional perception of pre-modern physicians and surgeons as uncaring and indifferent to pain is inaccurate.[22] It shows that sympathy played a far more important practical, social, and rhetorical function within pre-modern surgical practice than has generally been recognised.

As well as drawing on a rich vein of scholarship in the history of emotions, *Emotions and Surgery* is also firmly situated within the history and historiography of surgery. It is not unreasonable to suggest that the history of surgery has traditionally been something of a poor relation to the history of medicine, at least in terms of scale. Like much early work in the history of medicine, the history of surgery was once dominated by heroic accounts of innovation and progress.[23] This is perhaps even more true of surgery than of medicine, given the profession's enduring myth of a meteoric ascent from barbers to brain surgeons. As we shall see, this myth was largely constructed in the nineteenth century, when surgeons pointed to the achievements of pathological anatomy, anaesthesia, and antisepsis, innovations that found few rivals in the world of medicine, as evidence of the intellectual superiority and practical utility of their science. However, if popular histories of surgery still tend towards mythic triumphalism, the scholarly historiography of surgery has developed in sophistication and nuance since the early 1990s. This is due in no small part to the work of Christopher Lawrence, whose publications, including the path-breaking collection *Medical Theory, Surgical Practice:*

[21] For an overlap in terms of concepts and personnel, see Rob Boddice (ed.), *Pain and Emotion in Modern History* (Basingstoke: Palgrave Macmillan, 2014).
[22] Joanna Bourke, *The Story of Pain: From Prayers to Painkillers* (Oxford: Oxford University Press, 2014), ch. 8.
[23] For example, see Owen D. Wangensteen and Sarah D. Wangensteen, *The Rise of Surgery: From Empiric Craft to Scientific Discipline* (Minneapolis: University of Minnesota Press, 1978).

Studies in the History of Surgery (1992), opened up a whole new approach to the subject.[24] In time, this breach in the walls of surgical myth has been exploited by a number of scholars, including Carin Berkowitz, Clare Brock, Sally Frampton, and Thomas Schlich, all of whom have produced important accounts of surgical thought and practice from the late eighteenth to the early twentieth centuries.[25]

In drawing upon the historiography of surgery, this book is specifically indebted to two key studies. The first of these is Peter Stanley's *For Fear of Pain: British Surgery, 1790–1850* (2003). Stanley's book is a peerless general account of British surgery in the early nineteenth century, which uses an impressive range of sources to tell the history of surgeons and their patients in the 'final decades of painful surgery'.[26] However, Stanley's book, rich in content though it is, is a broad historical survey of the period whose approach is more descriptive than analytical, and more synoptic than specific. By contrast, *Emotions and Surgery* is focused on the particular role played by emotion in shaping surgical practice, identity, and experience. Unlike Stanley's book, it moves beyond the advent of anaesthesia to consider how the emotional landscape of surgery was reshaped by the epistemological upheavals of the late nineteenth century. Most importantly, *Emotions and Surgery* provides a rigorously analytical, interpretive, and explicatory account of the rise and fall of one surgical emotional regime and its supersession by another, situating these huge transformations within shifting constellations of social thought and cultural practice. The second book to which *Emotions and Surgery* speaks most directly is Lynda Payne's *With Words and Knives: Learning Medical Dispassion in Early Modern England* (2007). There is no need to say too much about the interpretive differences between our two books here, as these are discussed in detail in Chapter 2. Suffice it to say that whereas Payne emphasises the quality of surgical dispassion, a self-conscious act of emotional distancing from the sufferings of the patient, and presents this as the timeless quality of the surgical operator, I emphasise the historical mutability and contingency of surgical emotions, and put much greater emphasis on the place of emotional intersubjectivity within

---

[24] Christopher Lawrence (ed.), *Medical Theory, Surgical Practice: Studies in the History of Surgery* (London: Routledge, 1992). See also Roger Cooter, *Surgery and Society in Peace and War: Orthopaedics and the Organization of Modern Medicine, 1880–1948* (Basingstoke: Palgrave Macmillan, 1993).

[25] Thomas Schlich, *The Origins of Transplant Surgery. Surgery and Laboratory Science, 1880–1930* (Rochester, NY: University of Rochester Press, 2010); Carin Berkowitz, *Charles Bell and the Anatomy of Reform* (Chicago: Chicago University Press, 2015); Claire Brock, *British Women Surgeons and Their Patients, 1860–1918* (Cambridge, UK: Cambridge University Press, 2017); Sally Frampton, *Belly-Rippers, Surgical Innovation and the Ovariotomy Controversy* (London: Palgrave Macmillan, 2018).

[26] Peter Stanley, *For Fear of Pain: British Surgery, 1790–1850* (Amsterdam: Rodopi, 2003), p. 8.

the cultures of Romantic surgery.[27] And yet, despite the differences between our two approaches and arguments, and despite the fact that *With Words and Knives* is not a history of the emotions as conventionally conceived, it is important to acknowledge the significance of Payne's work in exploring the role of emotions in surgery, and in demonstrating what it can add to historical understanding.

Chronology and Concepts

Emotions and Surgery covers a period of huge social, cultural, and intellectual transformation. It begins in 1793, the year of John Hunter's death. As we shall see in Chapter 1, Hunter exerted a profound influence on early nineteenth-century surgery and his work was integral to the self-fashioning of surgeons as men of scientific credibility and social respectability. But, while Hunter's legacy lived on, his death also marked a shift in surgical culture. Payne suggests that Hunter cultivated a 'necessary inhumanity' in his emotional relationship with patients.[28] While there is reason to question how common this was among the practitioners of the later eighteenth century, what is certain is that the 1790s saw the rise of a new generation of surgeons who eschewed emotional dispassion, emphasising instead the importance of sympathy and compassion, and the necessity for effecting an emotional engagement with patients.[29] This marked the birth of what I call Romantic surgery. One of its early leading lights, arguably its founder, was the Scottish surgeon John Bell (1763–1820). Bell played a prominent role in constructing surgery as an emotionally 'authentic' science, one defined by its embodied qualities and by the surgeon's routine exposure to the extremes of pain, suffering, and distress.[30] He published his first major surgical text, the *Anatomy of the Bones, Muscles and Joints*, in 1793, which was also the same year as the start of war with France, a conflict that would continue, on and off, for over twenty years, and would cast a long shadow over early nineteenth-century Europe. Although *Emotions and Surgery* is not explicitly concerned with the practice of military surgery, it shows that war shaped the cultures and values of nineteenth-century surgery as a whole, a point that has been expounded in more detail elsewhere.[31]

---

[27] Lynda Payne, *With Words and Knives: Learning Medical Dispassion in Early Modern England* (Aldershot: Ashgate, 2007), pp. 1–2.

[28] Payne, *Words*, pp. 2, 6–7.

[29] Indeed, Payne suggests a similar model even for eighteenth-century surgeons like Percivall Pott. Lynda Payne, *The Best Surgeon in England: Percivall Pott, 1713–88* (New York: Peter Lang, 2017), p. 2.

[30] Michael Brown, 'Surgery, Identity and Embodied Emotion: John Bell, James Gregory and the Edinburgh "Medical War"', *History* 104:359 (2019), 19–41.

[31] Michael Brown, '"Like a Devoted Army": Medicine, Heroic Masculinity, and the Military Paradigm in Victorian Britain', *Journal of British Studies* 49:3 (2010), 592–622; Brown,

Emotions and Surgery begins by exploring the cultures of Romantic surgery and delineating the figure of the Romantic surgeon (as well as the Romantic patient). It is therefore imperative to clarify what I mean by the term 'Romantic'. Romanticism is a capacious concept that has found greater application in literary studies than in history. Indeed, it is rare to find historians using Romanticism as a chronological signifier at all. At the most general level, Romanticism can be defined as a cultural, intellectual, and artistic movement that originated in the very late eighteenth century and whose influence continued until around the middle of the nineteenth. While it is often seen as a reaction to Enlightenment rationalism, Romanticism displayed many marked continuities with earlier cultural forms, notably sensibility, that openness to the feelings of others that sentimental moral philosophers argued might regulate interpersonal conduct and improve social relations.[32] However, Romanticism reconfigured sensibility in distinct and important ways.[33] For instance, it devoted particular sentimental attention to the 'dependent', including women, children, animals, and the enslaved.[34] It also turned the emotional gaze inwards, lauding emotional introspection and self-reflection, and laying the groundwork for modern notions of psychic interiority.[35] Likewise, it placed great emphasis on emotional *experience*. Whether it be through an encounter with the natural world, the reading of a novel or poem, or an exposure to suffering, experience and introspection enabled the cultivation of a 'heartfelt' emotional authenticity that was held to be a hallmark of personal nobility, and that distinguished Romantic sensibility from the supposedly contrived and mannered artifice of the earlier period.[36]

'Wounds and Wonder: Emotion, Imagination, and War in the Cultures of Romantic Surgery', *Journal for Eighteenth-Century Studies* 43:2 (2020), 239–59; Christopher Lawrence and Michael Brown, 'Quintessentially Modern Heroes: Surgeons, Explorers, and Empire, c.1840–1914', *Journal of Social History* 50:1 (2016), 148–78.

[32] Norman S. Fiering, 'Irresistible Compassion: An Aspect of Eighteenth-Century Sympathy and Humanitarianism', *Journal of the History of Ideas* 37:2 (1976), 195–218; G. J. Barker-Benfield, *The Culture of Sensibility: Sex and Society in Eighteenth-Century Britain* (Chicago: Chicago University Press, 1992).

[33] Julie Ellison, 'Sensibility', in Joel Faflak and Julia M. Wright (eds), *A Handbook of Romanticism Studies* (Chichester: Wiley, 2012), 37–53.

[34] Debbie Lee, *Slavery and the Romantic Imagination* (Philadelphia: University of Pennsylvania Press, 2002); David Perkins, *Romanticism and Animal Rights* (Cambridge, UK: Cambridge University Press, 2003); Bailey, *Parenting*.

[35] For the move to an increasingly introspective, 'inwardly turned' self in the later eighteenth century, see Dror Wahrman, *The Making of the Modern Self: Identity and Culture in Eighteenth-Century England* (New Haven: Yale University Press, 2004).

[36] For the importance of emotional authenticity within Romantic sensibility, see Lionel Trilling, *Sincerity and Authenticity* (London: Oxford University Press, 1972); Tim Miles and Kerry Sinanan (eds), *Romanticism, Sincerity and Authenticity* (Basingstoke: Palgrave, 2010). On the issues of sensibility and artifice, see Markman Ellis, *The Politics of Sensibility: Race, Gender and Commerce in the Sentimental Novel* (Cambridge, UK: Cambridge University Press, 1996).

The relationship between Romanticism and science has been widely acknowledged.[37] This is particularly true for gas chemistry.[38] The English chemist Humphry Davy (1778–1829) was perhaps the quintessential Romantic man of science, melding sublime emotional experience and rigorous self-experimentation with a literary sensibility.[39] Likewise, Davy's friend Samuel Taylor Coleridge (1772–1834) combined the writing of Romantic poetry with scientific and philosophical pursuits.[40] Elsewhere, scholars have considered Romanticism in relation to the sciences of life, including debates over vitalism and the development of transcendental anatomy and cell theory.[41] And yet, with remarkably few exceptions, no study has yet addressed the impact of Romanticism on quotidian medical and surgical practice.[42] *Emotions and Surgery* does just this, demonstrating the profoundly important ways in which Romantic sensibility informed surgical practice and shaped surgical culture, both at the level of rhetoric and self-presentation, and at that of experience and identity. It argues that sympathy, compassion, and emotional intersubjectivity were central to an idealised Romantic relationship between surgeon and patient; these qualities were not simply culturally valued, allowing surgeons to shape resonant public identities as men of feeling, but were rooted in the conditions of pre-anaesthetic surgery, facilitating the emotional negotiation of death and distress, and functioning as a vital tool for the therapeutic regulation of bodily and mental health.

Given the centrality of the emotions within the cultures of Romanticism, it is perhaps somewhat strange that they have been subject to so little consideration in relation to contemporary surgery. Indeed, within the public consciousness,

---

[37] Andrew Cunningham and Nicholas Jardine (eds), *Romanticism and the Sciences* (Cambridge, UK: Cambridge University Press, 1990); Richard Holmes, *The Age of Wonder: How the Romantic Generation Discovered the Beauty and Terror of Science* (London: HarperCollins, 2008); Richard C. Sha, *Imagination and Science in Romanticism* (Baltimore: Johns Hopkins University Press, 2018).

[38] Mike Jay, *The Atmosphere of Heaven: The Unnatural Experiments of Dr Beddoes and His Sons of Genius* (New Haven: Yale University Press, 2009).

[39] Christopher Lawrence, 'The Power and the Glory: Humphry Davy and Romanticism', in Cunningham and Jardine (eds), *Romanticism*, 213–27; Jan Golinski, *The Experimental Self: Humphry Davy and the Making of a Man of Science* (Chicago: Chicago University Press, 2016).

[40] Trevor H. Levere, 'Coleridge and the Sciences', in Cunningham and Jardine (eds), *Romanticism*, 295–306; Nicolas Roe (ed.), *Samuel Taylor Coleridge and the Sciences of Life* (Oxford: Oxford University Press, 2001); Eric G. Wilson, 'Coleridge and Science', in Frederick Burwick (ed.), *The Oxford Handbook of Samuel Taylor Coleridge* (Oxford: Oxford University Press, 2009), 640–59.

[41] L. S. Jacyna, 'The Romantic Programme and the Reception of Cell Theory in Britain', *Journal of the History of Biology* 17:1 (1984), 13–48; Jacyna, 'Romantic Thought and the Origins of Cell Theory', in Cunningham and Jardine (eds), *Romanticism*, 161–68; Philip F. Rehbock, 'Transcendental Anatomy', in Cunningham and Jardine (eds), *Romanticism*, 144–60; Sharon Ruston, *Shelley and Vitality* (Basingstoke: Palgrave Macmillan, 2005).

[42] Robert Allard, 'Medicine', in Faflak and Wright (eds), *Handbook*, 375–90.

this era is typically reduced to caricature, a world of misery, gore, pain, and death in which patients reluctantly placed their lives in the callous(ed) hands of semi-literate butchers who were indifferent to their sufferings.[43] Even within the academic literature, the early nineteenth century is often conceived as little more than the prelude to surgical modernity, the last days of darkness before the dawn of anaesthesia and antisepsis. It would, of course, be disingenuous in the extreme to claim that surgery in this period did *not* involve a great deal of suffering, pain, and death. But, as this book demonstrates, it was precisely because of these conditions that surgeons shaped an extraordinarily rich and expressive emotional culture.

Having explored the emotional regime of Romantic surgery, *Emotions and Surgery* examines the transition to a new emotional regime between the second quarter of the nineteenth century and the first decade of the twentieth. In this period, I argue, emotion, both as a form of expression and as a way of conceptualising the patient, was increasingly marginalised within surgical culture. This process was facilitated by the emergence of new ways of talking and thinking about feeling within surgery, and the transformation of subjectivity and pain wrought by the introduction of inhalation anaesthesia. This transition from the Romantic to the techno-scientific, the pre-modern to the modern, was capped by Joseph Lister's application of germ theory to surgical practice in the mid-1860s, something that saw the patient, as an emotionally agentive presence, effectively disappear from surgery by the 1880s.[44] While I am cautious of giving the impression that this book adheres to a 'great man' view of history, the importance of Lister and antisepsis within this cultural transformation cannot be denied, and so the end date for the study is given as 1912, the year of Lister's death, and the moment at which modern techno-scientific surgery can be said to have come of age.

This book utilises a number of concepts and terms that are specific to the history of emotions and thus require some explanation. Perhaps the most important of these is emotional regimes. William Reddy defines an emotional regime as a 'set of normative emotions and the official rituals, practices, and emotives that express and inculcate them'.[45] Reddy's notion of the emotional regime is predicated on the theory of the 'emotive', which is the understanding that emotion is a 'speech act' (and also a gestural one) that not only gives expression to a feeling but also induces its sensation.[46] In other words, what it is possible to feel is, in large part, determined by one's ability to give

---

[43] For example, see Lindsey Fitzharris, *The Butchering Art: Joseph Lister's Quest to Transform the Grisly World of Victorian Medicine* (London: Allen Lane, 2017), prologue.
[44] As we shall hear, this has parallels with Jewson, 'Disappearance'.
[45] Reddy, *Navigation*, p. 129.
[46] Reddy, *Navigation*, p. 128.

expression to it. Emotional regimes, broadly speaking, constitute a culture within which certain emotions are expressible and meaningful, while others are less so. They are not fixed but mutable, and subject to change over time. Reddy's original formulation of emotional regimes was rather prescriptive, and his sense of their operation somewhat oppressive. This book therefore employs the concept in more of a heuristic than a purist way, to describe the historically contingent normativity of particular forms of emotional sensation and expression, and to distinguish the emotional cultures and practices of Romantic sensibility from those of scientific modernity. For this reason, while *Emotions and Surgery* generally employs Reddy's ideas, it occasionally references the work of other scholars, such as Barbara Rosenwein, whose concept of the emotional community allows for a more relational understanding of emotions as a system of feeling, connecting or defining a particular social or vocational group, such as surgeons.[47]

There has been a great deal of debate within the field about the role played by language in structuring our understanding of past emotions, and a suggestion that the terms we use might occlude, as much as enhance, our analysis. This is true even of the word 'emotion' itself, which, as Thomas Dixon has shown, has a particular intellectual history.[48] According to Dixon, emotion was not firmly established as 'a category of mental states that might be systematically studied' until the middle of the nineteenth century.[49] Nonetheless, he acknowledges that the word entered the English language in the eighteenth century, and was certainly in use by the early nineteenth to talk about sensations of feeling and mood. For example, in describing the effects of nitrous oxide in 1800, Humphry Davy wrote: 'My emotions were enthusiastic and sublime; and for a minute I walked around the room perfectly regardless of what was said to me'.[50] Moreover, Dixon credits Charles Bell (1774–1842), the younger brother of John Bell and one of the key figures in the early chapters of this book, with being the 'coinventor' of the modern concept of the emotions.[51] For this reason, and for the sake of terminological convenience, I have judged it appropriate to employ emotion as a descriptive shorthand for various sensations and expressions of mood, even if the sources do not always use precisely those terms. At the same time, however, I am sensitive to the historically contingent quality of emotion words, and I therefore avoid the term 'empathy', which is an early

[47] Rosenwein, *Emotional Communities*.
[48] Thomas Dixon, *From Passions to Emotions: The Creation of a Secular Psychological Category* (Cambridge, UK: Cambridge University Press, 2003); Dixon, '"Emotion"'.
[49] Dixon, '"Emotion"', p. 338.
[50] Humphry Davy, *Researches Chemical and Philosophical, Chiefly Concerning Nitrous Oxide or Dephlogisticated Nitrous Air and Its Respiration* (London: J. Johnson, 1800), p. 488.
[51] Dixon, '"Emotion"', p. 341.

twentieth-century neologism, using instead the actors' categories of sympathy and compassion. And yet, as we shall see, sympathy, which means 'suffering with', does not, in its modern sense at least, quite communicate the extent of imaginative projection into the other described by Romantic surgeons, and thus, when discussing the surgeon–patient relationship, I employ the modern concept of 'intersubjectivity', a term with less conceptual and moral baggage than empathy.

'Affect' is another contested term. For much of its history it communicated a variety of meanings related to mental sensation, including what we might call the cognitive aspects of feeling. Since the development of 'affect theory' in the 1960s, however, it has come to refer specifically to the physiological and pre-cognitive dimensions of emotional sensation and expression, such as a raised heart rate, sweating, or a flushed face. This technical use has increasingly moved out of psychology into the humanities. While some scholars, such as Barbara Rosenwein, reject the distinction, I generally use affect to describe the embodied aspects of feeling. At the same time, given that the concepts of emotion and affect are so inextricably intertwined, as are the mental and physical manifestations of feeling, they often function synonymously.[52]

As a last word on the topic of emotions, I should say that that, while this book mostly deals with emotions as conventionally understood, things such as anxiety, regret, anger, and joy, it also considers other, less easily categorisable, mental states and forms of bodily sensation and expression. Indeed, given that it is conceived, in large part, to trace the changing place of the patient within the cultures and practices of British surgery, *Emotions and Surgery* deals on occasion with much broader ideas of subjectivity and agency, including the embodied sensations of operative practice, the hallucinations of anaesthetised patients, or the unconscious movements of amputated limbs. These might not customarily be regarded as emotions strictly speaking, but they are nonetheless an essential element to consider in a phenomenologically sensitive account of surgical experience and embodiment.[53]

Having established the conceptual parameters of the term 'emotions', it is also necessary to define exactly what I mean by 'surgery'. This book is almost exclusively concerned with the practice of *operative* surgery, or with therapeutic practice of an explicitly surgical kind, often in anticipation of, as an alternative to, or in recovery from, operative intervention. As such, it focuses overwhelmingly on a group of men, sometimes called 'pure' surgeons, who were typically attached to large teaching hospitals, and who

---

[52] Barbara H. Rosenwein, *Generations of Feeling: A History of Emotions, 600–1700* (Cambridge, UK: Cambridge University Press, 2015), p. 7.

[53] Smith and Boddice, *Emotions*.

therefore performed surgical operations on a regular basis. Because of this, the story told here is one centred on the twin medical metropolises of London and Edinburgh. Outside of these and other major cities, the majority of men trained as surgeons actually practised as surgeon-apothecaries or, as they were increasingly known in the early nineteenth century, general practitioners. These men did not generally undertake a large number of operations, at least not 'capital' ones, the name given to major procedures such as amputations, lithotomies, or the excision of tumours. Much of their day-to-day work consisted of treating conditions that were essentially *medical* – that is, they were rooted in internal, constitutional complaints – or of performing minor surgical procedures like bleeding veins or removing superficial growths. In 1817, for example, a recently licensed surgeon by the name of John Wallace from Carshalton in Surrey wrote a letter to John Flint South (1797–1882), then a student at St Thomas' Hospital in London, in which he discussed his practice in 'the Country'.[54] He had seen two cases of hernia, he explained: 'two broken thighs and a broken arm the only other surgical cases of importance which have fallen to my lot'. For 'every surgical case', he remarked ruefully, 'there are 50 medical'.[55] While I am deeply sensitive to the importance of non-metropolitan medical cultures, and have written extensively about the role of the surgeon-apothecary and provincial practitioner in the ideological elaboration of the medical profession, when it comes to the cultures of operative surgery, there is ample justification for focusing on metropolitan surgeons.[56] After all, not only have they left behind the greatest volume of archival material, but they were also the principal operators, authors, and lecturers of the day, playing a prominent role in the shaping of surgical practice, culture, and identity. Of course, it could be suggested that this focus on metropolitan surgeons risks limiting the generalisability of the emotional regimes I reconstruct in this book. For example, in 1830, the Somerset surgeon Mr Valentine told Astley Cooper (1768–1841), one of the leading practitioners of the day, that 'It has fallen to my lot to perform many operations for a country practitioner amongst them fourteen for the stone 13 of which were successful'. Still, he claimed, 'I do it as a painful duty not with the indifference acquired by the extensive field of London practice'.[57] Here

---

[54] Carshalton is actually less than ten miles from central London.

[55] RCSE, MS0232/9, Letters to John Flint South and notes on his family, Letter from George Wallace to John Flint South, 8 February 1817.

[56] For example, Michael Brown, *Performing Medicine: Medical Culture and Identity in Provincial England* (Manchester: Manchester University Press, 2011); Brown, 'Medicine, Reform and the "End" of Charity in Early Nineteenth-Century England', *English Historical Review* 124:511 (2009), 1353–88.

[57] RCSE, MS0008/2/2/5, File of correspondence concerning cases including breast cancer and tumour, 1813–47, Letter from Mr Valentine to Astley Cooper, 24 August 1830.

we have a provincial surgeon articulating the idea that the routinisation of operative experience characteristic of London hospital surgery might induce a kind of emotional insensibility. As we shall see, however, the reality was that metropolitan surgeons in London and Edinburgh spoke just as openly about the emotional challenges of their work, suggesting that the values of Romantic surgical culture were widely shared.

I should perhaps add that, while this book adopts an emotions-centred approach, it is sensitive to the ways in which emotions intersect with categories of identity such as class, gender, and race. Gender plays a particularly prominent role in the story, though I have not engaged in any great depth with the entry of women into the medical and surgical professions in the late nineteenth and early twentieth centuries, both because this has been done so well elsewhere, and because the evidence suggests that women's impact on the emotional regime of surgery was, and in many ways continues to be, limited.[58] Likewise, while ideas about race and, more especially, ethnicity do feature in *Emotions and Surgery*, they are not employed as a framing device, in large part because another strand of the Surgery & Emotion project, and its resultant outputs, was conceived to address precisely these concerns.[59]

Sources and Structure

Emotions and Surgery is founded upon an extraordinarily rich body of primary source material. This includes thousands of pages of manuscript casebooks, letters, diaries, notes, and lectures, drawn from the personal papers of various nineteenth-century surgeons. As a case in point, the archive of Astley Cooper, the largest single collection of manuscript material consulted for this book, encompasses more than sixteen boxes of documents, and yielded nearly 3,500 digital images. This material alone took over six months to sort, transcribe, and code into an NVivo database. The majority of the archival materials consulted for this book are held by the Royal College of Surgeons of England, but *Emotions and Surgery* also makes use of material from other archives, including the Royal College of Surgeons of Edinburgh, the Wellcome Library, the National Library of Scotland, and the Cumbrian Archives Service. Moreover, *Emotions and Surgery* utilises a vast quantity of published texts, including medical journals, books, pamphlets, and newspapers. The richness, depth,

---

[58] See Brock, *British Women Surgeons*; Kim Peters and Michelle Ryan, 'Machismo in Surgery Is Harming the Specialty', *BMJ* 348 (2014), g3034 https://doi.org/10.1136/bmj.g3034 (accessed 06/10/21).

[59] James Kennaway, 'Celts under the Knife: Surgical Fortitude, Racial Theory and the British Army, 1800–1914', *Cultural and Social History* 17:2 (2020), 227–44.

and variety of this source material allow for an unprecedented insight into nineteenth-century surgical culture, practice, and identity, as well as the relationships between surgeons and their patients. Different sources offer different perspectives. Letters from patients and their medical representatives facilitate a unique understanding of their experience of surgical treatment, while casebooks can illuminate the place of emotion within hospital practice. Surgeons' diaries and correspondence allow us to explore the fashioning of surgical subjectivity, while lectures in both manuscript and printed form provide a useful way to gauge the cultural values and professional norms that surgeons sought to inculcate in their students. Likewise, journals provide a broad insight into the cultural politics of surgery, while surgical biographies and memoirs are highly suggestive of the image and identity that surgeons sought to construct of themselves and their profession.

A wide range of sources are employed throughout *Emotions and Surgery*, but different bodies of material are used to highlight particular issues. Chapter 1 lays the groundwork for our understanding of Romantic surgery as an avowedly 'scientific' practice, grounded in anatomy, but also as an embodied and performative one, in which the qualities of speed, dexterity, and decisiveness were balanced against an emotional assessment of the patient's needs. Using letters, lectures, journals, and books, it reconstructs the Romantic surgeon as an operative man of feeling, but also explores the contradictions and ambiguities of that persona in the form of perhaps the era's most contested figure, Robert Liston (1794–1847).

Chapter 2 focuses on the emotional interiorities and intersubjectivities of Romantic surgery. Drawing on diaries, letters, biographies, and other publications, it explores the cultures of Romantic emotional expression and introspection, countering the caricature of the early nineteenth-century surgeon as a callous or dispassionate butcher. It demonstrates the centrality of emotions not only in the shaping of the surgical self, but also in the affective management of the patient, and the regulation of bodily health and operative outcomes. Hence, it uses the extensive manuscript casebooks of Astley Cooper to open up the relationship between breast cancer and the 'emotion work' of gender within Romantic surgery.

Chapter 3 considers Romantic surgery from the patient's perspective. Using Cooper's rich archive of personal correspondence as well as his casebooks, it illuminates the importance of emotions as a form of agency both in the context of the private surgical relationship and within what, following Michel Foucault, we might consider the 'disciplinary' space of the hospital. Beyond the role of conscious emotional agency, it also demonstrates how this agency might be expressed through embodied acts, figuring the amputee's 'irritable' constitution and 'bad stump' as a site of ontological 'messiness' and as a form of unconscious resistance to surgical authority.

Chapter 4 uses a close reading of *The Lancet*, and its radical, charismatic editor Thomas Wakley (1795–1862), to delineate the 'high water mark' of Romantic sensibility as an emotional regime. It explores the ways in which Wakley and *The Lancet* leveraged the emotional politics of contemporary melodrama to attack the alleged nepotism and corruption of the London surgical elites. More especially, it analyses their campaign to expose instances of surgical incompetence at the city's leading teaching hospitals, demonstrating the ways in which this strategy weaponised the emotions of anger, pity, and sympathy, and considering its implications both for the cultural norms of an inchoate profession and for the ultimate stability of the emotional regime of Romantic sensibility.

Chapter 5 explores the beginning of the end of Romantic sensibility and the origins of surgical scientific modernity. Using a close reading of a wide range of published books, journals, pamphlets, and lectures, it elucidates the role of utilitarian thought in rendering the surgical body emotionally quiescent. It focuses on two distinct but interrelated historical episodes, namely the debates around anatomical dissection that preceded the passage of the Anatomy Act in 1832, and the introduction and early reception of inhalation anaesthesia in the mid to late 1840s. In the first instance, it demonstrates how an ultra-rationalist understanding of sentiment was set in opposition to popular 'sentimentalism' in order to divest the dead bodies of the poor of emotional value. Meanwhile, in the second, it considers how the subjectivity of the newly anaesthetised patient was swiftly tamed by the operations of a techno-scientific rationale.

Chapter 6 charts the ultimate triumph of the emotional regime of scientific modernity in the form of antisepsis, Joseph Lister's application of germ theory to surgical practice. Through an in-depth analysis of journal articles, reports, lectures, biographies, and visual images, it shows how antisepsis effectively eliminated the patient as an emotional presence in surgery. At the same time, however, it demonstrates how this 'new world of surgery' was configured in highly sentimentalised terms, constructing Lister, the ultimate scientific surgeon and the emotional template for surgical modernity, as a quasi-divine saviour.

Finally, the Epilogue builds on these collective insights to highlight the ways in which historical accounts of the Listerian 'revolution' have shaped our perception not only of surgical modernity, but also of the pre-antiseptic and pre-anaesthetic past, flattening the emotional landscape of the Romantic era and consigning it to a surgical 'dark age'. It suggests that these misunderstandings of the past have, in turn, shaped contemporary surgical culture, and it therefore considers how a more nuanced history might inform surgical practice today. As such, *Emotions and Surgery* will hopefully be of interest to a wide range of different readers, including students of the history of emotions and surgery, as well as those of nineteenth-century Britain more generally. Moreover, by challenging simplistic narratives of triumphant surgical progress, and by subverting much of the mythology that has grown up around this subject, it also speaks to a popular audience interested in the past in all of its complexity, as well as to current surgical practitioners, who may learn something new, unexpected, and possibly even provocative, about the historical origins of their profession and its cultures.

1   Between Art and Artifice
Emotion and Performance in Romantic Surgery

Introduction

Surgeons have long told stories about themselves and their history. As Christopher Lawrence has suggested, and as we shall see in this book, these stories often reveal more about the image that their tellers sought to project of themselves and their contemporaries than they do about the various mythical, half-remembered, and stereotyped pasts they invoked.[1] This tradition of story-telling, of historicising surgery in order to understand the present, had its roots in the writings of medieval surgeons such as Guy de Chauliac (c.1300–68), but, like historicism itself, it really came to prominence at the end of the eighteenth century and beginning of the nineteenth.[2] It was in this period, or so contemporary surgeons claimed, that surgery had become a fully fledged scientific discipline that had finally distinguished itself from its traditional associations with manual craft. This story had its institutional correlate in the split of the surgeons from the Barbers' Company (1722 in Scotland, 1745 in England) followed by the creation of the Royal College of Surgeons of Edinburgh in 1778 and the Royal College of Surgeons of London (later England) in 1800. Indeed, it was within these new institutional structures that surgery's mythical rebirth was most frequently, and most visibly, commemorated and rehearsed.

The first part of *Emotions and Surgery* is concerned, in large part, with exploring the professional cultures, identities, and ideologies of a generation of British surgeons that came of age in the very late eighteenth and early nineteenth centuries: a generation of *Romantic* surgeons. Perhaps the most prominent claim that this generation made for the transformation of their art in the fifty or so years prior to 1800 was its increasing scientific sophistication: the re-founding of surgical practice on the basis of sound anatomical knowledge,

---

[1] Christopher Lawrence, 'Surgery and Its Histories: Purposes and Contexts', in Thomas Schlich (ed.), *The Palgrave Handbook of the History of Surgery* (London: Palgrave Macmillan, 2018), 27–48. See also Christopher Lawrence, 'Democratic, Divine and Heroic: The History and Historiography of Surgery', in Christopher Lawrence (ed.), *Medical Theory, Surgical Practice: Studies in the History of Surgery* (London: Routledge, 1992), 1–47.

[2] Lawrence, 'Surgery', pp. 31, 37–40.

rather than mere empiricism. If the humanist surgeons of the sixteenth century had struggled to wrest learned surgery from the intellectual domain of the physician, then surgeons of the later eighteenth century had, it was claimed, made anatomical and physiological learning their own.[3] In fact, they had, to a significant degree, made *medical* knowledge their own. The eighteenth century produced a number of surgeons whom posterity would venerate as exemplars of this new-found theoretical and operative self-confidence. These included men such as William Cheselden (1688–1752) and Percivall Pott (1714–88).[4] However, by far the most iconic figure, and the man who, as Lawrence observes, would be 'shaped into the "father of scientific surgery"', was John Hunter.[5] It was Hunter whose name would, in 1813, be immortalised in the form of an annual oration at the Royal College of Surgeons of London, and it was his likeness, in the shape of Henry Weekes' (1807–77) statue of 1864, that would take pride of place in the College's Museum.[6] As Lawrence suggests, while English surgeons made Hunter their own, those in Scotland told a different story (somewhat ironically, given that Hunter was a Scot).[7] For Edinburgh chroniclers writing in the mid-nineteenth century, it was John Bell who was celebrated as 'the best surgeon that Scotland had then produced'[8] and 'the reformer of Surgery in Edinburgh, or rather the father of it'.[9] Indeed, the prowess of Scottish surgeons in the early to mid-nineteenth century, including the brothers John and Charles Bell, as well as Robert Liston and James Syme, allowed their contemporaries to imagine that Scottish surgery had initiated a revolution all of its own. Writing to his uncle from Edinburgh on New Year's Day 1833, the young Cumbrian surgical pupil Andrew Whelpdale spoke of 'the beauty of the modern School of Medicine in Edinbro [*sic*]'. 'I can assure you', he wrote, 'that there is as much difference between a surgeon of the Old School and one of the New as you can possibly imagine. We have here one of the best operators in the world Liston – A pupil of his is almost the equal, and indeed is far superior in some things to a practised surgeon of the old school'.[10]

In praising the 'new school' of Edinburgh surgery, founded by John Bell and raised to greatness by Liston, Whelpdale mocked the pretensions of the physician and asserted the claims of surgery to be the superior science. 'To

---

[3] Lawrence, 'Surgery', pp. 33–7.

[4] For a recent account of Percivall Pott's contribution to surgical knowledge, practice, and culture, see Lynda Payne, *The Best Surgeon in England: Percivall Pott, 1713–88* (New York: Peter Lang, 2017).

[5] Lawrence, 'Surgery', p. 38.

[6] L. S. Jacyna, 'Images of John Hunter in the Nineteenth Century', *History of Science* 21:1 (1983), 85–108.

[7] Lawrence, 'Surgery', p. 39.

[8] Henry Cockburn, *Memorials of His Time* (New York: D. Appleton and Company, 1856), p. 106.

[9] John Struthers, *Historical Sketch of the Edinburgh Anatomical School* (Edinburgh: Maclachlan and Stewart, 1867), p. 43.

[10] CAS-C, D HUD 17/90, Andrew Whelpdale to John de Whelpdale, 1 January 1833.

shew you the contempt in which the Doctors are held by the great men here', he wrote, 'I will relate a story about Liston'. This story, which involved Liston asking his students whether they thought 'there existed any one more ignorant than a Doctor?', was doubtless apocryphal. But Whelpdale also confided that his personal tutor in anatomy, the celebrated (and infamous) Robert Knox (1791–1862), had told him that he 'is sorry he graduated himself [i.e. became a physician] & would not let a son of his graduate'. 'Besides', Whelpdale concluded, 'no one gets on now but general practitioners. The surgeons seldom call in a Physician'.[11]

Whelpdale's letters nicely capture the sentiment, prevalent in the early nineteenth century, that the traditional balance of power between surgery and medicine was beginning to shift. Indeed, it is notable that he referred to this new 'School of *Medicine*' in purely surgical terms. This accords with an established historical narrative. Numerous historians have argued that it was during the nineteenth century that surgery came to prominence as a profession, eventually displacing medicine in the hierarchy of social and intellectual prestige. Indeed, within the historiography of medicine, surgeons are, like the middle classes of old, perpetually rising.[12] And yet, aside from a few examples, there is surprisingly little scholarship on what this process actually looked like or how it shaped British surgical culture.[13] This is certainly true when compared to the well-established historiography on the rise of surgery in France, which traces its influences through the eighteenth century to the clinical revolution of early nineteenth-century Paris.[14] *Emotions and Surgery* is not intended to function as a political history of surgical professionalisation in Britain, at least not as conventionally conceived. What it does seek to do is to provide a cultural historical account of nineteenth-century British surgery through a fine-grained analysis of surgical performance and identity at a time of remarkable transformation.

Emotions, this book contends, are critical for understanding nineteenth-century surgical culture, and they played an especially vital role in shaping

---

[11] CAS-C, D HUD 17/90, Andrew Whelpdale to John de Whelpdale, 18 November 1833, f. 12v.
[12] For a classic example, see Owen H. Wangensteen and Sarah D. Wangensteen, *The Rise of Surgery from Empiric Craft to Scientific Discipline* (Minneapolis: University of Minnesota Press, 1978).
[13] For example, see Christopher Lawrence and Michael Brown, 'Quintessentially Modern Heroes: Surgeons, Explorers, and Empire, c.1840–1914', *Journal of Social History* 50:1 (2016), 148–78.
[14] Erwin Ackerknecht, *Medicine at the Paris Hospital, 1794–1848* (Baltimore: Johns Hopkins University Press, 1967); Michel Foucault, *The Birth of the Clinic: An Archaeology of Medical Perception*, trans. A. M. Sheridan (London: Tavistock, 1973); David M. Vess, *Medical Revolution in France, 1789–1796* (Gainesville: University of Florida Press, 1975); Toby Gelfand, *Professionalizing Modern Medicine: Paris Surgeons and Medical Science and Institutions in the Eighteenth Century* (London: Greenwood Press, 1980); Matthew Ramsey, *Professional and Popular Medicine in France 1770–1830: The Social World of Medical Practice* (Cambridge, UK: Cambridge University Press, 1988).

Romantic surgical practice, experience, and identity. In his *Illustrations of the Great Operations of Surgery* (1821), Charles Bell claimed that 'it depends on the conduct of those who are now entering their Profession, whether Surgery will continue to be confounded with meaner arts, or rise to be the very first in estimation'. As we shall see in Chapters 2 and 3, he, like many of his contemporaries, framed the 'knowledge', 'honour', and 'abilities' of surgeons largely in terms of their capacity to act with, as well as to manage and manipulate, feeling.[15] This first chapter argues that one of the key features of the epistemic transformation that characterised the inheritance of Romantic surgery, namely a greater knowledge of human anatomy, was an increasing emphasis upon operative restraint and a caution against radical, dangerous, or so-called heroic procedures deemed likely to produce excessive suffering or even death to the patient. It is important to see this transformation not simply as an objective, epistemological phenomenon, but also as a subjective, ideological one. The deprecation of unnecessary or rash surgical intervention was the product not only of greater anatomical knowledge, but also of social and cultural change, the corollary of an emotional regime founded upon the values of sensibility, sentiment, and sympathy. As we shall see in successive chapters, these values had a profound impact on surgical identity and practice, as well as on patient experience. In this chapter, however, our focus is on their implications for the literal performance of surgery, for the manual skills and bodily dispositions deemed necessary for the cutting of one's fellow creatures: the 'hexis' and 'habitus', as it were, of Romantic surgery.[16] Thomas Schlich is one of the few historians of surgery to consider the place of manual skill and styles of operative performance in the shaping of surgical culture and identity.[17] Like other commentators, such as Peter Stanley, he characterises the early nineteenth century as an era defined largely by speed, something that was not only deemed necessary for the mitigation of pain, but also became central to the 'mystique of the heroic surgeon'.[18] Both Stanley and Schlich point to the existence of other operative ideals, notably grace, composure, and caution.[19] Moreover, Schlich rightly suggests that operative styles 'needed to be controlled by a moral framework to make sure that the surgeon's performance stayed within the limits of his patients' best interests'.[20] This chapter corroborates that suggestion

---

[15] Charles Bell, *Illustrations of the Great Operations of Surgery* (London: Longman, Hurst, Rees, Orme, and Brown, 1821), p. viii.

[16] On the concept of hexis and habitus, see Pierre Bourdieu, *The Logic of Practice* (Cambridge: Polity Press, 1990), pp. 42–51, 53–4, 74.

[17] Thomas Schlich, '"The Days of Brilliancy Are Past": Skill, Styles and the Changing Rule of Surgical Performance', *Medical History* 59:3 (2015), 379–403.

[18] Peter Stanley, *For Fear of Pain: British Surgery, 1790–1850* (Amsterdam: Rodopi, 2003), p. 64, quoted by Schlich, 'Brilliancy', p. 384.

[19] Stanley, *Pain*, pp. 224–9; Schlich, 'Brilliancy', pp. 384–5.

[20] Schlich, 'Brilliancy', p. 386.

but endeavours to go further, underscoring the moral complexity of Romantic surgical performance by suggesting that speed was far from being the principal attribute for which surgeons of the period were admired. Indeed, it argues that a new-found emphasis upon restraint actually had deeply ambiguous implications for the place of manual dexterity and operative flair in contemporary surgical culture and identity. On the one hand, physical dexterity and operative 'boldness' were praised as both practical necessities and signifiers of manual and mental aptitude, but, on the other, surgical commentators of the period increasingly expressed distrust of excessive flamboyance and self-regard, which they came to see as the expression of an inauthentic surgical persona.

With the expansion of hospital-based teaching in the late eighteenth and early nineteenth centuries, operations were performed with increasing frequency in front of sometimes large audiences of students and fellow practitioners. Schlich and others have suggested that such public performances encouraged surgical 'showmanship'.[21] As we shall see, especially in Chapter 4, surgeons were indeed scrutinised and judged for their operative performance, sometimes quite harshly. However, surgical performance in the Romantic operating theatre involved more than the mere display and evaluation of style and skill. The operating theatre was, in fact, a complex political and emotional space that required careful moral management.

If the performative dimensions of Romantic surgery were complex and ambivalent, then those qualities can be said to have crystallised in the form of one of the Romantic era's most celebrated operators, Robert Liston. Liston's renown as perhaps the greatest operative surgeon of the 1830s and 1840s was spread by contemporaries such as Andrew Whelpdale and has been sustained by subsequent generations of historians. And yet, while Liston is famed as a bold and skilful operator, and as the first surgeon to perform an operation under anaesthesia in Britain, he is often represented, especially in more sensationalist accounts of the history of surgery, as the last of the surgical old guard, a speed-obsessed showman whose rashness hints at the cruelty and brutality of the pre-anaesthetic era.[22] In her account of John Elliotson's (1791–1868) mesmeric demonstrations in the operating theatre at University College Hospital, Alison Winter remarks that 'insufficient historical study has been undertaken to recover the kinds of surgical displays that made Liston so immensely effective as a surgical performer'.[23] As we shall see in the final section of this chapter, the solution to that riddle is not necessarily straightforward. For one thing, Liston's performances, and their reception, were shaped by the twin demands

[21] Schlich, 'Brilliancy', p. 385.
[22] For example, Lindsey Fitzharris, *The Butchering Art: Joseph Lister's Quest to Transform the Grisly World of Victorian Medicine* (London: Allen Lane, 2017), pp. 10–15.
[23] Alison Winter, 'Mesmerism and Popular Culture in Early Victorian England', *History of Science* 32:3 (1994), 317–43, at p. 322.

of care and cure, demands that were not always easily reconcilable. Moreover, his reputation as an operator was not simply an objective corollary of his abilities, but was formed by a variety of complex social and political factors, not the least of which were the factious cultures of medical reform and the occasionally antagonistic relations of Anglo-Scottish surgery.

Anatomy, Science, and the Decline of Heroic Surgery

In order to understand how the notion of operative restraint became central to Romantic surgical identity, it is first necessary to consider how it came to be tied to a customary narrative of social, intellectual, and epistemological self-improvement. Surgeons of the period were profoundly conscious of their historically questionable status and of their associations with empirical, rather than scientific, practice. However, in their writings and lectures, they crafted a narrative of surgery as risen to respectability from humble origins in less than a hundred years. Speaking to his St George's Hospital class in 1820, Benjamin Brodie (1783–1862) claimed:

> In this and in many other Countries where surgery was first pursued as a separate profession, it was held in low estimation. Even in the beginning of the last century, the Surgeon was a subordinate person, who Trepanned and performed amputations, under the direction of the Physician. But since that time, our profession has made rapid strides towards its present dignified and honourable station. It has been adorned in this Country by Cheselden, Hunter, and Pott, and we may safely say, that at the present day, the Surgeon in the Metropolis, ranks in public estimation, at least as high as the Physician.[24]

As a lecturer at St George's, Brodie may have had good reason to single out William Cheselden and John Hunter as pioneers of modern surgery, as both men were closely associated with that hospital. Brodie's teacher, and fellow St George's Hospital surgeon, Everard Home (1756–1832) certainly had especial reason to celebrate the latter, as he was Hunter's brother-in-law and his former pupil, as well as the joint executor, together with Hunter's nephew Matthew Baillie (1761–1823), of his estate. Moreover, he was the direct inheritor of Hunter's intellectual legacy and benefited greatly from the association, although his reputation was tainted by his subsequent destruction of Hunter's personal papers, an act that gave rise to inevitable suspicions of plagiarism.[25] In 1811, some twelve years prior to this fateful decision, Home gave a series of lectures to his students at the Great Windmill Street Anatomy School, founded by John's older brother, William Hunter (1718–83); he chose to open in customary (and self-serving) fashion with some moral and historical instruction.

---

[24] RCSE, MS0470/1/2/5, Benjamin Brodie, 'Introductory lecture of anatomy and physiology' (October 1820), f. 4.
[25] N. G. Coley, 'Home, Sir Everard, first baronet (1756–1832)', *ODNB*.

'It is usual in beginning a course of lectures wither [*sic*] on Medicine or Surgery', he announced, 'to read an introductory Lecture, in which is given a short history of the art, its excellencies pointed out, & the sources from which the teacher derived his knowledge detailed'. He continued:

In the earlier times of physic, the art of Surgery was low and confined to the performance of manual operations, which were determined by the Physician. As the physicians professed no accurate knowledge of the structure of the human body, it was impossible that the art could be advanced under their direction. Surgery could not be improved till the practitioners had become acquainted with the different parts of the body; their use & connection with one another. With the progress of Anatomical Knowledge is to be traced the advancement of Surgery.[26]

Surgery's professional and social subordination was, then, according to Home, a direct product of the physician's ignorance of anatomy. However, even if the necessity of anatomical knowledge for improved surgical practice had long been acknowledged, 'the prejudices of mankind against dead bodies made it necessary that Anatomical pursuits should be followed in secret in the first instance'. This only began to change in the eighteenth century, Home alleged and, in a narrative that would become a staple of later hagiographic accounts, he held the personal achievements of the Hunters responsible for a greater national renewal:

In England, before the time of Dr Hunter, Anaty [*sic*] was superficially taught, & improvements in it confined to France. To the late Dr Hunter England is indebted for the rapid advancement she has since made in the Practice of Surgery. Dr Hunter not only made himself master of the anatomy of the human body but every thing concerned with that study by diligence & unwearied perseverance. His merit to his country however extended beyond these narrow limits. With infinite difficulty, notwithstanding the professional prejudices against it he instituted a practical School for Anatomical Dissections. He was hence not satisfied with being eminent himself, but desirous of making his pupils as capable as their master.[27]

Home's implication about the equivalence of master and pupil was clear enough. However, in case anyone in his audience had missed it, and to ensure that he caught the full light of the Hunters' reflected glory, he added that his testimony was 'a just tribute to the memory of that great man who erected the walls by which we are now surrounded & it was from him that I received my first lesson'.[28]

While Home may have had a particularly close personal connection to William and John Hunter, he was far from alone in claiming a unique place for the brothers in the history of anatomy and surgery. As his lecture implies,

[26] WL, MS.5604, Lawrence W. Brown, 'Notes on Twelve Lectures by Everard Home on the Principal Operations of Surgery' (1811–12), ff. 7–8.
[27] WL, MS.5604, f. 8.   [28] WL, MS.5604, f. 8.

William's contributions to anatomical study were widely recognised by Romantic surgeons, but it was his younger brother John who, as the surgical sibling, was most commonly singled out for praise. Indeed, Stephen Jacyna has argued that he was deified by later eighteenth- and early nineteenth-century surgeons to an extent rivalled only by Isaac Newton's (1642–1727) idolisation in natural philosophical circles.[29] According to Jacyna, unlike Newton, or indeed other celebrated figures in the history of medicine such as William Harvey (1578–1657) and even his own erstwhile apprentice, Edward Jenner (1749–1823), Hunter did not lend his name to a single discovery or therapeutic innovation. Instead, his fame rested on his wholesale transformation of surgery from a manual occupation to a scientific one.[30] As the Guy's Hospital surgeon Astley Cooper pithily put it to his students, 'Surgery before his time was good mechanical but after it good scientific'.[31]

The principal locus for the mythologisation of John Hunter and the celebration of scientific surgery in the nineteenth century was the Hunterian Oration to the Royal College of Surgeons, established by Home and Baillie in 1813. This provided an opportunity for leading surgeons of the day to rehearse their history, and to cement Hunter's place in it as the man who transformed surgery into a science. What is important to note is that these orators, and others who lauded Hunter's legacy, did not celebrate the cultivation of scientific anatomy for its own sake. In a remarkable claim that swept away the achievements of Andreas Vesalius (1514–64) and Ambroise Paré (1510–90) among others, William Norris (1757–1827) stated:

since the time of the Greeks, very many ponderous volumes, of pompous title and bombastic promise, on the subjects of Anatomy and Surgery have been published; but they contained little that was of any value, save what was purloined or imperfectly translated from their predecessors. The surgery therefore which prevailed in this country, even at the beginning of the eighteenth century, except in the treatment of a few diseases, could hardly be said to be an improvement upon that of Hippocrates, 2,200 years before![32]

What was different about Hunter and his contemporaries, Norris and others proposed, was that their knowledge of anatomy and pathology was fundamentally applicable to *practice*. This was not the classical anatomy of the

---

[29] One of the few dissenting voices was that of Jesse Foot (1744–1826), whose *Life of John Hunter* (1794) was, according to Jacyna, characterised by a 'quite extraordinary spite'. Jacyna, 'Images', p. 91.

[30] Jacyna, 'Images', p. 88.

[31] RCSE, MS0232/3, John Flint South, 'Lectures on the Principles and Practice of Surgery delivered by Astley Paston Cooper Esq, F.R.S. & Benjamin Travers Esq. F.R.S. in the Anatomical Theatre at St Thomas' Hospital between the years 1816 & 1818 Vol. 1', f. 8.

[32] William Norris, *The Hunterian Oration Delivered before the Royal College of Surgeons* (London: T. Cadell and W. Davies, 1817), pp. 26–7.

physician, concerned predominantly with structure and form, but rather a *surgical* anatomy, which enabled the surgeon to treat disease and injury with greater confidence and with better results for the patient. According to Norris:

This preliminary knowledge necessarily produced a more rational pathology; and that the comforts and safety to mankind from thence derived became apparent, and were properly appreciated, is seen by the high degree of estimation in which those who exercised the Art and Science of Surgery were held. The easy and effectual method of restraining haemorrhage by the ligature – the general adoption of simple and superficial applications to wounds and sores – the practice of saving as much skin as possible in operation – and even the bringing into contact the divided muscles from the opposite sides of a stump immediately after amputation, so that they occasionally unite by the first intention, are a few of the very many improvements that had taken place.[33]

As we have suggested, if John Hunter became *the* model of the scientific surgeon for London's practitioners in the early nineteenth century, the picture in Edinburgh was somewhat different. The reception of Hunter's legacy in Scotland in general, and Edinburgh in particular, is a topic that invites further study. Despite being a Scot, Hunter moved to London at an early stage in his career and stayed there until his death. As such, he remained indelibly associated with England's capital. Moreover, both brothers were born in Lanarkshire and had close ties to Glasgow. The latter was especially true of William, who studied at the university there, and it was to that institution that he left his anatomical collections after his death. Both men were therefore outside of the orbit of the Edinburgh medical and surgical elite, and neither could be comfortably assimilated into a collective narrative of Scottish surgical self-improvement.

If there was no one figure of equivalent stature to John Hunter in early nineteenth-century Edinburgh, there were a number of individuals associated with the development of surgical anatomy in that city. In his historical account of the Edinburgh anatomical school, published in 1867, John Struthers (1823–99) opens with the three generations of the Monro family who occupied the chair of anatomy at the University of Edinburgh between 1725 and 1846.[34] Alexander Monro primus (1697–1767) studied at Leiden, but did not take a degree and only received an honorary MD from Edinburgh in 1756.[35] By contrast, his son Alexander Monro secundus (1733–1817) and grandson Alexander Monro tertius (1773–1859) were both physicians and taught anatomy in a classical manner, predicated on medical rather than surgical requirements.[36] Indeed, Monro

[33] Norris, *Hunterian Oration*, pp. 42–3.   [34] Struthers, *Historical Sketch*, pp. 19–37.
[35] Anita Guerrini, 'Monro, Alexander, primus (1697–1767)', *ODNB*.
[36] Lisa Rosner, 'Monro, Alexander, secundus (1733–1817)', *ODNB*; Lisa Rosner, 'Monro, Alexander, tertius (1773–1859)', *ODNB*. Christopher Lawrence, 'The Edinburgh Medical School and the End of the "Old Thing" 1790–1830', *History of Universities* 1 (1988), 259–86, at pp. 265–7.

secundus actively opposed the Royal College of Surgeons' attempts to institute a professorship of surgery, thereby 'preventing the establishment of a course of surgery in Edinburgh for thirty years'.[37] For Struthers, then, the true 'father' of surgical anatomy in Edinburgh was John Bell. As he writes:

Among the crowd of students in Mono's class-room, there was one remarkable for his keen eye, intelligent countenance, and small stature. It struck this youth that, although Monro was an excellent anatomist and teacher, the application of anatomy to surgery was neglected. He saw this opportunity and took his resolution accordingly. This was John Bell [...] As Monro had never been an operating surgeon, the deficiency in his teaching would, we might suppose, be evident enough; but the merit of John Bell's early surgical discrimination is appreciated only when we remember that there was no surgical anatomy, as now understood, in the Edinburgh school till he introduced it by himself.[38]

Bell explained, in his own words, the inadequacy of a classical anatomical education for the practising surgeon:

It is an actionable and most dangerous occupation, to attempt to benefit the human race by acquiring skill, or learning anatomy, on any thing but CORK and WOOD! unless it be upon LIVING BODIES. In Dr Monro's class, unless there be a fortunate succession of bloody murders, not three subjects are dissected in a year. On the remains of a subject fished up from the bottom of a tub of spirits, are demonstrated those delicate nerves, which are to be avoided or divided in our operations; and these are demonstrated once at the distance of one hundred feet! nerves, and arteries, which the Surgeon has to dissect, at the peril of his patient's life.[39]

Bell began lecturing in 1786, first at the College of Surgeons and then, from 1790, at his own purpose-built anatomical school in the college grounds; he soon became one of the most popular extra-mural teachers in Edinburgh. According to Struthers, 'the position which John Bell exemplified and defended, was one which no man will now venture to dispute, that surgery must be based on anatomy and pathology, a doctrine for which there was at that time, in "the windy and wordy school of Edinburgh", neither acceptance nor toleration'.[40] As Bell himself put it, 'ANATOMY serves to a Surgeon, as the sole theory of his profession, and guides him in all the practice of his art'.[41]

John Bell is a central figure in the development of Romantic surgery, not least, as we shall see, because he was the most articulate advocate for a surgical identity founded upon sensibility and compassion and rooted in the embodied

---

[37] Rosner, 'Monro, Alexander, tertius'.   [38] Struthers, *Historical Sketch*, p. 37.
[39] John Bell, *Letters on Professional Character and Manners: On the Education of a Surgeon, and the Duties and Qualifications of a Physician* (Edinburgh: John Moir, 1810), p. 579.
[40] Struthers, *Historical Sketch*, p. 41.
[41] Bell, *Letters on Professional Character*, p. 548.

experience of operative practice.[42] For our immediate purposes, what is important to note is that Bell's scientific surgery, like that of John Hunter, was not only said to have transformed surgical practice in terms of its sophistication and efficacy. It was also said to have made surgeons more cautious, encouraging them to adopt a less heroic and interventionist approach to operations. Indeed, Bell, like many of his contemporaries, castigated the surgery of the past as rash and cruel, precisely because of its relative ignorance of human anatomy and pathology:

> We have now leisure to observe, how slowly diseases have been understood, or operations invented or improved; we can remark how slowly and imperfectly anatomy has been applied even to this day; at this moment we are employed in rooting out the prejudices and barbarous practices of those Gothic times! For the practice of the older surgeons was marked with all kinds of violence; and indifference about the simple cure of diseases; and a passion for operations, as the cutting off of limbs, the searing of arteries, the sewing of bowels, the trepanning of sculls [sic] round and round, and all the excesses and horrors of surgery.[43]

In this new age of scientific surgery, it became increasingly common for practitioners to trust to the curative powers of nature. In a lecture to his St Bartholomew's Hospital class in October 1818, for example, John Abernethy (1764–1831) considered the treatment of inflammation:

> The Question then comes, should I open the abscess? – What would be the use of it; nature is her own Surgeon, and knows better how to do it than any of us, she removes the superincumbent parts and sets up such disorder in them that they are the last to heal – but if we stick in our knives, in a short time the wound becomes united and this is the way to make a Fistula by interfering with natures [sic] processes.[44]

Of course, such a transformation did not happen overnight, and many surgeons doubtless continued to intervene while others were inclined to watch and wait. 'The truth is', Bell wrote, reiterating his earlier point, 'that the practices and the prejudices of the old times mix themselves with the more orderly and perfect operations of the present day'.[45] Even so, by the early decades of the nineteenth century it had become commonplace for surgeons to deprecate what Robert Liston called the 'old meddlesome surgery', the 'eternal pokings and probings of wounds, abscesses, and sinuses'. 'Nature', he argued, 'well and

---

[42] Michael Brown, 'Surgery, Identity and Embodied Emotion: John Bell, James Gregory and the Edinburgh "Medical War"', *History* 104:359 (2019), 19–41; Michael Brown, 'Wounds and Wonder: Emotion, Imagination, and War in the Cultures of Romantic Surgery', *Journal for Eighteenth-Century Studies* 43:2 (2020), 239–59.

[43] John Bell, *The Principles of Surgery* (Edinburgh: T. Cadell Jr and W. Davies, 1801), p. 10.

[44] RCSE, MS0232/1/1, John Flint South, 'Lectures on the Principles of Surgery delivered by John Abernethy Esq. FRS in the Anatomical Theatre at St Bartholomew's Hospital in the years 1818 and 1819', ff. 70–1.

[45] Bell, *Principles*, p. 10.

judiciously assisted, instead of being thus thwarted, tampered, and interfered with [...] will generally bring matters to a speedy and happy conclusion'.[46]

This increasing emphasis upon operative restraint was not simply a consequence of greater anatomical and pathological knowledge; it was also an expression of surgery's growing professional self-confidence and of the kinds of culturally resonant identities that Romantic surgeons sought to craft for themselves. For one thing, from the later eighteenth century onwards, what Owsei Temkin famously called 'the surgical point of view' had become increasingly central to the ways in which medical practitioners as a whole thought about the body and disease.[47] The effects of this were felt most powerfully in France, where the Parisian clinical 'revolution' of the early nineteenth century was predicated on a surgical sensibility that saw disease as located in the anatomical structures of the body, and where the traditional hierarchies of medicine, which placed the physician above the surgeon, were collapsed into the figure of the *officier de santé*.[48] In Britain, the manifestations of this process were not quite so dramatic, but they were no less transformative. After all, the notable expansion of the medical market in this period took place not so much among the ranks of the physician as among those of the surgeon-apothecary or general practitioner. These men may have been of lower status than the physician or the 'pure' surgeon, and many may have endured economic insecurity, but they were, in many ways, the vital force of early nineteenth-century medicine and, as Andrew Whelpdale's letter quoted earlier suggests, they commanded an increasing share of the market for medical services. What was notable about these men is that they were trained not as physicians, but rather as surgeons; they therefore viewed the diseased body, and the world it inhabited, through the eyes of the surgeon, albeit one acutely conscious of his subordination to the Council of the Royal College.[49]

In light of this, many surgeons were increasingly overstepping the traditional boundaries of their practice.[50] This was true not simply for general practitioners, but also for those among the surgical elite. John Abernethy, for example,

[46] Robert Liston, *Practical Surgery* (London: John Churchill, 1837), pp. 33, 199–200.
[47] Owsei Temkin, 'The Role of Surgery in the Rise of Modern Medical Thought', *Bulletin of the History of Medicine* 25:3 (1951), 248–59, at p. 255.
[48] Maurice Crosland, 'The *Officiers de Santé* of the French Revolution: A Case Study in the Changing Language of Medicine', *Medical History* 48:2 (2004), 229–44. As Crosland points out, it is important not to confuse the Revolutionary-era use of the term with its later derogatory application to provincial practitioners with limited qualifications.
[49] Irvine Loudon, *Medical Care and the General Practitioner* (Oxford: Oxford University Press, 1986).
[50] Christelle Rabier, building on a wealth of historical scholarship on early modern European surgery, suggests that this is a process that had been underway for some time. Christelle Rabier, 'Medicalizing the Surgical Trade, 1650–1820: Workers, Knowledge, Markets and Politics', in T. Schlich (ed.), *Handbook*, pp. 71–94.

was celebrated as a surgical lecturer but was, by all accounts, an indifferent operator. Astley Cooper, who otherwise regarded him as 'an amusing companion' with 'an excellent private character', stated that he 'would have made a good physician, but never was a perfect surgeon, and never would have been, had he lived a hundred years'.[51] Even his own biographer admitted that 'we have very little desire to rest any portion of his reputation on this branch of our duty', adding that as Abernethy 'advanced in life, his dislike to operations increased'.[52] We shall come to consider the reasons why Abernethy so disliked the operative aspects of surgery in Chapter 2. For the moment, it will suffice to observe that his aversion to the knife may have influenced the nature of his practice, which, in line with Cooper's observation, was very similar to that of a fashionable metropolitan physician.[53] Though his biographer was at pains to deny it, Abernethy's lectures speak to the fact that he saw the health of the digestive system as being at the root of many disorders, and it was this belief that led him to concoct his 'blue pill', something that Cooper believed 'did him harm'.[54] Even so, it would be inaccurate to conceive of Abernethy's practice purely in terms of his praxial limitations or intellectual idiosyncrasies. Rather, his reluctance to regard surgery 'merely as an operative art' was part of a broader ideological commitment to uniting medicine and surgery in the management of disease.[55] Never a political radical, Abernethy nonetheless invoked the radicalism of French medicine when he famously told his students that 'surgery and medicine are essentially, what the French Republic was declared to be, "one and indivisible"'.[56] 'The physician must understand surgery and the surgeon the medical treatment of disease', he informed the audience at his Hunterian Oration of 1819.[57]

---

[51] Bransby Blake Cooper, *The Life of Sir Astley Cooper, Bart.*, vol. 2 (London: John W. Parker, 1843), p. 472.

[52] George Macilwain, *Memoirs of John Abernethy*, vol. 2, 2nd ed. (London: Hurst and Blackett, 1854), pp. 202–4.

[53] L. S. Jacyna, 'Abernethy, John (1764–1831)', *ODNB*.

[54] Macilwain, *Memoirs*, vol. 2, p. 282; Cooper, *Life*, vol. 2, p. 472. For an example of the centrality of the stomach in Abernethy's surgical system, see RCSE, MS0232/1/1. For a scientific context for Abernethy's views on the stomach, see Ian Miller, *A Modern History of the Stomach: Gastric Illness, Medicine, and British Society, 1800–1950* (London: Pickering and Chatto, 2011), pp. 14–16.

[55] RCSE, MS0232/1/5, John Flint South, 'Lectures on Natural and Morbid Anatomy and Physiology, delivered by John Abernethy Esq. FRS in the Anatomical Theatre at St Bartholomew's Hospital in the years 1819 & 1820, Vol. 4th', f. 98.

[56] *Lancet* 3:54 (9 October 1824), p. 5. On Abernethy's political and theoretical orthodoxy, see Adrian Desmond, *The Politics of Evolution: Morphology, Medicine, and Reform in Radical London* (Chicago: University of Chicago Press, 1992), pp. 117–18; Jacyna, 'Abernethy'; Sharon Ruston, *Shelley and Vitality* (Basingstoke: Palgrave Macmillan, 2005), pp. 38–63.

[57] John Abernethy, *The Hunterian Oration for the Year 1819* (London: Longman, Hurst, Rees, Orme, and Brown, 1819), p. 30.

Even if the desire to stress competencies other than the manual can be seen as part of Romantic surgery's designs on the sphere of medicine, it might nonetheless appear odd that surgeons of the early nineteenth century sought to distance themselves from the one aspect of their practice that rendered them unique. After all, from the middle decades of the nineteenth century onwards, surgeons were apt to emphasise their physical capacities as heroic men of action, and by the later decades, operative surgery had become, in the words of Thomas Schlich, the 'technological fix' for the ills of the modern body.[58] In order to make sense of this rhetorical and political strategy, it is important to reiterate that it did not constitute a wholesale repudiation of embodied skill per se. Rather, it deprecated the kind of rash and heedless operative intervention that was represented not only as the marker of a more ignorant past, but also, on occasion, as the preserve of other surgeons whose abilities and temperament one might seek to call into question. Take, for example, John Bell's attack on the *System of Surgery* (1783–8) of the (unrelated) Edinburgh surgeon Benjamin Bell (1749–1806), written under the pseudonym 'Jonathan Dawplucker':

The difference betwixt your description and that of a bold operator, is just that which distinguishes an assassin from a brave man! You write bloodily, though not boldly: you speak not like a regular surgeon [...] but like a desperate man, careless of everything, and afraid only of being affronted, or, in other words, "embarrassed" in the midst of a public exhibition! You write like one who had been often caught and entangled in difficulties from which he had no other way of disengaging himself than by a slap-dash stroke of the knife [...] You are enfuriated [*sic*] by opposition! the words adhesion, stricture, gut, and sac, excite proportioned fury! and you exclaim, tear, cut, clip, destroy – Tear the adhesions, cut every thing; - surgery consists in cutting! and the best surgery is to cut every thing!!![59]

As this quotation suggests, Bell sought to represent his rival as a man whose operative 'boldness' was in actual fact a cover for vanity, anger, and incompetence. His implication was not that operative skills were unimportant; far from it. Rather, as we shall now see, Bell and others were beginning to suggest that not only were exquisite manual skills and a deep knowledge of anatomy

[58] Thomas Schlich, 'The Technological Fix and the Modern Body: Surgery as a Paradigmatic Case', in Ivan Crozier (ed.), *The Cultural History of the Human Body in the Modern Age* (London: Bloomsbury, 2010), 71–92. For the surgeon as man of action, see Christopher Lawrence, 'Medical Minds, Surgical Bodies: Corporeality and the Doctors', in Christopher Lawrence and Steven Shapin (eds), *Science Incarnate: Historical Embodiments of Natural Knowledge* (Chicago: Chicago University Press, 1998), 156–201; Delia Gavrus, 'Men of Dreams and Men of Action: Neurologists, Neurosurgeons, and the Performance of Professional Identity, 1920–1950', *Bulletin of the History of Medicine* 85:1 (2011), 57–92; Lawrence and Brown, 'Quintessentially Modern'.
[59] Jonathan Dawplucker [John Bell], *Number Second, Being Remarks on the First Volume of Mr Benjamin Bell's System of Surgery* (London: 1799), pp. 53–5.

essential to the effective practice of surgery, but so too was a particular kind of emotional disposition. Shaping a professional identity within the emotional regime of Romantic sensibility, these men sought to craft an image of the modern surgeon not simply as a cerebral and scientific practitioner, but also as a *moral* one: self-confident, composed, and utterly dedicated to his patient's safety and well-being.

Embodied Knowledge, Dexterity, and the Moral Surgeon

Speaking to his surgical class at St Thomas' Hospital in 1815, Astley Cooper defined the embodied qualities of the surgeon in a phrase that would become a veritable cliché in later years. 'With regard to operations', he stated, 'a few acquisitions are necessary. It has been said that an Operator should have a[n] Eagle's eye, a Lion's heart and a Lady's hand'.[60] This common proverb can be found as early as the mid-eighteenth century and, doubtless, has its origins even further back than that.[61] Even so, among his students and acolytes at least, it became closely associated with Cooper, a man widely regarded as the greatest English surgeon of the early nineteenth century and, alongside Liston, possibly the best operative surgeon of the pre-anaesthetic era. The phrase is remarkable for a number of reasons, not least the framing of haptic skill as feminine. As we shall see in Chapter 2, the culture of sensibility allowed for a more fluid gendering of surgical skill than was common in the latter part of the century, although surgery remained a resolutely masculine practice until that time.[62] What is also suggestive about it is the insight that it provides into the habitus of the Romantic surgeon: the melding of perceptual, physical, and emotional/affective qualities. We shall explore the emotional/affective aspects shortly, but first it is necessary to consider the other two dimensions.

It is notable that, in introducing these necessary qualities, Cooper refers to them as 'acquisitions', suggesting that they were things that could be taught and learned. This is not an unproblematic assumption. If we are to take his animal metaphor seriously, we might question whether the lion *learned* to be courageous or whether the eagle *acquired* excellent eyesight. It would surely be more accurate to suggest that these qualities (even as culturally constructed) are innate to those creatures. Certainly, there was a good deal of debate in this

---

[60] WL MS.1860, William Hamilton Brown Ross, 'Lectures on Surgery by Mr A. A. Cooper [*sic*]' (1815), unpaginated. The same phrase occurs in various other notes of Cooper's lectures, including RCSE, MS0232/3.

[61] For example, see Robert Campbell, *The London Tradesman: Being an Historical Account of all the Trades, Professions, Arts, Both Liberal and Mechanic*, 3rd ed. (London: T. Gardner, 1747), pp. 48–9.

[62] Claire Brock, *British Women Surgeons and Their Patients* (Cambridge, UK: Cambridge University Press, 2017).

period about whether the true surgeon was born or made. According to an anonymous correspondent to *The Lancet*, the public, thinking surgery a

mere mechanical operation [...] conclude that frequent practice, with a proper knowledge of anatomy, must make them perfect performers:- but this is not the case; daily practice upon a musical instrument will never make some people good players [...] nor will all the opportunities of operating in an [*sic*] hospital make a good operator of the man who has neither the eye [...] nor the dexterity of finger which are the necessary prerequisites for such a performer.[63]

The St Bartholomew's Hospital surgeon Frederic Skey (1798–1872) likewise maintained that the 'dexterity of hand' or 'the power of entire command over its movements, which should be at the same time firm, but light and graceful [...] can only prevail in perfection, in men naturally gifted by its possession'.[64] And yet there were few surgeons indeed who would have claimed to be perfect operators. Even Astley Cooper admitted that he was 'never a good operator where delicacy was required' and that 'for the operation of cataract he was quite unfitted by nature'.[65] Cooper's reference to surgical dexterity as being akin to the 'lady's hand' offers a suggestion as to how this paradox concerning nature and nurture might be resolved. After all, it was generally assumed in this period that women had an innate propensity for delicate handicraft. And yet, women's education (across the social spectrum) still put great store by cultivating and honing those skills.[66] By the same token, it might be assumed that an aspirant surgeon, even one possessed of the natural gifts of good eyesight and dextrous hands, would still need to be trained in order to realise their potential. As John Bell put it, 'Though the qualifications of a surgeon are not to be acquired, yet assuredly they may be improved'.[67]

Unfortunately for the historian, the sources of embodied surgical education are not readily accessible, and it remains difficult for us to fully grasp, using the conventional materials of historical research, the exquisite haptic repertoire of Romantic surgical performance, or the ways in which those skills were inculcated in the novice. As Mark Jenner and Bertrand Taithe have argued, 'Professional historians are deeply suspicious of modes of representation based upon bodily practices such as those followed by re-enactment societies' and 'rarely seek theatrically to recapture and master the manipulative techniques, the precision of hand, and other *non-verbal* embodied skills which were at the

[63] *Lancet* 2:48 (28 August 1824), p. 277.
[64] Frederic Skey, *Operative Surgery* (London: John Churchill, 1850), pp. 4–5.
[65] Cooper, *Life*, vol. 2, p. 474.
[66] Rozsika Parker, *The Subversive Stitch: Embroidery and the Making of the Feminine*, revised ed. (London: I. B. Taurus, 2010); Johanna Ilmakunnas, 'Embroidering Women and Turning Men: Handiwork, Gender, and Emotions in Sweden and Finland, c. 1720–1820', *Scandinavian Journal of History* 41:3 (2016), 306–31.
[67] Bell, *Principles*, p. 12.

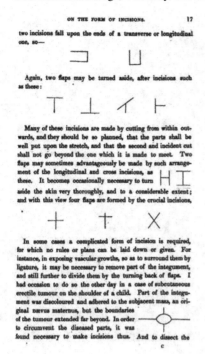

Figure 1.1 Haptic hieroglyphics: Robert Liston's guide to incisions from his *Practical Surgery* (London: John Churchill, 1837), p. 17. Public Domain Mark. Bodleian Library, Oxford via Google Books

core of much medical practice'.[68] However, if many of the praxial dimensions of surgical education remain lost to posterity (at least in terms of their depth and sophistication), we can nonetheless appreciate something of the importance of manual training to surgical practice through what textual forms are available to us. After all, most surgeons offered at least some basic advice in their lectures on the correct way of handling the knife, and of making incisions. It should perhaps come as no surprise, given his reputation in the operative dimensions of surgery, that one of the fullest such accounts can be found in the works of Robert Liston, notably his *Practical Surgery* (1837). This offered a reasonably compressive guide to operative technique, even within the constraints of the textual form (Figure 1.1).

[68] Mark S. R. Jenner and Bertrand O. Taithe, 'The Historiographical Body', in Roger Cooter and John Pickstone (eds), *Companion to Medicine in the Twentieth Century* (London: Routledge, 2003), p. 187.

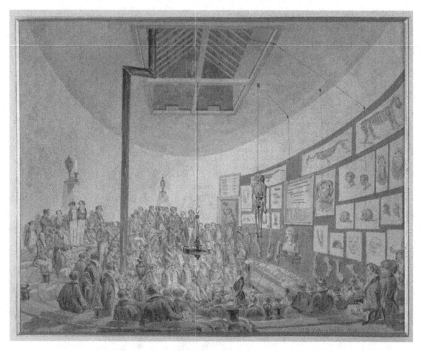

Figure 1.2 Robert Blemmel Schnebbelie, *A Lecture at the Hunterian Anatomy School, Great Windmill Street, London*, watercolour (1839). Wellcome Collection. Attribution 4.0 International (CC BY-NC 4.0)

Nevertheless, the principal lesson that such written accounts taught the student of surgery was that operative skills could be acquired only by doing, not reading. According to Charles Bell, 'words alone will never inform the young Surgeon of the things most necessary to a safe operation'.[69] For Astley Cooper, then, 'the first object to become a good Surgeon is anatomy', for 'a person may operate well without it, but it is only by chance'.[70] In order to learn anatomy, as we have heard, students conventionally attended lectures in which the forms and functions of the body might be elucidated, either through illustrations and preparations or the dissection of a corpse by an anatomical demonstrator (Figure 1.2). However, by the early nineteenth century the dictates of surgical anatomy, such as practised by John Bell in Edinburgh and in the private medical schools of London, ensured that students were increasingly provided access to their own (often illicitly acquired)

---

[69] Bell, *Illustrations*, p. iv.   [70] RCSE, MS0232/3, f. 5.

corpses.[71] Such forms of hands-on dissection were deemed increasingly essential to the training of operative surgeons, and specialist publications such as *The London Dissector* (1811) sought to guide the student through the process. 'Dexterity in the manual operation of dissection', it argued, 'can only be acquired by practice':

This species of knowledge will afford him the most essential assistance in his future operations on the living subject; in which indeed it is so necessary that we are perfectly astonished to see persons rash enough to use the knife without possessing this information; but we view the hesitation, confusion, and blunders by which such operators betray their ignorance to the bystander, as the natural result, and the well-merited but too light punishment, of such criminal temerity.[72]

By dissecting the dead human form, then, aspirant surgeons might familiarise themselves not only with the anatomy of the body, but also with its haptic presence, the resistance provided by flesh and bone to knife and saw. They might also guard against future disgrace. Dissection, according to John Bell,

gives a dexterity of hand, and acuteness of sight; a manner of searching for and seizing, with the most delicate of hooks and other instruments, parts almost invisible to one not trained to dissection: And that dexterity and acuteness of sight, gives presence of mind in the moment of operation [...] [it] renders scenes of danger familiar by anticipation; and inspires by degrees that address and courage, which enables a Surgeon to bear up undismayed, against alarms and accidents, when his own reputation is at stake; and, what is more distracting, while the life of a fellow-creature is endangered: Of a fellow-creature who has, at his suggestion, submitted to a dangerous operation, and is fainting in his hands, from pain and loss of blood.[73]

Bell's comments, and those of the *London Dissector*, are notable for their deployment of emotion: their evocation of the tribulations and anxieties of operative surgery, and of the personal costs of failure, especially in front of an audience. This should come as little surprise. After all, while it might promote familiarity with the intricacies of the human frame and the use of surgical instruments, the dissection of a dead body (or even ten dead bodies, for that matter) could never truly prepare the student for the realities of operating upon a living, breathing, writhing patient. Surgical pupils were therefore encouraged to attend operations by eminent practitioners and become acquainted with the realities of operative practice. For example, Home stated

[71] For an excellent account of anatomical education in the early nineteenth century, see Carin Berkowitz, *Charles Bell and the Anatomy of Reform* (Chicago: Chicago University Press, 2015), ch. 2. For a classic account of London hospital teaching, see Susan Lawrence, *Charitable Knowledge: Hospital Pupils and Practitioners in Eighteenth-Century London* (Cambridge, UK: Cambridge University Press, 1996).
[72] *The London Dissector; Or, a System of Dissection Practised in the Hospitals and Lecture Rooms of the Metropolis*, 3rd ed. (London: John Murray, 1811), pp. 1–3.
[73] Bell, *Letters on Professional Character*, p. 548.

that the student 'should add to his own information by the practice of others. Public Hospitals are so many Seminaries for this part of Education, whose Operations are performed under all circumstances & varied according to the Knowledge & dexterity of the Surgeons'.[74] Students might even gain direct personal experience by paying to assist in operations, a position known as a 'dresser'. Nonetheless, it was perfectly common to qualify as a surgeon without ever having performed an operation, let alone a capital procedure such as amputation or lithotomy.

In her ethnographic study of contemporary American surgical education, Rachel Prentice states that 'Surgeons must teach both skills and meaning'. Most of the surgeons she worked with spoke of technical skill as constituting a mere 20 per cent of surgical education, 'falling lower in importance than difficult-to-quantify qualities of wisdom, judgement and experience'.[75] Such was also the case for the early nineteenth century. Indeed, confronted by the prospect of a sentient patient in extraordinary pain, such considerations were even more important. Thus, Astley Cooper claimed that 'the quality which is considered of the highest order in surgical operations, is self-possession; the head must always direct the hand, otherwise the operator is unfit to discover an effectual remedy for unforeseen accidents that may occur in his practice'.[76] Over thirty years later, Frederic Skey's advice was similar: 'He should possess great firmness of purpose [...] to be acquired only by previous thought and preparation, and a self-possession which no accident, however unlooked for, can disturb or alienate'.[77]

At one level, this emphasis upon self-possession was a reaction to the practical challenges of pre-anaesthetic surgery. But it was also much more than this. In the early nineteenth century, surgical lecturers increasingly emphasised the moral and emotional aspects of the surgical persona, in contradistinction to the traditional emphasis on manipulative skill and operative dexterity. 'If I were to judge of a Surgeon's abilities', Cooper told his students, 'I would not judge him by his manner of performing the operation for the stone or the amputation of a limb, but would form my opinion of him according as he possesses a power of encountering unexpected dangers with calmness. It is this quality above all others [...] which you should endeavour to make yourselves masters of'.[78] In delivering his Hunterian Oration in 1826, meanwhile, the Westminster

---

[74] WL MS.5604, f. 10.
[75] Rachel Prentice, 'Drilling Surgeons: The Social Lessons of Embodied Surgical Learning', *Science, Technology and Human Values* 32:5 (2007), 534–53, at p. 535; Prentice, *Bodies in Formation: An Ethnography of Anatomy and Surgery Education* (Durham, NC: Duke University Press, 2013).
[76] *Lancet* 1:1 (5 October 1823), p. 4.
[77] Skey, *Operative Surgery*, p. 6.   [78] WL MS.1860, unpaginated.

Hospital surgeon Anthony Carlisle (1768–1840) argued that 'The *operative* practice of surgery is a mere mechanical art' and that 'if it be exercised with daring temerity, unchecked by moral or by scientific reflection, it becomes a desperate if not a mischievous calling'. The 'vain pretender brandishing his knife over the affrighted victims of his violence, may become a popular surgeon', he claimed, 'and by early good luck may reach his way to vulgar fame; but his career is most dangerous, and the result unenviable'.[79]

Frederic Skey was similarly sensitive to this delicate balance between the moral and manual qualities of surgery. 'To write a work on Operative Surgery, which should consist of merely mechanical rules for the performance of an amputation', he observed:

would be to leave the work more than half unfinished, simply because the knowledge, which determines the necessity of the undertaking is far more valuable [...] than that which is required to qualify a surgeon for its performance. The one qualification involves both the moral feeling and intellect of the surgeon. The other demands the exercise of his physical functions only[80]

This 'moral feeling', Skey maintained, 'is more involved in the establishment of a just reputation than the world at large imagines'.[81] This was because the operating surgeon was 'not a mechanic, but the agent through whose instrumentality is carried into action the highest principles of scientific medicine'.[82] Skey's sense of the primacy of 'moral feeling' over manual skill was such that, even in a book dedicated to the subject of operations, he proclaimed:

I have endeavoured as an English metropolitan surgeon to carry into execution at least one primary object, viz., to strip the science of Operative Surgery of a false glare, mistaken by the ignorant for the brightness of real excellence, to check a spirit of reckless experiment and to repress rather than encourage the resort to the knife as a remedial agent.[83]

Operative Surgery (1850) was published only a few years after the introduction of ether and chloroform, but it was fundamentally a product of the pre-anaesthetic era; Skey had studied under John Abernethy and his career had been forged in the 1820s. Indeed, Skey's distrust of what he called the 'brilliancy' and 'éclat' of operative performance had deep roots in the cultures of Romantic surgery, which can be traced back to John Bell. Bell's elaboration of a Romantic surgical persona at the turn of the nineteenth century was shaped by contemporary anxieties about the dangers of artifice and the

---

[79] *Lancet* 5:129 (18 February 1826), p. 690. Emphasis in original.
[80] Skey, *Operative Surgery*, p. iv.   [81] Skey, *Operative Surgery*, pp. vi–vii.
[82] Skey, *Operative Surgery*, p. viii.   [83] Skey, *Operative Surgery*, pp. x–xi.

importance of emotional sincerity and personal authenticity.[84] For Bell, the truly authentic surgical man of feeling rejected ostentation, artifice, and self-promotion in favour of a selfless and compassionate dedication to his patient's well-being. Thus, in his *Principles of Surgery* (1801) he argued that 'boldness is a seducing word, and the passion of acquiring character in operations is surely full of danger'. 'We are but too apt', he continued, 'to allow the audax in periculis [boldness in danger] to be the character of a good surgeon. But this is a temper of mind and a line of conduct which can benefit nothing but the character of the surgeon himself; for as to his patient, this shameless thirst of fame! this unprincipled ambition, is full of danger'. In place of such self-centred exhibitionism, Bell proposed the following:

Should not then the present suffering of the patient, and sense of his own duty, and above all the trust that is reposed in him, occupy the surgeon's mind too much to leave room for vain or selfish thoughts? Yet we every day see surgeons cutting out harmless tumours with affected and cruel deliberation, and in the same hour plunging a gorget among the viscera with unrelenting harshness.

Believe me, those qualities which relate to operations and other public exhibitions of skill, are of a very doubtful kind, while the duties of humanity and diligence are far more to be prized; they are both more amiable and more useful.[85]

According to Bell, then, operative flair was not simply an affectation that, in many cases, concealed as much as it revealed; it was a morally repugnant act that put the practitioner's desire for esteem ahead of his patient's interests. Charles Bell certainly inherited his brother's sensibility in this, as in many things, writing that 'Any thing [*sic*] like a flourish on such an occasion, does not merely betray vanity, but a lamentable want of just feeling. It is as if a man said – Look at me now – see how unconcerned I am, while the patient is suffering under my hand!'[86] Moreover, John Bell's arguments had a lasting impact far beyond his own family. John Struthers praised the *Principles of Surgery* as an 'undying book', while *The Lancet* claimed that it 'may be fairly considered the most interesting, if not the most useful, that has ever appeared on the subject of surgery [...] a work which may make a man proud of his calling'.[87] Indeed, if Skey's comments suggest something of Bell's influence, in other cases the intellectual inheritance was even clearer. For example, in lecturing to his students at the Aldersgate Street Medical School in the early 1830s, James Wardrop (1782–1869) quoted directly from the above passage of 'the late Mr John Bell' before adding his own coda:

---

[84] Brown, 'Surgery, Identity'.   [85] Bell, *Principles*, p. 12.
[86] Bell, *Illustrations*, p. vii.
[87] Struthers, *Historical Sketch*, p. 43; *Lancet* 7:166 (4 November 1826), p. 139.

Some of you may have heard of instances where surgeons, in other respects deservedly eminent, forgetting the duties of civilized life, have attempted a kind of theatrical effect in performing operations, for no other purpose than to give bystanders a false impression of their dexterity, coolness, and presence of mind [...] that affectation of dexterity, or doing operations quickly, is but a pitiful ambition in those who use it [...] but you will invariably observe that none except those who are deficient in moral courage [...] find it necessary to resort to such conduct; and that a man who feels himself equal to the task he undertakes proceeds deliberately and calmly, steadily bearing in mind the grand object – relief to the patient.[88]

Clearly, then, Romantic surgical culture militated against the idea of excessive, ostentatious, and unrestrained operative display. However, the very fact that surgical writers and lecturers of the early nineteenth century felt the need to caution against flamboyance and *theatricality* hints at another important dimension of operative practice. We have already heard from publications such as *The London Dissector* that surgery was often performed in front of an audience and that surgical skill was increasingly subject to scrutiny. Now we shall discover that this 'public' quality had profound implications for surgical performance, both literal and metaphorical.

The Operating Theatre as Performative and Emotional Space

The nineteenth-century Scottish author John Brown (1810–82) is now not much remembered. But in his lifetime he was a celebrated essayist and man of letters and was invariably mentioned in conjunction with his most well-known story, *Rab and His Friends* (1859). Essentially a paean to the nobility of dogs, this is a semi-autobiographical work in which surgery plays a central role.[89] Brown studied surgery in Edinburgh in the late 1820s, was apprenticed to James Syme, and served as a dresser and assistant at Syme's Minto House Hospital.[90] The story begins in 1825 with Brown as a teenage boy witnessing Rab, a large grey mastiff, kill a crazed bull terrier on the Cowgate. It resumes six years later with Brown a student at Minto House. He is now close to Rab and is acquainted with the dog's owner, a simple carter by the aptronymous name of James Noble. One day, James brings his wife, Ailie, to the hospital with what he refers to as 'trouble in her breest [*sic*]'. On examination, her breast is found to be 'hard as stone, a centre of horrid pain', and Syme opines that the advanced nature of the cancer means that she must be operated on urgently.[91]

---

[88] *Lancet* 20:514 (6 July 1833), p. 454.
[89] The story was seemingly based on a real episode. John Chiene, *Looking Back 1907–1860* (Edinburgh: Darien Press, 1908), p. 19.
[90] He later practised as a physician. A. C. Cheyne, 'Brown, John (1810–82)', *ODNB*.
[91] John Brown, *Rab and His Friends*, 8th ed. (Boston: Colonial Press, 1906), pp. 20, 24.

The operation takes place the following day and the students, eager to wit-ness the procedure, rush into the theatre. 'Don't think them heartless', Brown cautions his readers; 'they are neither better nor worse than you or I; they get over their professional horrors, and into their proper work – and in them pity – as an emotion, ending in itself or at best in tears [...] lessens, while pity as a motive is quickened'. 'The operating theatre is crowded', he continues;

much talk and fun, and all the cordiality and stir of youth. The surgeon with his staff of assistants is there. In comes Ailie: one look at her quiets and abates the eager students. That beautiful old woman is too much for them [...] These rough boys feel the power of her presence [...] The operation was at once begun; it was of necessity slow; and chloroform – one of God's best gifts to his suffering children – was then unknown. The surgeon did his work [...] [Finally] it is over: she is dressed, steps gently and decently down from the table, looks for James; then turning to the surgeon and the students, she courtesies, – and in a low, clear voice, begs their pardon if she has behaved ill. The students – all of us – wept like children.[92]

Brown's story provides a linking thread between the conventions of Victorian sentimentality and those of Romantic sensibility, linkages that are now increasingly recognised by historians.[93] Even so, it explicitly represents a pre-anaesthetic emotional regime in which the sufferings of the patient constituted a moral drama at the heart of surgical performance. Brown begins by asking his readers not to judge his fellow students for their enthusiasm or jocularity, suggesting that emotional restraint is a central aspect of surgical character and education. And yet, when confronted by the nobility of this woman, they are moved, ultimately, to tears. Neither is it just the students who express emotion. Syme himself is recorded as addressing Ailie in 'a kind way, pitying her through his eyes'.[94] This is not incidental. Such affective engagement is central to the story's purpose, for as Brown notes, 'there is a pleasure, one of the strangest and strongest in our nature, in imaginative suffering with and for others'.[95]

As we shall see, Brown's representation of the emotional and moral politics of the pre-anaesthetic operating theatre was an idealised one. Nevertheless, it captures something vital about this space as one of noise, confusion, and occasionally irreverence, which had, somehow, to be managed and disciplined. It also reminds us of the theatrical aspects of surgery in this period. Romantic surgery was not only an intense drama, it also often had a stage and actors, as well as an audience. In Chapter 4, we shall consider in more detail the ways in which a theatricalised sensibility shaped the radical scrutiny of surgical

[92] Brown, *Rab*, pp. 25–8.
[93] For example, see Rebecca Bedell, *Moved to Tears: Rethinking the Art of the Sentimental in the United States* (Princeton: Princeton University Press, 2018).
[94] Brown, *Rab*, p. 30.   [95] Brown, *Rab*, p. xi.

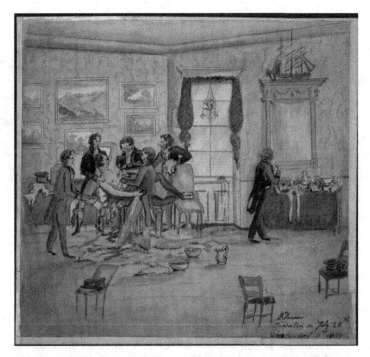

Figure 1.3 'A surgical operation to remove a malignant tumour from a man's left breast and armpit in a Dublin drawing room', watercolour (1817). Wellcome Collection. Attribution 4.0 International (CC BY 4.0)

practice. For the moment, we are concerned with the general cultures of the operating theatre and its impact on surgical performance.

Before considering the theatrical dimensions of Romantic surgery, it is important to note that many operative procedures in this period were undertaken in private residences by fee-paying patients. Aside from the occasional textual reference, or images such as the well-known 1817 watercolour of an operation to remove a tumour, undertaken in the otherwise salubrious surrounds of a Dublin drawing room (Figure 1.3), we know relatively little about how such homes were arranged, or rearranged, for the purposes of medical and surgical procedure. By contrast, we know rather more about how the operative spaces of public institutions were appointed. Most hospitals, including small provincial ones, had some kind of discrete space for the performance of operations. With the expansion of surgical education in the later decades of the eighteenth century, however, teaching hospitals, such as those in London, built larger rooms to accommodate students. Few operating theatres from this period

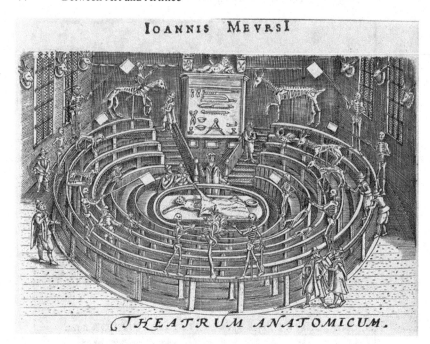

Figure 1.4 Leiden anatomical theatre (1596), from Johannes van Meurs, *Athenae Batavae* (1625). Wellcome Collection. Public Domain Mark

survive. The best example in Britain is that of the old St Thomas' Hospital, originally built in 1822 before being rediscovered and partially reconstructed in the late 1950s. From this survival, as well as from contemporary sources, we know that operating theatres of the period traced their spatial lineage back to the anatomical theatres of the Renaissance.[96] The oldest of these was built at Padua in 1594, followed by a similar structure at Leiden in 1596 (Figure 1.4). As Jonathan Sawday observes, these spaces 'combined elements from a number of different sources, drawing together different kinds of public space in order to produce an event that was visually spectacular'. 'In the construction of these theatres', he states, 'we can discern outlines of the judicial court, the dramatic stage, and, most strikingly, the basilica-style church or temple'.[97] What is perhaps most characteristic about these structures is their steep terraced sides, often with a balustrade and handrails to allow the audience to gain as unobstructed a view as possible. Enhancing the visuality of the proceedings

[96] For an overview of the history of operating room architecture, see Annemarie Adams, 'Surgery and Architecture: Spaces for Operating', in Schlich (ed.), *Handbook*, 261–81.
[97] Jonathan Sawday, *The Body Emblazoned: Dissection and the Human Body in Renaissance Culture* (London: Routledge, 1995), p. 64.

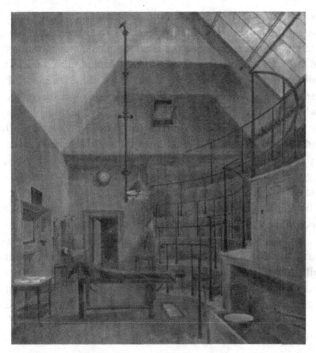

Figure 1.5 F. M. Harvey, *The Old Operating Theatre at The London Hospital, Demolished in 1889* (1889), oil on canvas. Barts Health NHS Trust Archives

was not simply about observation, however. The spatial arrangement of the theatre also focused the audience on the moral dimensions of the performance. In her work on the anatomical demonstrations of Alexander Monro primus, Anita Guerrini coins the term 'moral theatre' to describe the ways in which anatomical dissection functioned as a 'public performance intended to induce in its audience such emotions as awe, fear, and compassion – emotions similar to those provoked by religious practices'.[98]

However, while the operating theatre of the early nineteenth century had its antecedents in the anatomical theatres of the Renaissance, they were not identical structures. Most operating theatres built in this period had a more proscenium than amphitheatrical quality, with the audience facing the 'stage', so to speak, more or less front on (Figure 1.5). In part, this reflected wider shifts in theatrical architecture, but it also coincided with a fundamental shift in purpose. Early modern anatomical dissection was, to a great extent, a public

[98] Anita Guerrini, 'Alexander Monro Primus and the Moral Theatre of Anatomy', *Eighteenth Century* 47:1 (2006), 1–18, at p. 1.

spectacle. Artists attended to view the form and articulation of the body, while others sought spiritual succour in the wonders of divine creation. By the early nineteenth century, however, routine public anatomical demonstrations had all but died out. Such practices increasingly moved behind closed doors as their rationale shifted from quasi-religious revelation to utilitarian medical education. The same is true of the operating theatre. These spaces were located in hospitals, which, during the course of this period, were transitioning from quasi-public civic spaces into professional institutions dedicated to the construction and dissemination of medical knowledge.[99] Members of the public occasionally continued to attend operations in the first half of the century, but there was a growing consensus that these were professional spaces that should be accessible only to practitioners and students.

To say that the early nineteenth-century operating theatre was a more tightly policed space than its forebears is not to say that it was any less moral or dramatic. Indeed, one might say that, as the space was shorn of its spiritual connotations, it became ever more akin to a theatre in the literal sense. In almost all the hospitals of the metropolis, it was necessary to be either a practitioner, or a student in possession of a ticket, in order to attend an operation. The behaviour of this audience also resonated with the experience of play-going. The St Thomas' Hospital surgeon John Flint South recalled that, as a young student:

The operation day was Friday, and in the earlier part of my hospital life it was very rare to have less than two or three operations. The operating theatre was small, and the rush and scuffle to get a place was not unlike that for a seat in the pit or gallery of a dramatic theatre; and when one was lucky enough to get a place, the crowding and squeezing was oftentimes unbearable, more especially when any very important operation was expected to be performed.[100]

Chaotic though such scenes might appear, there was, in principle at least, a semblance of order. Generally speaking, the space immediately around the table was occupied by the surgeon, his assistants, and dressers. The seats closest to the front were reserved for the house surgeons and eminent visitors, while those behind were taken up by fee-paying students. Other, less prestigious visitors, meanwhile, were relegated to the back. These arrangements were subject to a delicate politics. In 1844, for example, Joseph Rogers (1820–89) decided to attend an amputation of the thigh undertaken by James Moncrieff Arnott

---

[99] Michael Brown, 'Medicine, Reform and the "End" of Charity in Early Nineteenth-Century England', *English Historical Review* 124:511 (2009), 1353–88. See also Brown, *Performing Medicine: Medical Culture and Identity in Provincial England* (Manchester: Manchester University Press, 2011), pp. 138–40.

[100] John Flint South, *Memorials of John Flint South* (London: John Murray, 1884), p. 27.

(1794–1885) at his *alma mater*, the Middlesex Hospital. On entering the theatre, he 'walked into the front row, where I found two old pupils, like myself' and was reassured by a notice 'to the effect that former house-surgeons, old pupils who came as visitors, and the dressers to the other surgeons, were allowed to stand there'. However, on entering the theatre, Arnott 'turned upon me, saying [...] "You have no business here – go out"'. Humiliated, Rogers 'withdrew, (observing as I went, "I am an old pupil",) and then took my station at the top of the theatre, amidst the tittering of the students who doubtless thought me an intruder'.[101]

In many ways, the atmosphere of the operating theatre was in keeping with the broader cultures of medical student life, as described by Keir Waddington and Laura Kelly.[102] Concern about student behaviour, according to Waddington, 'fed on a rich vein of anxiety about moral decay, crime, and intemperance associated with urbanization [...] [and] its visible display of playhouses, pleasure gardens [and] prostitutes'.[103] For the most part, however, it resembled little more than schoolboy pranks or the limited licence of the apprentice. Thus, in 1823 a former Edinburgh student complained to *The Lancet* about the conduct of those awaiting Astley Cooper's lecture at St Thomas' Hospital. 'What an interesting spectacle', he wrote, 'to see a body of young men assembled for the purpose of acquiring professional knowledge, actively engaged in discharging masticated paper and apple into each other's faces; or employed in the no less intellectual occupation of twirling around the Lecturer's table, or sprinkling dirt on the heads of those who happen to sit under them'.[104] At other times such rowdiness could serve more political ends, as students sought to defend their perceived rights and interests. This was especially notable in the aftermath of the acrimonious collapse of the so-called United School of Guy's and St Thomas' in 1825.[105] Bransby Cooper (1782–1853), Astley Cooper's nephew and protégé, had been appointed professor of anatomy to the new school at Guy's and when he attempted to attend a lithotomy at St Thomas', undertaken by Joseph Henry Green (1791–1863), he was forced 'out again immediately, several of the pupils having expressed their disapprobation of his presence by hisses'.[106]

[101] *Lancet* 44:1107 (16 November 1844), p. 245.
[102] Keir Waddington, 'Mayhem and Medical Students: Image, Conduct, and Control in the Victorian and Edwardian London Teaching Hospital', *Social History of Medicine* 15:1 (2002), 45–64, Laura Kelly, *Irish Medical Education and Student Culture, c.1850–1950* (Liverpool: Liverpool University Press, 2017).
[103] Waddington, 'Mayhem', p. 48. [104] *Lancet* 1:11 (14 December 1823), p. 381.
[105] Michael Brown, '"Bats, Rats and Barristers": *The Lancet*, Libel and the Radical Stylistics of Early Nineteenth-Century English Medicine', *Social History* 39:2 (2014), 182–209, at p. 194.
[106] *Lancet* 13:325 (21 November 1829), p. 290.

Much of the time, the disordered scenes in metropolitan operating theatres were merely the product of students endeavouring to get the best possible return on their fees. In 1828, a pupil at St George's Hospital wrote to *The Lancet* complaining that

I have heard, occasionally, the voice of the surgeon as he addresses the patient; I have seen, occasionally, the gleam of the knife in the operating theatre of this establishment, and have been electrified by the scream of the patient, and edified by the remonstrating voice of the surgeon; but I have rarely seen or heard more [...] I have never had a fair and distinct view of an operation on the regular day of operating, since I have had the happiness of being attached to this establishment. That portion of the theatre where the patient is placed, is, upon the arrival of the operating surgeon, instantly filled by friends, dressers, surgeons, house surgeons, etc.; all these literally club their sagacious heads together, and – but need I say more? the pupils in the first row endeavour to overtop them, those in the second or third row follow their example, and the rest are under the necessity of standing on the rails, bars, posts, etc. to obtain a casual glance at what is going forward.[107]

With its reference to the electrifying 'scream of the patient', this letter reminds us of the intense pathos at the heart of such scenes. Likewise, another correspondent evoked the 'weeping and cries' of Mary Hayward, a 25-year-old woman who had come to St Bartholomew's to have a tumour removed from her knee. In the midst of the procedure she pleaded with the operator, imploring him to '"let it alone, let it alone! don't pull it about any more [...] plaster it up! I won't let you cut it any more, I won't, I won't, I won't"'. These expressions were combined with 'cries of "heads! heads!"' from the back of the theatre as the students endeavoured to catch sight of proceedings, followed by hisses when their requests were ignored. It was, according to the correspondent, an unedifying scene that 'entirely did away with the ordinary view and benefit derived from the performance of operations in this theatre'.[108] Needless to say, many commentators were aware that such an atmosphere can have done little to improve the patient's emotional state. Writing to *The Lancet* in 1827, for example, a student at the Borough hospitals of Guy's and St Thomas' argued that 'The mode in which operations were conducted at both hospitals was shameful' and that 'during the performance of the operation there was a continual cry of "hats off, heads", etc., which was not only annoying to the more gentlemanly students, but also tended to render the patient more fearful'.[109]

We shall see in Chapter 2 how surgeons sought to render the experience of operations more emotionally palatable to the patient, and in Chapter 4 we will

---

[107] *Lancet*, 10:254 (12 July 1828), p. 464.   [108] *Lancet*, 12:298 (15 May 1829), p. 220.
[109] *Lancet*, 8:213 (29 September 1827), p. 828.

consider the political consequences of their failure to do so adequately. For the moment, however, it is important to recognise that the atmosphere of the operating theatre also had a profound impact on surgical conduct. For one thing, the audience members did not always limit themselves to watching the procedure or interacting only with each other. As with the contemporary dramatic theatre, which had yet to be 'rationalised' by the efforts of reformers and the effects of the Theatres Act of 1843, there was often a permeable boundary between 'pit' and 'stage'.[110] In an incident at St Bartholomew's in 1834, for example, Eusebius Lloyd (1795–1862) and William Lawrence (1783–1867) were tying an arterial aneurysm when they were surrounded by several other surgeons, one of whom 'actually took the knife and forceps from MR. LLOYD'S hand and proceed coolly to satisfy his doubts by actual dissection'.[111] Such direct interference was rare and greatly frowned upon. Nonetheless, the routine throng of participants and observers could be intensely distracting, as in the case of Mary Hayward's operation, where the crowd around the operator was such that he was forced to 'raise his head and shoulders above those of others (thus indecorously conducting themselves) to perform parts of the operation with his arms completely extended before him', or in another instance at Guy's where an actual fight broke out between a pupil and a dresser over the former's obstructed view.[112]

In light of this, it is perhaps unsurprising that the Romantic ideal of operative performance should involve calm and considered deportment. Surgery was always a challenging affair, full of risks and unforeseen eventualities, but in as intense an atmosphere as the hospital operating theatre, there was all the more necessity to practice with a focused precision, unperturbed by the goings-on around. Moreover, one's actions were subject to constant scrutiny by the audience, even down to the smallest gesture. As such, operators were discouraged from talking to their assistants unless absolutely necessary, directing their actions with nothing more conspicuous than a discreet glance or motion of the hand. At one level, while it might not necessarily accord with the conventional image of the pre-anaesthetic surgeon as a flamboyant showman, this cool-headedness was, as Stephanie Snow has suggested, a form of showmanship in itself:

---

[110] Marc Beer, *Theatre and Disorder in Late Georgian London* (Oxford: Clarendon Press, 1992); Elaine Hadley, *Melodramatic Tactics: Theatricalized Dissent in the English Marketplace, 1800–1885* (Stanford: Stanford University Press, 1995); Jim Davis and Victor Emeljanow, *Reflecting the Audience: London Theatregoing, 1840–1880* (Iowa City: University of Iowa Press, 2001); Jacky Bratton, *The Making of the West End Stage: Marriage, Management and the Mapping of Gender in London, 1830–1870* (Cambridge, UK: Cambridge University Press 2011).

[111] *Lancet*, 23:581 (18 October 1834), p. 144.

[112] *Lancet*, 12:298 (15 May 1829), pp. 220–1; 23:585 (15 November 1834), pp. 299–300.

By the late 1840s, 'modern' surgeons had constructed their professional identity upon attributes such as coolness and decisiveness. It was an image with elements of show-manship; the surgeon was the oasis of authority among the bodily confusion of severed flesh and bones, and the disarray of minds.[113]

There is much truth in this statement, but there is also much more to be said, for, as we have suggested, by practising with a self-contained composure, operative surgeons not only demonstrated their intellectual and praxial author-ity, they also set a moral example, disciplining and ennobling their audience through calm and measured dedication to the patient's well-being. As John Bell argued earlier in the century:

A man of science never proceeds without due reflection: The whole plan of his opera-tion is perfect in his own mind: He communes with his assistant rather by signs than words, and his manner commands that stillness which is due to a moment of suffer-ing, and essential to his self-possession and success: He is formed by education, and qualified, from the first moment in which he takes those public duties upon him, to give impressive lessons to the younger members of the profession: They are awe-struck with the first horrors of incisions and blood, but depart with gratified feelings, when they see the scene closed with entire relief to the sufferer, and happy prospect of success; and they learn to love and respect their profession, and to study it with emulation.[114]

In this way, even the conventional signifiers of public and professional appro-bation were to be discouraged. In 1835, for example, *The Lancet*, commenting on the lithotomy of a 6-year-old child at Westminster Hospital, stated:

We are sorry to have to animadvert on the bad taste which has lately been frequently exhibited amongst the visitors at this theatre, and exemplified in the highly injudi-cious practice of applauding the operator in the course or at the conclusion of his labours [...] Even putting out of sight the inhumanity of such demonstrations at a time when the patient is writhing in acute agony, the ill effect which any expression of feeling by an assembly must produce upon the nerves of the most intrepid surgeon at a critical moment, must be obvious to every reflecting mind, superadding, as it does, to the natural difficulty of the surgeon's duty, the intense excitement of a public exhibition.[115]

On occasion, the surgeon was even required to exercise a vocal emotional and moral authority over the space of the operating theatre. Generally speak-ing, surgeons were discouraged from addressing the audience, or offering instruction, until after the operation was over and the patient removed. A remarkable exception to this took place at St Bartholomew's where William Lawrence, having amputated the cancerous penis of a 60-year-old man, 'turned

[113] Stephanie Snow, *Operations without Pain: The Practice and Science of Anaesthesia in Victorian Britain* (Basingstoke: Palgrave Macmillan, 2006), p. 129.
[114] Bell, *Letters on Professional Character*, p. 559.
[115] *Lancet*, 23:594 (17 January 1835), p. 597.

his back to the patient, and immediately began dissecting the part that had been removed'. Upon this, 'the poor man raised himself up, took the handkerchief from his eyes, and was permitted to sit looking over the dissector's shoulder for four minutes'. 'At length', the patient requested to know 'what was to be the fate of this once important part', to which Lawrence replied, '"Oh! It shall be taken care of, my friend, it shall be taken care of"', a comment that 'occasioned much laughter throughout the theatre'.[116]

Doubtless, on this occasion the degree of jocularity permitted to Lawrence and his audience stemmed from the patient's age and gender, as well as his active participation in the process. But in other instances, where the politics of sensibility demanded due reverence to suffering, especially that of women and children, the 'voice of the surgeon', as the St George's correspondent quoted earlier put it, was to be edifying and remonstrative. In 1831, for example, during an operation to remove a tumour from the neck of a young boy, Joseph Henry Green admonished his rowdy audience at St Thomas', telling them that 'I am astonished that any set of persons calling themselves gentlemen should pass their *jokes* in this place, especially when a human being is suffering, putting myself out of the question, though I am not likely to perform a nice and delicate dissection the better by hearing such noises'.[117] Likewise, in 1840, Robert Liston had just commenced an operation to remove a piece of necrosed bone from the heel of a child at University College Hospital when

a person in the theatre, because the poor little sufferer began to *cry*, burst out into a loud laugh; whereupon Mr. LISTON instantly turned round, and asked, "if the offender belonged to that hospital?" He then remarked that "such unfeeling conduct was disgusting and disgraceful in the extreme." The honourable gentleman also alluded, in strong terms of reprehension, to a similar exhibition of cruel misbehaviour a few days since [...] This well-timed and excellent rebuke appeared to give great satisfaction to the gentlemen present. The operation was quickly executed, in Mr LISTON'S admirable and unrivalled style.[118]

While this scene offers a stark contrast to Brown's idealised representation of the emotional dynamics of the operating theatre in *Rab and His Friends*, it nonetheless presents Liston as a model of the Romantic surgeon, performing with great skill while also exercising moral authority and demonstrating a compassionate concern for his patient's well-being in the face of callous indifference to suffering. However, as we shall see in the final section of this chapter, Liston's reputation was not always so straightforward and serves as a reminder of the complexity and ambiguities of Romantic surgical culture.

[116] *Lancet*, 12:301 (6 June 1829), p. 319.   [117] *Lancet* 17:428 (12 November 1831), p. 229.
[118] *Lancet*, 35:896 (31 October 1840), p. 215.

Robert Liston: The Making of an Ambivalent Icon

In 1912, the American-born pharmaceutical entrepreneur Henry Wellcome (1853–1936) commissioned the Bristol artist Ernest Board (1877–1934) to paint twenty-six images of important events from the history of science and medicine. One of these images portrays Robert Liston performing the first operation carried out in Britain under inhalation anaesthesia at University College Hospital on 21 December 1846 (Figure 1.6). That Wellcome should have chosen this event is testament to its mythic place in the history of British surgery. As we shall discover later in this book, by the time Wellcome commissioned these paintings the introduction of anaesthesia was well established in professional and popular consciousness as a pivotal moment in the shift from a squalid, barbaric past to a clean, pain-free surgical modernity. But if the value of that particular historical moment was, and remains, largely unquestioned, the identity of its key protagonist was, and still is, less clearcut. Though indelibly identified with the first use of ether in Europe, Robert Liston is something of a liminal figure, standing at the threshold of this new age while never being truly a part of it. To a large extent this is due to the fact that he died of an aneurism of the aorta less than a year later, at the peak of his career. But it also derives from his rootedness in the operative cultures of the pre-anaesthetic era. Indeed, within the historiography he is often portrayed as the literal embodiment of the physical prowess, manual dexterity, and, most especially, operative speed that came to prominence in the decades immediately before surgery's supposed transfiguration. However, as if to serve as a cautionary exemplar of the horrors of surgery's *ancien régime*, this operative celerity is frequently represented as both 'a gift and a curse'.[119]

The roots of Liston's modern representation as an 'incorrigible bustler' are readily traced and demonstrate the ease with which spurious anecdote can pass into historical fact.[120] Take, for example, Lindsey Fitzharris' popular history of Joseph Lister, *The Butchering Art* (2017); her reference to Liston as 'the fastest knife in the West End' and her account of an apocryphal operation in which his obsession with speed supposedly led to the deaths of the patient, an assistant, and a bystander are taken, virtually word for word, from a book written by the anaesthetist and *Doctor in the House* author Richard Gordon (1921–2017).[121] This book, *Great Medical Disasters* (1983), which contains a brief three-page sketch of the man, is the source of much modern Liston folklore. For example, Gordon's claims that Liston 'sprung across the bloodstained

---

[119] Fitzharris, *Butchering*, p. 10.

[120] Richard Gordon, *Great Medical Disasters* (New York: Stein and Day, 1983), p. 19.

[121] Fitzharris, *Butchering*, pp. 10–12. Either that or Wikipedia, whose entry on Robert Liston is heavily reliant on Gordon's book: https://en.wikipedia.org/wiki/Robert_Liston (accessed 11/05/22).

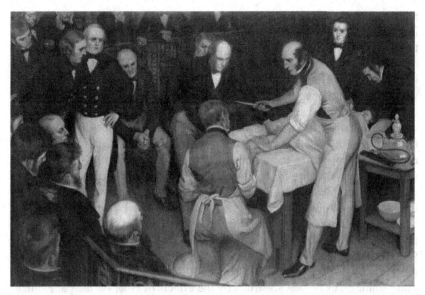

Figure 1.6 Ernest Board, *Robert Liston Operating* (1912). Wellcome Collection. Attribution 4.0 International (CC BY 4.0)

boards upon his patient like a duelist [*sic*], calling "Time me gentlemen, time me!'" and that 'To free both hands, he would clasp the bloody knife between his teeth' are often repeated in popular accounts.[122] Gordon's sources, other than his own imagination, are two articles in the *University College Hospital Magazine*, one of which is a general biographical account of Liston, written by Percy Flemming (1863–1941) in 1926.[123] This is the principal source for the assertion that Liston would hold the knife between his teeth.[124] Flemming likewise maintains that Liston 'would begin an operation by exclaiming, "time me, gentlemen, time me"'.[125] In turn, this claim is an extrapolation from the second of Gordon's sources, an account of Liston's first use of ether, written by F. William Cock (1858–1943) and published in 1911.[126] A contemporary

---

[122] Gordon, *Disasters*, pp. 19–21. For example, see Wendy Moore, *The Mesmerist: The Society Doctor Who Held Victorian Society Spellbound* (London: Weidenfeld and Nicolson, 2017), pp. 94–5.

[123] Percy Flemming, 'Robert Liston', *University College Hospital Magazine* 11.4 (September 1926), 176–85.

[124] Flemming, 'Liston', p. 177.   [125] Flemming, 'Liston', p. 179.

[126] F. William Cock, 'The First Operation under Ether – The Story of Three Days', *University College Hospital Magazine* 1:4 (February 1911), 127–44. One recent account refers to Cock as 'a member of the audience', even though he was born over ten years after these events took place: Harold Ellis, *A History of Surgery* (London: Greenwich Medical Media, 2000), p. 85.

article in *The Lancet* states that 'Dr Cock's restrained, but vigorous, writing invests the narrative with due fascination'.[127] Meanwhile, Flemming refers to the events of 21 December 1846 as having been 'graphically described by my old friend F. W. Cock'.[128] Indeed, on inspection it is clear that Cock's article is largely a work of fiction, embellishing the known details of the operation with imagined dialogue, including Liston's request to be timed.[129] It is also one of the principal accounts to claim that Liston referred to anaesthesia as a 'Yankee dodge' that 'beat mesmerism hollow'.[130] Despite Alison Winter's attribution of this quotation to Liston's assistant William Squire's (1825–99) account of the operation published in *The Lancet* in 1888, there is no evidence of such a phrase, either in this article or in his later recollections published in the *British Medical Journal* in 1896.[131] It is true that, in an account published at the end of the nineteenth century, John Russell Reynolds (1828–96) claimed to remember Liston uttering these words 'as if it were yesterday', but it is odd that no such phrase appears before around 1872, some twenty-six years after the fact.[132] Indeed, what is consistent in Squire's reports, and in most other first-person accounts, is that Liston either made 'few remarks' or said 'nothing', as he was so struck by the effects of ether on the patient that 'he could scarcely command himself sufficiently to address even a few words to the spectators'.[133]

While Liston's ambivalent historical reputation, awkwardly poised between hero and villain, is largely a product of the early twentieth century and owes little to his contemporary public and professional identity, the irony is that his place within the cultures of Romantic surgery was no less ambiguous or contingent. He was, by almost all accounts, a somewhat difficult man who lacked the easy manner and social graces of Astley Cooper, a surgeon who, as we shall see in Chapter 2, conformed more readily to the culturally resonant ideal of the man of feeling. Even Liston's obituary in *The Times* notes that 'His manner in ordinary society was sometimes complained of as harsh or abrupt'

---

[127] *Lancet* 177:4573 (22 April 1911), p. 1093.   [128] Flemming, 'Liston', p. 183.

[129] Cock, 'Ether', p. 137. Earlier accounts do suggest that he was timed at thirty-two seconds, but not that he asked to be, e.g. *British Medical Journal* 2:1868 (17 October 1896), p. 1140.

[130] Cock, 'Ether', pp. 137–8.

[131] Alison Winter, *Mesmerised: Powers of Mind in Victorian Britain* (Chicago: Chicago University Press, 1998) p. 180, n. 48. Fitzharris, *Butchering*, p. 7, uses the same quotation, citing a number of secondary sources, including Winter. *Lancet* 132:3408 (22 December 1888), 1220–1; *British Medical Journal* 2:1868 (17 October 1896), 1142–3.

[132] John Russell Reynolds, *Essays and Addresses* (London: Macmillan, 1896), p. 274. The 1872 reference comes from another University College Hospital alumnus, George Vivian Poore (1843–1904). Poore refers to Liston describing ether as a 'Yankee dodge' that was 'better than mesmerism': *Lancet* 100:2563 (12 October 1872), p. 521.

[133] *Lancet* 132:3408 (22 December 1888), p. 1221; *British Medical Journal* 2:1868 (17 October 1896), pp. 1140, 1143.

and that he was 'rather backward or indifferent in his address'.[134] In this sense, he more closely resembled John Abernethy, who was said to have been occasionally rough in his manner, or John Bell, who, despite his literary appeals to sensibility, had a dubious interpersonal reputation, even within his own family.[135] Certainly, Liston's directness, rudeness even, is evident in his correspondence with his former assistant, James Miller (1812–64).[136] However, his obituary was at pains to aver that, despite this, he was still a man of tender compassion, claiming that 'in the chamber of the sick – he was gentle as he was resolute', and that 'into the scene of suffering he never brought a harsh word or an unkind look and the hand which was as hard as iron and true as steel in the theatre of operation, was soft as thistledown to the throbbing pulse and aching brow'.[137] As this quotation suggests, if Liston's professional character and demeanour were ambiguous, then much of that ambiguity centred, then as now, on his operative performance. And in its reference to 'thistledown', it also indicates how much of this ambiguity also derived from his identity as a Scot practising in the English metropolis.

As we have suggested in the case of the Edinburgh student Andrew Whelpdale, Liston's fame in the early nineteenth century was spread, in part, by his pupils and acolytes. But it was, at a fundamental level, made by an expanding and increasingly vital medical press. There is a growing body of literature on the culture and politics of the early nineteenth-century medical press, but if there is one journal that has received the greatest attention, it is *The Lancet*, founded in 1823 by the radical surgeon Thomas Wakley.[138] *The Lancet* was significant not simply because it was one of the first journals to be published weekly, nor simply because it had by far the largest circulation of any medical journal, but also because of its literary style, which, by embracing the radical conventions of 'democratic celebrity', played a vital role in the making and unmaking of medical and, more especially, surgical reputations.[139]

---

[134] *Times*, 20 December 1847, pp. 8–9.
[135] Macilwain, *Memoirs*, vol. 2, pp. 184–92; Jacyna, 'Abernethy'. The best insight into John Bell's vexatious relationship with his family, especially his brothers, is provided by RCSEd, GD82, Bell family archive, Box 1/2, Handwritten notes and memoranda by George Joseph Bell (1770–1843).
[136] WL, MSS.6084–6094, Original letters from Robert Liston to James Miller.
[137] *Times*, 20 December 1847, pp. 8–9.
[138] Mary Bostetter, 'The Journalism of Thomas Wakley', in Joel H. Wiener (ed.), *Innovators and Preachers: The Role of the Editor in Victorian England* (London: Greenwood Press, 1985); William F. Bynum, Stephen Lock, and Roy Porter (eds), *Medical Journals and Medical Knowledge: Historical Essays* (London: Routledge, 1992), Debbie Harrison, 'All the *Lancet's* Men: Reactionary Gentleman Physicians vs. Radical General Practitioners in the *Lancet*, 1823–1832', *Nineteenth-Century Gender Studies* 5:2 (2009), www.ncgsjournal.com/issue52/harrison.html (accessed 14/10/21); Brittany Pladek, '"A Variety of Tastes: *The Lancet* in the Early Nineteenth-Century Periodical Press', *Bulletin of the History of Medicine*, 85:4 (2011), 560–86; Brown, '"Bats, Rats"'; Sally Frampton and Jennifer Wallis (eds), *Reading the Nineteenth Century Medical Journal* (London: Routledge, 2021).
[139] Brown, '"Bats, Rats"'.

Nowhere was the role of *The Lancet* in shaping surgical reputations more obvious than in the case of Robert Liston. One of his earliest appearances in its pages was in connection with an operation performed by his cousin, friend, and soon to be bitter rival, James Syme, in 1823. This procedure, the amputation of the leg at the hip joint, undertaken on a 19-year-old by the name of William Fraser, was what Syme called 'the greatest and bloodiest operation in surgery' and had yet to be performed in Scotland.[140] Liston assisted in the operation, covering 'the numerous cut arteries with his left hand and compress[ing] the femoral in the groin by means of his right'.[141] *The Lancet* reprinted the *Edinburgh Medical and Surgical Journal*'s initial report in early February 1824 without comment.[142] At the end of the month, however, it ran a highly critical editorial on the (ultimately fatal) procedure. Wakley was enraged by the idea that 'the northern [i.e. Scottish] journals' sought to use the incident 'for the purpose of casting a shade upon the splendour of London surgery', particularly in the way they 'sarcastically compared the time occupied by Mr. SYMES [*sic*] to that occupied by Sir A. COOPER when he recently performed a similar operation at Guy's Hospital'. Whereas Cooper 'required *twenty* minutes to remove the limb', Syme 'according to his own account, was contented with ONE minute'.[143] As we shall see in Chapter 4, Wakley and *The Lancet* were nothing if not London centric, and the journal's attitude towards Scottish (and Irish) medicine was deeply ambivalent. Moreover, Cooper had been Wakley's tutor at St Thomas' and so he was doubtless jealous of the great man's reputation, as much for his own sake as for that of London surgery. Thus, rather than 'throwing scandal upon the operation of Sir ASTLEY', Wakley suggested that such reports seemed 'to inculcate the pernicious principle that manual dexterity is the most important desideratum in the performance of surgical operations'. That the amputation was 'performed with expertness, all must readily admit', he claimed; 'but that it was executed with judgement will be universally denied'. 'We sincerely hope that MR. SYMES [*sic*] will never expose a patient to similar risk, nor himself to a repetition of such dreadful anxiety', he concluded. As for Liston, who had 'grappled with and squeezed the arteries [...] this circumstance is so truly ludicrous and anti-surgical, we are almost inclined to believe that the assistant operator was Mr. LISTON of Drury-lane theatre'.[144]

The Lancet's comments on this matter, including its reference to the celebrated actor John Liston (c.1776–1846), illustrate the ways in which that

---

[140] *Edinburgh Medical and Surgical Journal* 21:78 (1 January 1824), p. 27. For the original report, see *Edinburgh Medical and Surgical Journal* 19:77 (1 October 1823), pp. 657–8.
[141] *Edinburgh Medical and Surgical Journal* 21:78 (1 January 1824), p. 23.
[142] *Lancet* 1:19 (8 February 1824), pp. 199–200.   [143] *Lancet* 1:22 (29 February 1824), p. 291.
[144] *Lancet* 1:22 (29 February 1824), pp. 291–3.

journal would frequently characterise Edinburgh surgery as theatrical, self-promotional, and heedlessly ostentatious, in contrast to the more considered and humane surgery of the metropolis. And, as Edinburgh surgery's leading light, as well as a man whose 6 ft 2 in. frame and physical strength shaped his identity as a surgeon, these associations stuck most closely to Liston. For example, in a quite remarkable 'sketch' written by 'Scotus' in 1830, Liston is characterised as a man 'whose brains are obviously not contained in his cranium, but, by original conformation have been deposited, or what perhaps is more probable, have been transuded into his muscular system, by virtue of that physiological law which apportions energy to parts according to the demands of exercitation'. 'Scotus' figures Liston as a man utterly defined by his physicality and almost entirely lacking in sensibility and compassion: 'He has brought [to the practice of surgery] a breadth of shoulder, muscularity of arm, and a merciful indifference to the tortures of the knife, seldom, if ever equalled by the coolest and most corpulent cultivators of that sanguinary art'. In the public space of the operating theatre, 'Scotus' claims, this all-consuming physicality allows for an effortless, yet inherently cynical, display of coolness:

His entrance into this arena of his most favourite avocations, is never marked by those concomitants of perturbed expression, which characterise the appearance of his contemporaries [...] Instead of that self-collected contour, or compound expression of difficulty, arrangement, and responsibility of serious undertaking, which the workings of the mind impress on the countenance on those occasions, Mr. Liston's muscular system alone evinces symptoms of emotion. A sort of vermicular movement is quite obvious throughout his prehensile apparatus, which is busily engaged in knotting his apron-strings, adjusting his sleeve wrists, manipulating some instrument, as if familiarising his fingers with the peculiarities of its form and extent of its mechanical powers; or his brawny arms and shoulders are thrown into repeated preparatory contractions, as if measuring their strength, or modulating their tone to the present undertaking. Now and then, indeed, a half-suppressed smile of self-complacency plays around his lips [...] It could not be well expected that one who reserves his services for more important objects to the patient, should waste any portion of his useful energies in empty condolence; Mr. Liston consequently seems to take little interest in the feelings of those upon whom he operates, and reduces the reluctant and refractory to obedience, more by his cool, commanding and confident demeanour, than by the persuasive eloquence of compassionate address.[145]

There is much in here to sustain extended analysis. For one thing, it speaks to Thomas Dixon's observations about changing ideas of the emotions in the early nineteenth century: about what they were and where they resided.[146] It also has much to tell us about developing ideas of physicality within a culture

[145] *Lancet* 13: 334 (23 January 1830), pp. 364–5.
[146] Thomas Dixon, '"Emotion": The History of a Keyword in Crisis', *Emotion Review* 4:4 (2012), 338–44.

of Romantic sensibility and its relationship to professional identities. At a time when surgeons were seeking to obvert their historical association with manual trade, it seems hardly surprising that such profuse physicality would be construed as problematic. And yet there is ambivalence here, for while Liston is represented as incapable of care, in terms of compassion at least, he is nonetheless physically capable of cure. Thus, 'his incisions are invariably steady, rapid, and scientifically directed, costing the subject of them as little suffering as is, perhaps, consistent with the necessity of their performance'. The question of whether this Liston is a good or a bad surgeon is not entirely clear, but the overall perception is certainly negative. Hence, while 'Mr. Liston's merits [...] are of the first order of excellence', they are 'degraded by a mannerism bordering on buffoonery'. Moreover, they are critically undermined by his self-conscious theatricality, for '[e]ven with the scalpel in his hand, his vanity of his own qualifications is putting forth its tenacula in a thousand impertinent fopperies, to receive the laudatory alms of the spectators on which it feeds'.[147]

The literally monstrous figure 'Scotus' conjures is an extreme, yet entirely consistent, example of *The Lancet*'s representation of Liston during the 1820s and early 1830s. The occasional piece published in this period might allude to his operative skills. Nevertheless, most other editorials and articles either refer to him, in the characteristic language used by Wakley to describe office holders and 'monopolists', as 'the *northern* BAT', criticise him for his conceit and 'indifference to the vulgar notion, of the difficulty of the operation', or sarcastically characterise his tenure at the Edinburgh Royal Infirmary as one of callous indifference, where 'the patients (or sufferers) are treated with great mildness and humanity; the infliction of a few blows to render them docile, obedient, and quiet during painful operations being intended and calculated for their benefit'.[148]

All this was soon to change, however. In 1833, Liston's rivalry with Syme reached its peak as the latter was appointed to the Chair of Clinical Surgery at the University of Edinburgh, Liston having refused to pay the incumbent, James Russell (1754–1836), the £300 a year he had stipulated.[149] As a result, Liston left Edinburgh for London in 1834, having accepted the post of surgeon to the newly founded North London Hospital (soon to be University College Hospital). The following year, he was also appointed Professor of Clinical Surgery at its parent institution, London University (soon to be University College London). As Adrian Desmond has shown, London University was

---

[147] *Lancet* 13: 334 (23 January 1830), p. 365.
[148] *Lancet* 8:196 (2 June 1827), p. 276; 10:242 (19 April 1828), p. 84; 11:289 (14 March 1829), p. 757; 12:314 (5 September 1829), p. 726.
[149] Robert Paterson, *Memorial of the Life of James Syme* (Edinburgh: Edmonston and Douglas, 1874), p. 57.

a Benthamite project, headed by the leading Scottish Whigs, James Mill (1773–1836) and Henry Brougham (1778–1868). As such, it drew heavily upon the rationalist traditions of Scottish medical and scientific education and consciously imported many of its leading lights from north of the border. For its conservative critics, this was yet another example of "'Scotch" jobbery'.[150] But even for those attached to the institution it could cause tensions. This was notable in Liston's fractious relationship with his fellow surgeon Samuel Cooper (1780–1848), but more especially so after Liston's death, when the appointment of Syme as his successor led to Cooper's resignation in the face of hostility from the Scottish Professor of Anatomy and Physiology William Sharpey (1802–80) and the Irish Professor of Descriptive Anatomy Richard Quain (1800–87). On that occasion, Wakley and *The Lancet* were trenchant in their opposition to the 'Scottish influence' at University College London, but on the appointment of Liston in 1834/5 they were surprisingly tight-lipped, especially given their previous criticisms.[151]

By the end of 1835, moreover, something remarkable had occurred. Its first flowerings are evident in an editorial concerning Charles Bell's appointment as Chair of Surgery at the University of Edinburgh, in which Wakley expressed his pleasure that Liston had not accepted the offer himself, claiming that 'Within the short space of time that he has already resided in the Metropolis, Mr. LISTON has succeeded in establishing here a reputation equally well founded with that which he had previously acquired by the exercise of his scientific attainments in Edinburgh'.[152] However, it only came into full bloom following Liston's attendance, together with Wakley, at a meeting of the medical students of London, held on 18 January 1836, calling for the formation of a 'Central Students Association' and a change to the way in which candidates were examined for medical licences and degrees. 'Mr. LISTON', the report in *The Lancet* observed, 'was the only hospital surgeon in London who supported the cause of the students'. More than this, he and Wakley volunteered to lead the deputation sent to the Chancellor of the Exchequer to pass the resolutions of the meeting to government.[153]

From this point on, and with his radical credentials secured, Liston could, in the eyes of Wakley and *The Lancet* at least, do no wrong. Indeed, in its annual 'Account of the London Hospitals and Schools of Medicine' in 1836, *The Lancet* claimed that Liston 'has for some time been renowned as the first

[150] Desmond, *Evolution*, pp. 33–41.
[151] For its criticism of the 'Scottish influence', see *Lancet* 51:1271 (8 January 1848), pp. 48–51.
[152] *Lancet* 25:642 (19 December 1835), p. 470.
[153] *Lancet* 25:647 (23 January 1836), pp. 668–680. Liston was also a member of the radical London-based British Medical Association (not to be confused with the 1855 successor to the more moderate Provincial Medical and Surgical Association). *Lancet* 27:699 (21 January 1837) pp. 593–608.

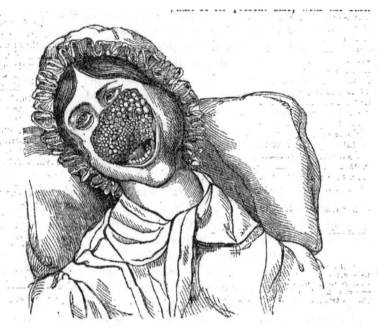

Figure 1.7 Mary Ann Griffiths, *The Lancet* 27:688 (5 November 1836), p. 237. Public Domain Mark

operator among British surgeons' and that 'If the justly-distinguished, and far-famed ASTLEY COOPER is ever to have a successor, in this metropolis, Mr. LISTON will be that man'.[154] Thus, while in 1824 Liston's operative style had been derided as 'ludicrous and anti-surgical' and actively contrasted with Cooper's, by the mid-1830s it was presented as the latter's rightful inheritor. Indeed, what is remarkable about *The Lancet*'s *volte-face* with regard to Liston is the fact that the very qualities of boldness and operative dexterity that had initially rendered him problematic now functioned as the grounds on which his fame and reputation were most vigorously defended. For example, in November 1836 *The Lancet* reported on the case of Mary Ann Griffiths, a 20-year-old woman suffering from a horribly disfiguring tumour of the superior maxillary bone (Figure 1.7). It described Liston's excision of the bone and its tumour, which took only seven minutes and twenty seconds, as 'one of the most splendid triumphs that operative surgery has ever achieved'.[155] Meanwhile, within the very same month, it reported on a similar, though more

---

[154] *Lancet* 27:682 (24 September 1836), p. 20.
[155] *Lancet* 27:688 (5 November 1836), pp. 236–40.

tragic, case of a 24-year-old shoemaker, known simply as 'W. B.', whose face had been injured by a blow from a cricket ball and who had likewise developed a tumour of the superior maxilla bone. In this instance, however, the patient died several hours after the operation. Though the case 'was unfortunate with regard to the suffering patient', the report claimed that it 'furnishes a useful lesson to young practitioners' that 'success after operations cannot be *ensured*'. Moreover, it 'must prove of still greater value for Mr. LISTON himself':

The reputation of that gentleman as an operator stands unrivalled, and the dexterity which he possesses is a subject of astonishment with surgeons who have visited the continental hospitals. The public, therefore, on discovering that an operation may occasionally be followed by fatal consequences even when it is performed by the most distinguished of our surgeons, will shrink in dismay from the thought of entrusting their lives [...] to half-instructed bunglers, who, under the system of nepotism, obtain the office of surgeon in our old endowed hospitals. The issue of the case of the patient E. B. [*sic*], proves, beyond question or dispute, that capital operations in surgery cannot be undertaken, with safety to the reputation of the practitioner, unless by such a man as Mr. LISTON, – a surgeon of undoubted skill and established fame.[156]

Here, then, *The Lancet* sought to use Liston's failure to further illuminate his reputation and castigate the shortcomings of others. Such rhetorical contortions were not lost on Wakley's opponents. The moderate reforming journal the *Medico-Chirurgical Review* claimed that 'a more bungling attempt to protect a friend could scarce be made'. Questioning the wisdom of Liston's actions in both cases, it maintained that 'The day indeed for flashy operations is gone by. The refinement of our manners is disgusted at the exhibition of what wears more the aspect of clever butchery than science'. This was especially true, it argued, of those operations that, like that upon W. B., are of 'so disgusting and revolting an appearance, that an eye-witness declares that of "upwards of two hundred spectators present, many became faint, and some were carried out of the theatre – such was the scene"'.[157]

While the *Medico-Chirurgical Review* thought Liston's propensity to operate an unseemly instance of 'clever butchery', a correspondent to *The Lancet* signing himself 'A WELLWISHER TO TALENT AND TRUTH' endeavoured to refute its imputations. Though he denied that 'therein lies his *forte*', this correspondent acknowledged that Liston's operative dexterity was 'naturally the most striking' aspect of his surgical identity 'and the first to be canvassed'. He claimed that most of Liston's critics were 'envious spirits' who 'strive to represent the matter to others in a disparaging point of view' and argued that, if by 'flashy' the *Review* meant 'tinsel, a gaudy, empty show', then they were

[156] *Lancet* 27:691 (26 November 1837), p. 344.
[157] *Medico-Chirurgical Review* 26:51, new series (1 January 1837), pp. 276, 271.

correct, for 'this is not the time for such displays'. However, if by that word they meant to impugn all surgical novelty, then they were mistaken. Moreover, he challenged the idea that Liston's actions were inhumane, asking

is not the surgeon who dextrously and safely removes a hideous swelling […] and thereby restores his patient to health, comfort and happiness […] better 'informed' and more 'humane' than the surgeon who […] with a wide shrug of the shoulders, and a scientific shake of the head, expresses pity for the suffering of the patient, but leaves the disease to run its course unmolested, and the fellow-being unassisted, to drag out a miserable existence, harassed by his fell destroyer.[158]

Not all were convinced by such protestations. In particular, the conservative *London Medical Gazette*, Wakley's *bête noire*, thought that it detected more than a little favouritism in *The Lancet's* reporting of Liston. Contrasting Liston's hallowed status with that of Wakley's former friends and allies, John Elliotson, Professor of the Principles and the Practice of Medicine at University College London, and William Lawrence, the former radical and *Lancet* contributor turned conservative 'placeman', it wrote:

Mr Liston, the present idol of Wakley's attachment is, we believe, the only person of any standing in the profession in London, who is desirous of the good opinion of the honourable member for Finsbury [Wakley was MP for Finsbury from 1835]; he has not been ashamed to be present at, and to take part in, meetings where Wakley has been prominent: hence, naturally, the reciprocal feeling on the part of the latter. The great attraction now at the North London Hospital is Mr Liston: Mr Liston is all in all, just as it used to be with Dr Elliotson, who at present seems to be completely thrown overboard. Why is this? […] Are we right in attributing it to the mortal hatred that subsists between Dr Elliotson and the *great surgeon* of the North? […] Mr Liston is held up as the model of surgeons – the greatest after Sir Astley Cooper, and so forth. How is this, when we have Mr Lawrence still amongst us in all his pristine vigour and ability […] But Mr Lawrence shook off the patronage of Wakley, and hence the rival that has been set beside his throne.[159]

Conclusion

The case of Robert Liston clearly demonstrates that Romantic surgical identities were shaped not simply by words and deeds, but also by the politics of representation. Likewise, it suggests that issues such as manual skill and operative dexterity, as well as compassion and humanity, could be used to both sustain and undermine surgical reputations. Indeed, what is perhaps most evident from Liston's fame (and infamy) is that Romantic surgical identities were dependent on a delicate balance between physicality and sensibility, action and

[158] *Lancet* 27:701 (4 February 1837), p. 674.
[159] *London Medical Gazette* (1 October 1836), p. 25.

judgement. While some might question Liston's decision to proceed with a 'disgusting and revolting' operation, even if it was 'not one which [he] undertook from choice, but on account of the urgent solicitations of the patient', others clearly thought that trusting to nature in a case where death was almost certain was no more compassionate or humane than resorting to the knife.[160]

This balance between doing and thinking, force and feeling, was not unique to the practice of surgery; nor was it static. As Joanne Begiato has argued, while masculinities are always determined by a combination of these qualities, the Romantic era saw a particularly acute set of tensions develop between them. If the age of sensibility and the deprecation of artifice created the conditions for the Romantic man of feeling, open to the authentic emotions of embodied experience, then the shadow of war and revolution also demanded virile male bodies capable of violence.[161] Even so, if surgery was not alone in this regard, it nonetheless provided a particularly vital arena for the playing out of these issues. After all, surgeons of the early years of the nineteenth century were acutely aware of the need to divest themselves of their traditional associations with brute physicality and shape identities as gentlemen of refined sensibility. By the 1830s and 1840s, on the other hand, it was perhaps becoming somewhat easier to combine physicality and vigour with morality and emotion.[162] Thus, Liston's body could become a site of conflict not simply for competing political agendas but also for changing social attitudes, as the image of a showy and vulgar physicality depicted by 'Scotus', which allowed no room for sensibility, gave way to 'Wellwisher's' man of action for whom pity and sympathy were not enough. Without wanting to push our analysis too far, we might even conceive of Liston as a metonym for Scottish national identity more generally, in its shift from 'savage' warriors, though Enlightenment men of feeling, to the 'heroic' warriors of the Victorian imagination.

While such semiotic considerations are clearly vital to understating his place in the cultures of Romantic surgery, it is important to note that Liston's own relationship with the knife was equally complex, ambivalent, and conditional. Thus, in his *Elements of Surgery* (1831), he dismissed healing by what he called 'the pure force of surgery', asking: 'Who will question, that there is more merit in saving one limb by superior skill, than in lopping of a thousand with the utmost dexterity?' Despite his occasional representation as a rough handler of patients, he also maintained that 'It is of utmost importance to attend

---

[160] *Lancet* 27:691 (26 November 1837), p. 343.
[161] Joanne Begiato, *Manliness in Britain, 1760–1900: Bodies, Emotions and Material Culture* (Manchester: Manchester University Press, 2020), pp. 10–11; Begiato, 'Between Poise and Power: Embodied Manliness in Eighteenth- and Nineteenth-Century British Culture', *Transactions of the Royal Historical Society* 26 (2016), 125–47.
[162] Begiato, *Manliness*, pp. 40–1.

to the state of the patient's mind and feelings'.[163] By the time of his *Practical Surgery* (1837), however, he was perhaps more confident with his operative reputation, claiming that 'a dexterous surgeon, like a man skilful in the use of weapons, will not enter rashly into difficulties, but being engaged from conviction, will bring himself through with courage'. He even took a swipe at the *Medico-Chirurgical Review*, arguing that while surgeons 'are too often asked to admit, that operations are the opprobria of their art [...] it is unjust to sneer at this department of the profession, as is done by some, affecting to consider the dexterous and successful operator as little better than a "clever butcher"'.[164] And yet, two years later, he wrote to James Miller telling him that he was engaged in 'lots of cutting at present', adding 'awful I am sick of it. Operations every day at the Hospital – 4 or 5 for today – amputations – 2 thighs – arm and great toe [...] also disarticulation of the jaw in very pretty young woman'.[165] Meanwhile, in another letter sent the following month, he questioned his public and professional reputation, writing that 'They begin to find that I am not as much given to cutting as they thought'.[166] Such comments are suggestive, for as we shall see in Chapters 2 and 3, emotions were no mere counterpoint to operative performance; rather, they shaped the very experience of surgery for surgeon and patient alike.

---

[163] Robert Liston, *Elements of Surgery*, vol. 1 (London: Longman, Orme, Brown, and Green, 1831), pp. x, xii.
[164] Liston, *Practical Surgery*, pp. 436, 210.
[165] WL MS.6089 2/1, Robert Liston to James Miller, 25 January 1840.
[166] WL MS.6089 3/1, Robert Liston to James Miller, 4 February 1840. My thanks go to Sally Frampton for directing me towards these particular letters, making the trawl through Liston's semi-legible handwriting that much easier.

2   Anxiety and Compassion
Emotional Intersubjectivity and the Romantic Surgical Relationship

Introduction

In the introduction to his *Illustrations of the Diseases of the Breast* (1829), Astley Cooper writes that the 'difference between the experienced and scientific, and the ignorant and unobserving member of the profession', is his ability to determine 'the distinctive character of disease as soon as it is presented to his attention'. Such knowledge, he claims, enables the scientific surgeon to 'discriminate curable from incurable cases; the dangerous from the slight; those which require surgical operations from those which do not demand them; and such as admit of a trifling operation from those which call for one of extreme severity'. Nowhere, Cooper suggests, is this essential quality 'more fully exemplified [...] than in the diseases incidental to the female Breast'. Cooper's first volume of the *Diseases of the Breast* is concerned with non-malignant growths (the second volume on malignant tumours was never published). In this regard, the ability of the surgeon to determine the nature of a swelling, through 'a very careful and nice manipular examination of the complaint', combined with experience of pathological presentations and a 'minute history of the case', was vital. Otherwise, 'the uninformed Surgeon is too apt to fall in with the opinion of the vulgar, and to confound all the swellings of the breast under the general term of Cancer', when in fact 'a great number of genera of tumours actually exist', ranging from the acute to the chronic and the malignant to the benign. He continues:

The result of such knowledge is frequently the source of great security and happiness to a person afflicted with a disease in the breast, as well as of great satisfaction to the Surgeon. I have scarcely witnessed a stronger expression of delight than that which has illuminated the features of a female – perhaps the mother of a large family dependent upon her for protection, education, and support – who, upon consulting a Surgeon for some tumour in her bosom, and expecting to hear from him a confirmation of the sentence she has pronounced upon herself, receives, on the contrary, an assurance that her apprehensions are unfounded. Pale and trembling, she enters the Surgeon's apartment, and baring her bosom, faintly articulates – Sir, I am come to consult you for a Cancer in my breast; – and when, after a careful examination, the Surgeon states, he has the pleasure of assuring her that the disease is not cancerous – that it has not the character of malignancy – that it is not dangerous, and will not require an operation; the sudden transformation from apprehension to joy brightens her countenance with the smile of gratitude; and the happiness of the moment can hardly be exceeded when she returns with delighted affection to the family, from whom she had previously considered herself destined soon to be separated by death, with the alternative only of being saved by a dubious and painful operation.[1]

There is perhaps no better introduction to the emotional dynamics of the Romantic surgical encounter than this passage. In the midst of a brief and otherwise functional introduction, Cooper intrudes a highly wrought literary vignette. He draws on his extensive first-hand experience to present the reader with the figure of an unspecified woman, and to encourage our pity and sympathy by imagining her as the mother of a large, dependent family. At the same time, he evokes her delight at his being able to dispel the despondency, fear, and anxiety she has mistakenly imposed upon herself in thinking her condition cancerous. Cooper is not content with this, however, and provides an intensely dramatic rendering of the same essential narrative, evoking an embodied transformation from the pale, trembling woman who can barely articulate her self-diagnosis to one brightened by a joyful countenance of relief and happiness. What is more, he proceeds beyond the bounds of the consultation room, and indeed of his personal experience, to imagine her return to her family and their collective joy at the news of her relative good health.

At one level, this passage is a straightforward account of a woman's deliverance from the fear and anxiety of a malignant and fatal disease and from the possibility of having to undergo an intensely painful, and frequently unsuccessful, surgical procedure. At another, however, it is suggestive of a more complex dynamic. Cooper begins by establishing the twin poles of the emotional relationship between patient and practitioner; for the patient, surgical knowledge brings 'happiness', while for the surgeon, it brings 'satisfaction'. Superficially at least, this passage is concerned with the former, with the patient's relief and happiness. Yet it is clear by inference that the 'satisfaction' of the practitioner is of equal, if not greater, importance. After all, the whole scene is ultimately intended to stir feelings in the surgical reader as to the emotional rewards of clinical knowledge and experience. This passage should, then, be viewed through the prism of paternalism, not to say patriarchy. There is an evident power relationship here. It is not straightforward; after all, the consultation is most likely a private one in which the patient is patron. Nevertheless, the imbalance of expertise and the gendered dynamics of the relationship serve to cast Cooper in the dominant role. We might call this passage melodramatic, not simply because of its appeal to emotion, but because it accords with many of the conventions of melodrama, notably an inert and

---

[1] Astley Cooper, *Illustrations of the Diseases of the Breast*, vol. 1 (London: Longman, Rees, Orme, Brown, and Green, 1829), pp. 1–4.

suffering woman in need of male rescue.[2] She enters weak, vulnerable, and supplicatory, and leaves happy and grateful.

This passage testifies to the importance of emotion in the Romantic surgical relationship and in the cultures of surgical performance and self-fashioning more generally. But it also poses questions about the sorts of cultural work that these kinds of emotional expressions performed. As we saw in Chapter 1, early nineteenth-century surgeons were increasingly promoting a culture of operative restraint, based on claims to superior anatomical and pathological knowledge. Certainly, such concerns are evident here, as Cooper deploys emotions to underscore an epistemological and professional authority founded upon extensive experience at a prestigious metropolitan hospital and a familiarity with the Parisian clinical method. This knowledge and experience, he makes clear, allow him to distinguish between a truly cancerous tumour requiring caustic treatment, or perhaps an operation, and one requiring much milder remedies. In the hands of another, 'uninformed Surgeon', this patient might have been subject to a dangerous, painful, and ultimately unnecessary treatment when she should instead have been sent home to her family.

What this chapter demonstrates is that, as well as serving a rhetorical function, emotions also played a more vital role in the shaping of Romantic surgery. Within the cultures of Romantic sensibility, feelings and expressions of anxiety, pity, sympathy, and compassion could serve to shape a culturally resonant image of the surgeon as a genteel man of feeling, in keeping with surgery's social aspirations and far removed from its traditional associations with brute physicality and manual trade. Yet emotions shaped not only surgical *identities*, but also *experiences* and *subjectivities*. The issue of phenomenology in the history of the emotions is a vexed one. Needless to say, it would be naïve to assume that early nineteenth-century surgeons' emotional expressions can be taken at face value. And yet, at the same time, it would be reductive to assume that such expressions were merely the product of cultural convention or professional self-interest. As we shall see, surgeons of the period gave expression to their emotions in a variety of contexts and settings, from public lectures to more private letters and diaries. Drawing on the emotive theory of William Reddy, we might see these expressions as a form of 'navigation', an attempt to reconcile lived experience and inward feelings with the dictates of the dominant emotional regime of the period, in this case Romantic sensibility.[3] Hence, when we are

---

[2] Katherine Newey, 'Melodrama and Gender', in Carolyn Williams (ed.), *The Cambridge Companion to English Melodrama* (Cambridge, UK: Cambridge University Press, 2018), 149–62. For the broader political and social resonances of the 'melodramatic mode', see Chapter 4.

[3] William M. Reddy, *The Navigation of Feeling: A Framework for the History of the Emotions* (Cambridge, UK: Cambridge University Press, 2001). For a case study of the emotives of Romantic surgery, see Michael Brown, 'Wounds and Wonder: Emotion, Imagination and War in the Cultures of Romantic Surgery', *Journal for Eighteenth Century Studies* 43:2 (2020), 239–59.

told that Astley Cooper burst into tears when a child about to undergo an operation 'smiled very sweetly upon him', we might think of this both as an authentic
emotional response and as a culturally conditioned performance.[4]

In many ways, the authenticity of surgical emotion was rooted in the embodied experience of operative practice.[5] As will be shown, compared to the later
nineteenth century, when surgeons shaped identities as heroic miracle workers
and carried out operations with the assistance of anaesthesia and antisepsis,
Romantic surgeons were acutely aware of the limitations of their art and were
consistently exposed to the suffering, misery, and death that disease and injury,
as well as their surgical treatment, could cause. If this shaped surgical subjectivities, encouraging anxiety, fear, reflection, and regret, then it also shaped
what I call an 'intersubjectivity' between surgeons and their patients. Indeed,
one of the defining characteristics of the Romantic surgical relationship was the
emphasis that surgeons placed on their ability to project themselves, through
acts of imagination, into their patient's position, so that they might assess their
state of mind and manage their condition more effectively.

Of course, this display of emotional acuity resonated with the cultures of
sensibility and shaped the surgeon's public identity as a sympathetic and compassionate individual. But it also did more than this. Early nineteenth-century
understandings of the relations between body and mind placed great emphasis
upon the importance of mental states in the propagation and progress of disease. In the absence of a concept of post-operative infection, many surgeons
were unable to account for the post-operative deaths of patients, even those
who had borne the procedure well, in terms other than what James Wardrop
called 'moral depression'.[6] In this context, then, an ability to read and manage
the patient's emotions was not simply the marker of a refined sensibility, it was
an essential clinical skill, allowing the surgeon to understand, prognosticate,
and treat their patient's illness or injury.

This chapter begins with a discussion of surgeons' emotional expressions
and reflections, including their attitudes towards the trials of operative surgery
and clinical practice. It demonstrates how, within the cultures of sensibility,
expressions of anxiety, fear, pity, and regret could shape surgical identities

[4] John Flint South, *Memorials of John Flint South* (London: John Murray, 1884), p. 56.
[5] Michael Brown, 'Surgery, Identity and Embodied Emotion: John Bell, James Gregory and the
Edinburgh "Medical War"', *History* 104:359 (2019), 19–41.
[6] *Lancet*, 20:516 (20 July 1833), p. 521. The use of the word 'moral' in this case derived from
the French *le moral* and pertained to mental states, in a manner similar to the later synonym
'morale'. In his history of this latter concept, Daniel Ussishkin completely neglects the extensive
use of the term 'moral' in medical discourse of the later eighteenth and early nineteenth centuries, perhaps the most famous example of which was the system of 'moral therapy' pioneered
at the York Quaker lunatic asylum, The Retreat. *Morale: A Modern British History* (Oxford:
Oxford University Press, 2017), pp. 12–13.

and subjectivities in powerful ways. It then considers how those emotions were managed and harnessed and how, through the mechanisms of emotional intersubjectivity, it was imagined that the patient's sufferings might be alleviated. Finally, it returns to the subject of our opening remarks by considering the nature of Astley Cooper's relationship with his patients, particularly those women he treated for breast cancer, demonstrating the importance of gender relations, identities, and ideologies in shaping the emotional dynamics of the therapeutic relationship. As can be seen, this chapter is predominantly concerned with the emotional perspective of the surgeon. Although patients are a near-constant presence, their voices, experiences, and agency are considered in more detail in Chapter 3.

Expressing Surgical Emotions

In 1759, the Scottish moral philosopher Adam Smith (bap. 1723, d. 1790) published his *Theory of Moral Sentiments*, a foundational text for the culture of sensibility, which asserted the importance of sympathy and intersubjectivity in the shaping of social relations. 'As we have no immediate experience of what other men feel', he writes:

we can form no idea of the manner in which they are affected, but by conceiving what we ourselves should feel in the like situation. Though our brother is on the rack, as long as we ourselves are at our ease, our senses will never inform us of what he suffers. They never did, and never can, carry us beyond our own person, and it is by the imagination only that we can form any conception of what are his sensations.[7]

Smith's example of the rack was a fanciful historical allusion, for it, together with all other forms of judicial torture, had been phased out in Britain over one hundred years before his book was published. Nonetheless, if torture no longer provided a convenient occasion for sympathetic projection, there was another spectacle of human suffering far more readily available to Smith and his contemporaries: operative surgery. Thus, in his discussion of pain and suffering, Smith suggests that 'Some people grow faint at the sight of a chirurgical operation, and that bodily pain which is occasioned by tearing the flesh, seems, in them, to excite the most excessive sympathy'.[8] Meanwhile, for Smith's friend and intellectual ally David Hume (1711–76), the mere anticipation of an operation was enough to provoke a powerful emotional response. 'Were I present at any of the more terrible operations of surgery', he writes in his *Treatise on Human Nature* (1740), ''tis certain that even before it began, the preparation of the instruments, the laying of the bandages in order, the

---

[7] Adam Smith, *The Theory of Moral Sentiments* (London: A. Miller, 1759), p. 2.
[8] Smith, *Sentiments*, p. 57.

heating of the irons, with all the signs of anxiety and concern in the patient and assistants, wou'd have a great effect upon my mind, and excite the strongest sentiments of pity and terror'.[9] For Smith, however, 'Nothing is so soon forgot as pain' and, once removed from the scene, he alleges, it becomes almost impossible for an individual to imagine themselves back into a state of agony.[10] Indeed, compared to Hume's first-person evocation of sympathetic feeling, Smith's phrase 'Some people' suggests a certain distancing from the 'excessive sympathy' of the surgical witness; he even goes so far as to suggest that 'One who has been witness to a dozen dissections, and as many amputations, sees, ever after, all operations of this kind with great indifference, and often with perfect insensibility'.[11]

In her account of eighteenth-century surgical emotion, *With Words and Knives* (2007), Lynda Payne makes no mention of the moral philosophy of Smith or Hume, nor indeed of the cultures of sensibility and sentiment. Her interpretation of the surgeon's emotional disposition nonetheless approaches Smith's notion of a habituated 'insensibility'. She argues that 'Objectivity was necessary to render a professional judgement' and asks: 'did objectivity preclude having sympathy for the suffering patient?' Her answer is that on balance, it did, and that, to quote William Hunter, surgeons of the period were encouraged to develop 'a sort of necessary inhumanity'. 'Losing pity and gaining control went hand in hand', she argues; 'Hardening or dampening emotions led to heightened perception, knowledge, rationality and a new sensibility – dispassion'.[12]

However, even if Payne's observations are true for the eighteenth century (and there is reason to believe that she overstates her case), they do little justice to the emotional cultures of Romantic surgery. This might be accounted for in part by the cultural shift from the public and stylised figurations of sensibility in the Enlightenment towards the internalised and emotionally self-reflective modes of the Romantic era. Certainly, as we shall see, surgeons of the early nineteenth century were far more apt to give expression to their feelings than Payne's reading of the earlier period suggests. But, at a more fundamental level, this disjuncture between Payne's dispassionate stoics on the one hand, and the surgeon as man of feeling on the other, derives from her very conceptualisation of the emotions and their action. She opens her book by stating that 'In practice, physicians, and especially surgeons, have always had to learn some type of detachment […] in order to cope with the more revolting aspects of their art', and her foundational premise is that 'medical dispassion, or […]

---

[9] David Hume, *A Treatise of Human Nature*, vol. 3 (London: Thomas Longman, 1740).
[10] Smith, *Sentiments*, p. 56.   [11] Smith, *Sentiments*, p. 58.
[12] Lynda Payne, *With Words and Knives: Learning Medical Dispassion in Early Modern England* (Aldershot: Ashgate, 2007), p. 153.

clinical detachment, has existed throughout the history of medicine'.[13] Such presentism occludes historical understanding. While it is certainly true to say that emotions have always been, to a greater or lesser extent, managed, Payne's adoption of a modern notion of clinical detachment, which tends to regard emotions as a contaminant of rational decision-making, blinds her both to the culturally and historically relative nature of emotional experience and expression, as well as to the varied forms of work that such emotions might perform, including the exercise of clinical judgement.[14]

In order to reach a nuanced understanding of the historical relationship between surgery and emotion, it is therefore necessary to adopt a more inclusive approach, one that is capable of acknowledging complexity and ambivalence. Hence, while this book argues for the centrality of emotions in the shaping of Romantic surgical culture, it is important to note that, whatever the realities of surgeons' emotional sensations and expressions, it was a relative commonplace of early nineteenth-century popular discourse that surgeons were unfeeling. As Benjamin Brodie told his students in 1820, 'It has been a matter of complaint against our profession that the being perpetually present at scenes of woe tends to blunt the feelings of our nature, and to render us less capable of sympathizing with the sufferings of others'.[15] Likewise, nine years earlier, Everard Home told his audience that 'Operations in Surgery have in general been considered as acts of cruelty, & Surgeons have been accused of want of humanity'.[16] Such ideas were given powerful visual expression in the rich satirical traditions of the period, notably in such famous images as Thomas Rowlandson's *Amputation* (1793) (Figure 2.1), which portrays a gaggle of corpulent and decrepit surgeons, with such names as 'Benjamin Bowels', 'Launcelot Slashmuscle' and 'Samuel Sawbone', surrounding a terrified patient, who is about to have his leg bisected by a fearsome-looking bone saw.

As we saw in Chapter 1, surgeons of the Romantic era were actively seeking to challenge such stereotypes of their profession. It should therefore come as little surprise that both Brodie and Home referred to popular prejudices only to dispute them. However, if we are to push beyond the boundaries of rhetoric and approach something closer to subjective emotional experience, it might be worth starting with the diary of Henry Robert Oswald (1790–1862).

[13] Payne, *Words*, pp. 1–2.
[14] Michael Brown, 'Redeeming Mr Sawbone: Compassion and Care in the Cultures of Nineteenth-Century Surgery', *Journal of Compassionate Healthcare* 4:13 (2017), https://doi.org/10.1186/s40639-017-0042-2.
[15] RCSE, MS0470/1/2/5, Benjamin Brodie, 'Introductory lecture of anatomy and physiology' (October 1820), f. 20.
[16] WL, MS.5604, Lawrence W. Brown, 'Notes on Twelve Lectures by Everard Home on the Principal Operations of Surgery' (1811–12), f. 12.

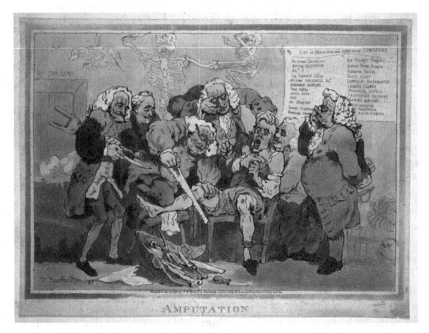

Figure 2.1   Thomas Rowlandson, *Amputation* (1793). Wellcome Collection.
Attribution 4.0 International (CC BY 4.0)

Unlike most of the surgeons featured in this book, Oswald was not a leading
practitioner. Indeed, he lived and died in relative obscurity, although his son,
Henry Robert Oswald (1827–92), became Surgeon General of India, while
his grandson, also confusingly called Henry Robert Oswald (1852–1940),
became a leading coroner.[17] Nonetheless, his diary offers a revealing insight,
not only into the emotional life of this particular surgeon, but into the cultures
of Romantic introspection more generally.

Oswald was born in Fife and educated in Edinburgh, where he was apprenticed to the surgeon George Bell (1777–1832). He joined the Inverness-Shire
Militia, but resigned his commission after less than a year, having 'seen
much of the envy and selfishness of the world'.[18] With the assistance of Bell
and the Professor of the Practice of Physic at the University of Edinburgh,
James Gregory (1753–1821), he subsequently secured a post as 'Government
Surgeon' to John Murray, 4th Duke of Atholl (1755–1830) and Governor

---

[17] *Times*, 15 March 1940, p. 11.
[18] NLS, MS 9003, Diary of H. R. Oswald Snr, describing his first six months as surgeon to the 4th
Duke of Atholl, Governor General of the Isle of Man (1812–13), f. 1r.

General of the Isle of Man. Oswald moved to Douglas, where he remained for the rest of his life, despite being divested of his post on the Duke's death in 1830.

Oswald began his diary in 1812 with the intention of recording 'such things and thoughts therein as may be useful and a lesson to me in future life'.[19] His entries suggest that he was a highly sensitive man, racked by doubts and anxieties concerning his place in society, his relations with others, and his own state of mind. Thus, one of the earliest entries reflects on his relationship with his former master, particularly the fact that during his apprenticeship he was required to sit at dinner in total silence, Bell being 'affectedly distant in his manner'. Oswald worried that the 'long habit of silence in that family at table has given a turn to my manners which may hurt me in future society'. At the same time, he maintained that he 'was not an inattentive observer when in that situation and had many visionary conjectures about the nature of the human heart'. Though Oswald wrote that he could now only 'wonder that I submitted to the senseless affected and cold freaks of that family', an interleaved note, written at some later date, offered an apology for his earlier sentiments:

The page regarding my situation in Mr Bell's family arose more from the Diseased state of my feelings than reality [...] it requires the intellect watching over the mind and the feelings to prevent their being led astray by the appearances that in fact have [...] nothing worthy of being considered real in them. Still that was the state of my feelings and therefore it ought to be recorded.[20]

Sadly for Oswald, things were not to improve on Mann. The Duke's stand-offishness mirrored his experience with Bell and caused him great consternation. So too did his subordinate status and his relations with others on the island. Indeed, at times he worried that he was losing his mind. For example, in January 1813, after having been called upon to attend a 'melancholic maniac', he reflected on his own sanity:

Did not reason tell me that the many wild imaginations and ridiculous notions that daily pass through my mind, were foolish, and prevent me from noting them down here. I might justly consider myself a mad man; indeed at some futurity, if I live, when I look over this diary I believe I will consider myself a silly fellow.[21]

Oswald was consumed by the 'strange notion' that his actions were unwittingly the 'cause of great inquietude [sic] and vexation to some unknown persons'. 'Even I myself consider them foolish and indicate a derangement of the imagination', he wrote: 'would not others if I mentioned them do the same'.[22] Somewhat later, he also developed the notion that his stomach

[19] NLS, MS 9003, f. 1r.   [20] NLS, MS 9003, ff. 4v–6r.
[21] NLS, MS 9003, ff. 33r, 36v.   [22] NLS, MS 9003, f. 39r–v.

complaints were the result of being poisoned by unknown parties, who were adulterating his food. 'Such wild ideas', he confided to his diary; 'They are those of a melancholic man. Away with them. Let me be content with things as they are and be thankful that they are not worse. I would blush if these thoughts were to come to the knowledge of any one, they would condemn me for a mad man'.[23]

Oswald's self-reflections may indicate his personal idiosyncrasies, but they also cast light on the broader cultures of contemporary surgery. In part, his anxieties about his relations with others stemmed from his tenuous social position and the very real risks of disgrace and ruin. At one point, for example, he was called upon to attend a gravely ill patient who was already in consultation with two senior practitioners, a perilous professional situation. As he reflected in his diary:

I believe there is no profession which harbours so much mean and mercenary jealousy and hypocritical ill nature as the medical. One reason is that we are almost universally very fond of money and another is that we are public men and our actions have gravity [...] so that every unfortunate or unlucky action goes a great way to break our reputations. This is not the case with other professions. A Physicians [sic] success depends almost altogether on popular fame. A few malevolent insinuations unless he is a man of ability and address is sufficient to blot his character forever: for of nothing is a man more anxious about than his health.[24]

Oswald alludes to the physician here, and his practice was certainly more akin to that of the surgeon-apothecary or general practitioner than to the 'pure' operating surgeon of the metropolis. Even so, there is reason to believe that surgeons were particularly vulnerable to shame and disgrace. According to Benjamin Brodie:

The diseases, concerning which the Surgeon is usually consulted are such as are visible to the eyes, and sensible to the touch, and their nature, or something respecting their nature, is known to everyone. The treatment of the Surgeon is known also, and the effects of it are evident to those who stand by [...] The professional character of a Surgeon is continually open to discussion. Where he acts with judgement or skill his merit can seldom fail of being known; where he displays ignorance or folly, the subterfuges and evasion to which weak minds are disposed to resort, will seldom be capable of concealing his defects.[25]

Whereas the physician dealt with the interior of the body, an invisible domain whose management might be regarded as arcane, the surgeon, Brodie suggests, dealt with conditions that were highly visible and whose mitigation or aggravation was equally apparent. It is important to remember that the fear of disgrace was probably one of the most consistent emotions experienced by surgeons.

---

[23] NLS, MS 9003, unnumbered ff. between ff. 53 and 54.
[24] NLS, MS 9003, ff. 32v–33r.   [25] RCSE, MS0470/1/2/5, ff. 7–8.

As we shall see, this was particularly true in this period, given the potential for quite literally spectacular forms of failure in the operating theatre. But even in the case of the surgeon-apothecary, professional humiliation, though perhaps of a less dramatic kind, was still an ever-present anxiety.

Despite this, Oswald's emotional reflections on his professional life were by no means entirely self-interested. In fact, his diary is full of pity for the sufferings of others, such as in the case of an 'Infant Patient', a 'Poor Little Dear' who 'suffered much from dry cough and Restlessness' and who was 'long gone before I saw it'.[26] Perhaps most poignantly, in March 1813 he was called upon to attend a young girl from Castletown who was 'very ill' and 'very extraordinarily impressed with the Idea that she is to die'. He spent that night in her home, observing:

To see a father very highly affected with the prospect of losing a daughter [...] is no easy task. He groaned in Spirit and writhed with anguish. These are the scenes which medical men are obliged to behold in apparent coolness whatever may be their inward pain. Perhaps by seeing them so frequently they make less impression on them than others but people are not aware of the anxiety we suffer when a patient is suffering severely and approaching to death, and when every effort of art is in vain. Then we must suppress all feeling appear composed and endeavour to comfort if we do not wish to produce mischief by adding to the alarm which others experience. Though I am sensible of this yet from the distressing nature of these scenes and from the embarrassing uncertainty of the medical art I have often wished that some other profession had fallen to my lot: I have myself to blame: it was my own wish.[27]

Oswald's entry beautifully encapsulates the emotional demands of practice and the tensions between sensation and expression in the clinical encounter. Clearly, given his deep concerns about recording his reflections on his mental state for posterity, there is no indication that he intended such thoughts to reach a public audience. Rather, his diary might best be interpreted as a private act of *Bildung*, an attempt to reconcile heart and mind in the formation of the self. Because of its private nature, however, it provides a highly suggestive insight into both his personal subjectivity and his public identity. As is evident, one of the central motifs of Oswald's diary is the distinction between emotions that are inwardly felt and those that are outwardly expressed. Again, we might invoke Reddy's concept of emotional navigation, the attempt to reconcile felt sensations with the cultural conventions of emotional expression. For Reddy, this can lead to emotional 'suffering', as there is often a disjuncture between what is felt and what can be expressed.[28] This was certainly the case for Oswald, whose emotional agony centred around his inability to fully

[26] NLS, MS 9003, f. 61r.   [27] NLS, MS 9003, ff. 71r–v.
[28] Reddy, *Navigation*, pp. 123–30.

express his all-consuming anxieties, even in such an ostensibly private arena. But as well as causing him suffering, such emotional introspection was also central to his sense of self, and to his identity as an authentic man of feeling. As he wrote, 'A man can only be truly polite who had acute feelings and a cultivated understanding. With these he will never go far wrong, nor do an uncivil action'.[29] Indeed, for Oswald, such suffering was ultimately a price worth paying. 'I wish I could subdue every such passion', he reflected; 'But this I would do at the risk of having the character of a cold hearted humdrum. Nor would I wish to overcome the fair and honourable feelings and I am afraid that if the spirit were overcome character must also suffer'.[30]

There is a relative paucity of ego documents equivalent to Oswald's diary that might provide the basis for an extensive insight into the intimate elaboration of surgical selfhood. Even so, it is not uncommon to find Romantic surgeons expressing similar sentiments in more public contexts. John Bell, for example, echoes Oswald in his description of 'that silent humiliation in the presence of misery, which so well becomes one, who feels that he cannot alleviate the pangs, nor avert the changes, of the scene before him; while the afflicted look up to him for help'.[31] However, if the sufferings of patients in the clinical encounter, especially those for whom little could be done, were deeply affecting, the greatest emotional tribulation for the surgeon was undoubtedly that posed by operative practice. As we saw in Chapter 1, Romantic surgeons were avowedly inclined to reduce the frequency of operations and to diminish the role of operative performance in the shaping of surgical identities and reputations. They were also concerned to counter the popular stereotype of the rash and reckless sawbones with an idealised image of the surgeon as compassionate and selfless, always placing his patients' interests ahead of any desire to cultivate a reputation as a dextrous and skilful operator. These reformulations derived, in part, from claims to a greater understanding of anatomy and pathology, but they also stemmed from a recognition that, however advanced surgical knowledge had become, operative surgery remained a deeply imperfect art productive of occasionally unbearable suffering. The 'father' of scientific surgery, John Hunter, claimed that operations were 'a tacit acknowledgement of the insufficiency of surgery' and maintained that 'No surgeon should approach the victim of his operation without a sacred dread and reluctance'.[32] Such sentiments, albeit with a more emotionally reflective twist, were taken up by his acolytes, notably John Abernethy who, in 1827, told his own students that 'The necessary performance

[29] NLS, MS 9003, f. 9r.   [30] NLS, MS 9003, f. 75v.

[31] John Bell, *Letters on Professional Character and Manners: On the Education of a Surgeon, and the Duties and Qualifications of a Physician* (Edinburgh: John Moir, 1810), pp. 352–3.

[32] James F. Palmer (ed.), *The Works of John Hunter, F.R.S.*, vol. 1 (London: Longman, Orme, Brown, Green, and Longman, 1835), p. 210.

of an operation is, or ought to be, an humiliating reflection, since it contains a confession that our art is inadequate to the cure of disease'.[33]

For Abernethy, however, more so perhaps than for Hunter, the relative worth of operative surgery was measured not only by its scientific validity, nor simply by the suffering it caused the patient, but also by the emotional toll it exacted on the surgeon. Indeed, in this period patients and practitioners alike approached surgery as a shared tragedy and a mutual ordeal. Thus, Abernethy's mid-nineteenth-century biographer wrote that there was 'little in most of them [operations] to set against that repulsion which both his science and his humanity suggested'. He also claimed that Abernethy's 'benevolent disposition led him to feel a great deal in regard to operations', particularly 'when a patient bore pain with fortitude'. To support this point about the overwhelming force of Abernethy's sympathy, he recounted the case of 'a severe operation on a woman' that the patient bore 'with great fortitude'. In the midst of the procedure, she turned to Abernethy to ask him if it would take long, to which he replied 'No, indeed [...] that would be too horrible'.[34]

Abernethy's repugnance for operations was well known. Indeed, he famously, though possibly apocryphally, remarked, on being asked how he felt before an 'important operation', that 'I feel as if I was going to be hanged'.[35] Such expressions might seem peculiar coming from a leading metropolitan hospital surgeon, as these men were often thought to be inured to such sentiments. In actual fact, the notion that operative enthusiasm, perhaps even operative confidence, might be diminished by the effects of sympathy was widespread enough to constitute a cliché of surgical self-representation in this period. Even Cooper, whose reputation as an operative surgeon was virtually unrivalled at the peak of his career, reportedly said of himself that 'He felt too much before he began ever to make a perfect operator'.[36] One of the most expressive surgeons on this point was Charles Bell. Trained in large part by his older brother John, Charles left Edinburgh for London in 1804 because John's public dispute with James Gregory had rendered his professional position in that city untenable, at least for a period.[37] While in London he lectured at the Great Windmill Street anatomy school and, briefly, at London University.[38] During that time

---

[33] *Lancet* 8:197 (9 June 1827), p. 289.

[34] George Macilwain, *Memoirs of John Abernethy*, vol. 2, 2nd ed. (London: Hurst and Blackett, 1854), pp. 202–3.

[35] The likely source of this oft-repeated anecdote is James Miller, *Surgical Experience of Chloroform* (Edinburgh: Sutherland and Knox, 1848), p. 29.

[36] Bransby Blake Cooper, *The Life of Sir Astley Cooper, Bart.*, vol. 2 (London: John W. Parker, 1843), p. 474.

[37] Brown, 'Surgery, Identity'.

[38] For Bell's professional life in London, see Carin Berkowitz, *Charles Bell and the Anatomy of Reform* (Chicago: Chicago University Press, 2015); L. S. Jacyna, 'Bell, Charles (1774–1842)', *ODNB*.

he developed a reputation not only as an excellent teacher and experimentalist, but also as a highly capable surgeon. Indeed, Charles wrote in his extensive correspondence with his brother George Bell (1770–1843) that 'My hands are better for operation than any I have seen at work'.[39] However, Charles was also a man of great sensitivity and once told his wife Marion Bell (1787–1876) that 'I get wearied – exhausted by the sufferings of others'.[40] This sensitivity was so acute as to give rise to a profound malaise in anticipation of an operation, something he regularly referred to in his letters. In many cases this stemmed from an acknowledgement of the limitations of the surgical art in alleviating human suffering. Thus, in July 1824 he told George that 'I must do an operation to-morrow, which makes me to-day quite miserable [...] I have not only the conviction that great blockheads have enjoyed this before me, but that I am providing for a relay and continual supply of suffering'.[41] Similarly, in February 1826 he wrote: 'I have had operations both at the Hospital and in private, from which I suffer indescribable anxiety, so that I vote my profession decidedly a bad one – the more to do, the worse'.[42]

Charles' anxieties in advance of an operation, which were 'the greatest any man can suffer', hint at the enormous emotional demands of the procedure itself.[43] His brother John wrote that 'An operation is a distressing scene, even when conducted by men the best prepared for such awful duties'.[44] Indeed, for John the experience of operating was one that defined the surgeon's professional and affective character and distinguished him from the physician. In his dispute with James Gregory, for example, he claimed that as a physician, Gregory had 'never passed a sleepless night, reflecting what was to be done on the morrow; never witnessed the severities of the surgeon; never strained hard his breath, nor involuntarily clenched his hands at the sight of another's agony; nor blanched with fear, nor felt the palpitations of anxiety, in the midst of an eventful operation'.[45] As these comments suggest, the emotional challenges of operative surgery derived not simply from the infliction of pain and suffering, but also from the weight of responsibility and the capacity for things to become 'eventful'. Needless to say, surgical operations of the early nineteenth century

[39] Charles Bell to George Bell, 8 December 1835, *Letters of Sir Charles Bell* (London: John Murray, 1870), p. 346.
[40] Charles Bell to Marion Bell, 8 August 1841, *Letters*, p. 392. For more on Charles' emotional dispositions, particularly his relationship to the war wounded, see Brown, 'Wounds'.
[41] Charles Bell to George Bell, 28 July 1824, *Letters*, p. 285.
[42] Charles Bell to George Bell, 16 February 1826, *Letters*, p. 294.
[43] Charles Bell, *Illustrations of the Great Operations of Surgery* (London: Longman, Hurst, Rees, Orme, and Brown, 1821), p. vii.
[44] Bell, *Letters on Professional Character*, p. 535.
[45] John Bell, *Answer for the Junior Members of the Royal College of Surgeons of Edinburgh to the Memorial of Dr James Gregory* (Edinburgh: Peter Hill, 1800), Section II, p. 7; Brown, 'Surgery, Identity'.

were nowhere near as extensive or invasive as those of today. The limiting factors of shock and blood loss generally prevented surgeons from intruding too far into the body's main cavities of head, thorax, stomach, and abdomen until around the 1880s.[46] And yet, operations of this period were often far more sophisticated and complex than is generally assumed. Moreover, if intraoperative death is now an extremely rare occurrence (in the developed world at least), in the early nineteenth century it was, if not routine, then certainly a far more common experience. A particularly dramatic example of this can be found in the archives of Astley Cooper who, in late 1829 or early 1830, received from the Lancashire surgeon and obstetrician James Barlow (1767–1839) an account of an operation to remove a tumour from the neck of 'a delicate lady' named Mrs Beardsworth.[47] With the patient seated on a 'reclined chair', Barlow 'began by making two elliptical incisions with the scalpel from under the ear over the most prominent part of the tumour' when

a sudden and unexpected hissing noise issued obviously from a large divided empty vein and the patient instantly expired without either sigh, groan or struggle and every effort used to restore animation became fruitless. This unexpected event was truly appalling to all present for scarcely an ounce of blood was lost on the occasion.[48]

In this instance, what was especially notable and 'appalling' about the patient's sudden death was the lack of blood, for catastrophic operative failure was most often accompanied by a sanguinary effusion. Indeed, haemorrhage can rightfully be said, in the words of Peter Stanley, to have constituted 'the surgeon's greatest fear'.[49] John Bell claimed that to 'expire by successive haemorrhages is perhaps the least painful of deaths, and yet it is the most awful'. 'Is not this fear of haemorrhagy always uppermost in the minds of the young surgeon?' he asked; 'Were this one danger removed, he would go forward in his profession almost without fear'. This fear remained a constant presence, however, and in a typically embodied and affective description of operative practice, he wrote:

It is the dashing of the blood from the great arteries, and the fainting of the patient, that hurries our most important operations, and makes all the difference betwixt operating on the living body and dissecting the dead. It is this which unsteadies at times the hand of the boldest surgeon, and makes his heart, at the first alarm, sink within him.

---

[46] For an account of the controversies engendered by early attempts at invasive surgery, see Sally Frampton, *Belly-Rippers, Surgical Innovation and the Ovariotomy Controversy* (London: Palgrave Macmillan, 2018).

[47] RCSE, MS008/2/2/12, Notebook of notes on a case of the removal of a tumour from the cheek. A version of this account, where the patient is named, was subsequently published in *Medico-Chirurgical Transactions* 16 (1830), 19–35.

[48] RCSE, MS0008/2/2/12, unpaginated.

[49] Peter Stanley, *For Fear of Pain: British Surgery, 1790–1850* (Amsterdam: Rodopi, 2003), p. 222.

No surgeon nor spectator can keep the natural colour of his cheek when a patient is expiring, or in danger of expiring, by loss of blood; and the actual death of a patient must leave a lasting melancholy on the surgeon's mind.[50]

If haemorrhage challenged the resolve of even the 'boldest surgeon', then it was a particularly terrifying prospect for the surgical initiate. Hence, various lecturers regaled their students with cautionary tales of the dangers of blood loss, and of the importance of maintaining composure when faced with its appearance. In January 1820, for example, John Abernethy told his St Bartholomew's class of a student who opened the artery of a woman and 'when he saw the scarlet blood gush out, he had so little of the mind of a Surgeon that he said "Good God, what have I done, I have murdered you and ruined myself"'.[51] Meanwhile, several cohorts of Astley Cooper's St Thomas' surgical class heard the story of a hospital dresser who 'wished very much to perform an operation' and therefore convinced the hospital's 'surgery boy' Abraham, 'who had a bad leg', to consent to him performing an amputation. Upon making his incision, the dresser was confronted by a 'great discharge of blood' and so he 'cried out' to his assistant to '"Screw the tourniquet tighter"'. Unfortunately, however, the screw of the tourniquet broke:

At this unforeseen accident, the dresser lost all presence of mind; he jumped about the room, then ran to the sufferer, and endeavoured to stop the effusion of blood by compressing the wound with his hand, but in vain; his sleeve became filled with blood, and poor Abraham would have died in a very short time, had not a pupil accidentally called, who had the presence of mind to apply the key of the door to the femoral artery, and, by compressing it, stopped the bleeding.[52]

As both of these cases suggest, if fear and anxiety were a near-constant presence in the mind of the operative surgeon, their ultimate realisation was almost invariably accompanied by panic and professional disgrace. This was especially true given the highly 'public' nature of many surgical procedures, notably those undertaken in metropolitan teaching hospitals. Hence, in advocating for a rigorous anatomical education, John Bell wrote of the consternation of 'untaught men operating upon their fellow creatures' who

---

[50] John Bell, *The Principles of Surgery* (Edinburgh: T. Cadell Jr and W. Davies, 1801), pp. 141–2.

[51] RCSE, MS0232/1/5, John Flint South, 'Lectures on Natural and Morbid Anatomy and Physiology, delivered by John Abernethy Esq. FRS in the Anatomical Theatre at St Bartholomew's Hospital in the years 1819 & 1820, Vol. 4th', f. 243.

[52] *Lancet* 1:1 (5 October 1823), p. 6. A version of this anecdote appeared in Cooper's lecture in 1816, where the person applying the key is identified as 'Mr Forbes of Camberwell', possibly William Forbes (c.1753–1818); RCSE, MS0232/3, John Flint South, 'Lectures on the Principles and Practice of Surgery delivered by Astley Paston Cooper Esq, F.R.S. & Benjamin Travers Esq. F.R.S. in the Anatomical Theatre at St Thomas' Hospital between the years 1816 & 1818 Vol. 1', ff. 5–6. For William Forbes, see NA, PROB 11/1609/366, Will of William Forbes, Surgeon of Camberwell, Surrey (29 October 1818); *Gentleman's Magazine* 88 (July–December 1818), p. 471.

are seen agitated, miserable, trembling, hesitating in the midst of difficulties, turning round to their friends for that support which should come from within, feeling in the wound for things which they do not understand, holding consultations amidst the cries of the patient, or even retiring to consult about his case while he lies bleeding in great pain and awful expectation; and thus [...] incurring reproaches which attend them throughout life.[53]

Operative surgery was, then, a profoundly challenging experience, fraught with anxiety and fear. For Bell, it was one that could only truly be mastered by the surgeon whose capacity for emotional self-possession transcended the tribulations of the moment, enabling him to function to the best of his abilities and to see the operation to a successful conclusion, even in the most trying of circumstances. Indeed, it was that capacity, that inner resolve, which was for Bell, as for many of his contemporaries, the highest indication of professional surgical acumen.

However relieved by the successful termination of an operation a surgeon might be, the emotional trials of surgery did not necessarily end when the patient was removed from the table or chair. For some surgeons, such as Charles Bell, the strain of operating continued to resonate long after the knife was set down. In 1818 he wrote to his wife saying: 'I have just been performing a serious operation, and that, you know, is always severe upon me'. In order to clear his mind, Charles proposed to 'take a run to Box Hill tomorrow'. Nevertheless, in this case even the thought of a ride in the country quickly turned to despondency. 'Quick! quick! and get well, and come back again', he wrote. 'This is the most stupid life imaginable. I really have not interest enough in anything to drag me this way or that. If I were once set a running, I think I should run a long way'.[54] Charles' thoughts of quite literally running away were, as he recognised, fanciful, for the surgeon's life was far too busy for such indulgences. Indeed, the days and weeks following an operation often involved an anxious vigil, as the patient was monitored, either in person or by proxy, for signs of recovery or decline. Hence, in 1830, Charles told George that 'Last night I said I must sit down and write to you, because I found my spirits unusually light'. However, 'Just then I got a notice that one of my patients had altered very much for the worse in the last two hours, and so I was put again in the blue devils'.[55] Needless to say, the death of a patient, either during or after an operation, had the most profound emotional consequences. In 1823, for example, Charles wrote to George telling him that 'I have had a most miserable time since I wrote to you, from the failure of an operation, and the death of a most worthy man. I shall regret

---

[53] Bell, *Principles*, p. 6.
[54] Charles Bell to Marion Bell, 28 September 1818, *Letters*, pp. 261–2.
[55] Charles Bell to George Bell, 3 April 1830, *Letters*, p. 310.

it as long as I live. It is very hard, more trying than anything that any other profession can bring a man to'.[56]

Regret was a common motif of Romantic surgical discourse, albeit one that had to be carefully deployed. After all, a surgeon's living was highly dependent on his reputation and so any public admission of remorse risked drawing unfavourable attention. Nevertheless, it was not uncommon for surgeons to express regret, even to their students. Like many others in his position, John Abernethy would occasionally use such reflections as a means of discouraging students from certain modes of treatment or therapeutic management, such as when he told them, in relation to the delicate art of bone setting, that 'I have done much mischief by getting patients up to have their beds made, cramps come on, the Bone is moved and we have all to do over again'.[57] Abernethy's regrets testified to the lessons of occasionally bitter experience. As we shall see, breast cancer was one of the most emotionally challenging diseases for early nineteenth-century surgeons to deal with and often functioned as a source of regret. Its disfiguring virulence and almost inevitable recurrence meant that many experienced surgeons were despairing of cure and sceptical of the value of surgical excision. Looking back on his early experience with the disease, Abernethy recalled the case of 'a pretty girl' who

came to me with one of these tumours in her breast which she was desirous of having removed, I made a small elliptical incision to remove it, being anxious that there should be but a little scar and not knowing the disease well then; but it grew again, which was devilish vexatious and very disgraceful to a Surgeon.

Abernethy's experience of breast cancer, like that of most of his contemporaries, was grim. 'Having seen these cases turn out so unfortunately', he claimed, 'I began to be very much afraid of them'.[58]

In other instances, Abernethy's reflections gave rise to more mixed feelings: for example, in the case of a woman with an inguinal hernia that he decided to reduce by operation. On cutting into the sac he found it contained no bowel but merely the omentum. 'Here was a lesson for my vanity', he told his students. 'I went home exceedingly displeased with myself for having performed the operation'. The patient died a few days later, but on examining her body he found that she had a condition of the descending colon that would have complicated the procedure, 'so that I was as well pleased with myself as I was before displeased'.[59]

[56] Charles Bell to George Bell, 28 December 1823, *Letters*, p. 281.
[57] RCSE, MS0232/1/1, John Flint South, 'Lectures on the Principles of Surgery delivered by John Abernethy Esq. FRS in the Anatomical Theatre at St Bartholomew's Hospital in the years 1818 and 1819', f. 230.
[58] RCSE, MS0232/1/1, f. 105.   [59] RCSE, MS0232/1/5, ff. 201–2.

In most cases, however, the only consolation Abernethy could derive from reflecting on past mistakes was that he had done the best he could in the circumstances. Hence, in one of his lectures he stated:

I always regret not having sufficiently enlarged the wound in a poor boy who fell on a stick by which a wound was made in the abdomen and through it the viscera protruded in great quantities from vomiting – they had been much pummelled in the endeavour to return them – I measured the opening and put them in by degrees, but it was a long business and if I had made the wound larger it would have been better – he died – but I do not reproach myself for I did all that lay in my power and what I then believed to be best.[60]

What is clear is that such emotional self-reflection shaped Abernethy's surgical practice, encouraging him to operate in certain cases and discouraging him from doing so in others. Moreover, it also allowed him to pass on the fruits of his wisdom to his students. As we have seen, Abernethy, like most of his contemporaries, was painfully aware of the limitations of operative surgery. By sharing his experiences of such uncertainty, he sought to forewarn his pupils of what lay ahead, and reassure them that as long as they acted according to the best knowledge and practice and adhered to what he called the maxim of 'do as we would be done by [...] then we shall be acquitted in the grand tribunal'.[61] As he said of that most dangerous and invasive of procedures, lithotomy:

No blame can be attached to you if you lose a patient after the operation for the stone – we are called in to operate when the case is desperate – we do not solicit patients to let us perform this operation, we are urged by them to it – and in many cases like the coup de grace of the executioner [it] puts them out of their troubles at once.[62]

This comment might seem offhand, callous even. But in reality, such sentiments were less the product of emotional detachment or gallows humour than an acknowledgement of the inherent pathos of human suffering. They were also at one with Abernethy's social and professional identity. One of his former students claimed that he liked Abernethy's lectures 'because he is always so gentlemanly' and because he had 'a kind of unaffected respect for himself and his audience, which obliges one to pay attention to him, if it were only because you feel that a man of education is speaking to you'.[63] Through his lectures, Abernethy not only presented himself as a gentleman of great experience, capable of earnest reflection, he encouraged similar behaviour in his students.

60 RCSE, MS0232/1/5, ff. 115–16.   61 RCSE, MS0232/1/1, f. 240.
62 RCSE, MS0232/1/5, ff. 222–3.   63 Macilwain, *Memoirs*, vol. 2, p. 112.

As is clear, then, emotional expression played a vital role in shaping both professional identities and personal subjectivities. Contrary to Adam Smith's observation about the desensitising effects of exposure to suffering, the experiences of men like John Abernethy and Charles Bell suggest that the performance of operative surgery enhanced the intensity of emotional sensation, encouraging an emotional self-reflection that in turn determined future practice. However, as we shall now see, while emotional expression was a virtue, emotional incontinence was not, for the emotions of the surgical relationship had to be carefully managed, not only those of the surgeon but also those of the patient.

Managing Surgical Emotions

Perhaps the most vivid, and certainly the most famous, account of undergoing operative surgery in this period is that provided by Frances Burney (1752–1840). In 1810, during her time in France, she was diagnosed with a breast tumour and her husband, General Alexandre D'Arblay (1748–1818), secured the services of Antoine Dubois (1756–1837), consultant surgeon to the Imperial family, and Dominique Jean Larrey (1766–1842), surgeon-in-chief to the Imperial army. The relationship between Burney and these two men was structured, to a very significant degree, by feelings and expressions of emotion. For example, Larrey was 'so anxious [...] from his own fear lest he was under any delusion, from the excess of his desire to save me' that he asked Burney to consult with the anatomist and surgeon Francois Ribes (1765–1845).[64] Upon telling her that she would need an operation, Larrey 'had [...] tears in his eyes', while Dubois was almost 'unintelligible [...] from his own disturbance'.[65] Larrey was 'always melancholy' around Burney and 'so deeply affected [...] that – as he has lately told me, he regretted to his Soul ever having known me, and was upon the point of demanding a commission to the furthest end of France in order to force me into other hands'.[66] Indeed, so pronounced were these surgeons' emotions that during the procedure itself, Burney spoke only to assure them how much she pitied them, 'for indeed I was sensible to the feeling concern with which they all saw what I endured' and, when it was all over, she saw 'my good Dr Larry [sic], pale nearly as myself, his face streaked with blood, and its expression depicting grief, apprehension, and almost horrour [sic]'.[67]

---

[64] Frances Burney, 'Journal Letter to Esther Burney, 22 March–June 1812', in Peter Sabor and Lars E. Trodie (eds), *Frances Burney: Journals and Letters* (London: Penguin, 2001), pp. 433–4.

[65] Burney, 'Letter', pp. 434, 435.

[66] Burney, 'Letter', pp. 437, 438.   [67] Burney, 'Letter', p. 443.

It is hard to imagine quite such a degree of emotional expressiveness from British surgeons. As Reddy has shown, sentimentalism reached a peculiarly high pitch in France in the decades following the publication of Jean-Jacques Rousseau's (1712–1778) *Julie, ou la nouvelle Héloïse* (1761). During the period of the French Revolution, especially the Terror of 1793–4, profuse expressions of feeling came to function as a marker of moral and political virtue.[68] British observers were generally distrustful of such tendencies as, according to Markman Ellis, excessive displays of emotion had already come to be regarded as vulgar and disingenuous, even before their association with foreignness or political radicalism.[69]

In early nineteenth-century Britain, therefore, a somewhat more restrained form of emotional expression was *à la mode*. Moreover, for surgeons of this period, regardless of their nationality, there was a balance to be struck between the expression of feelings such as pity and sympathy and one's ability to operate effectively. In 1815, for example, Charles Bell attended the wounded after the battle of Waterloo. Referring to his experience with the French casualties, he described a situation in which 'All the decencies of performing surgical operations were soon neglected' as he amputated one man's thigh while 'there lay at one time thirteen, all beseeching to be taken next'. 'It was a strange thing', he recalled, 'to feel my clothes stiff with blood, and my arms powerless with the exertion of using the knife'. But it was 'more extraordinary still, to find my mind calm amidst such variety of suffering; but to give one of these objects access to your feelings was to allow yourself to be unmanned for the performance of a duty'.[70] In his history of tears and national character, *Weeping Britannia* (2015), Thomas Dixon uses this example to suggest that Charles was a surgeon (or rather, as he incorrectly states, a physician) who led a 'dual existence' as 'a man of feeling in private, but a resolute and apathetic stoic in his professional activities'.[71] In his work on Romantic military art, Philip Shaw likewise sees Charles as an exemplar of professional detachment, donning 'armour' in order to 'protect the core self from the intrusion of feminized affects'.[72] As we have suggested in relation to Payne's work, such dichotomies between the 'professional' and the 'private' self do little to capture the complexities of emotional navigation, nor do they acknowledge the role that emotions played in Romantic surgical culture more generally. After all, Charles' reaction to his ability to function

---

[68] Reddy, *Navigation*, chs. 5 and 6.
[69] Markman Ellis, *The Politics of Sensibility: Race, Gender and Commerce in the Sentimental Novel* (Cambridge, UK: Cambridge University Press, 1996), ch. 6.
[70] Charles Bell to Francis Horner, July 1815, *Letters*, p. 247.
[71] Thomas Dixon, *Weeping Britannia: Portrait of a Nation in Tears* (Oxford: Oxford University Press, 2015), p. 131.
[72] Philip Shaw, *Suffering and Sentiment in Romantic Military Art* (Aldershot: Ashgate, 2013), pp. 194–5.

in such circumstances was one of astonishment rather than professional 'apathy'. He acknowledged the danger that excessive pity and sympathy might prevent him from performing his duty adequately, but this danger was precisely due to the acuity of his sentiment, not its absence.[73] What this example demonstrates, then, is that though Romantic surgeons might be emotionally affected by their exposure to suffering, they nonetheless had to manage those emotions in order to be of use, even if, as in Charles Bell's case, it was contrary to their inclinations.

If the emotions of battlefield surgery ran particularly high, then those of civil surgery were equally in need of careful management. As we heard earlier, in 1820 Benjamin Brodie told his class of aspirant surgeons of the public's belief that 'being perpetually present at scenes of woe' tended to 'blunt the feelings of our nature'. However, as he continued,

It appears to me, that the prejudice of some persons on this point is very unfounded. Undoubtedly a Surgeon does not sympathise with the bodily pain of the patient as an ordinary bystander would do: but this is not because he is deprived of feeling, but because his mind is occupied by other considerations; because he is engaged in adopting means for his patients relief.[74]

Here, the surgeon's focus on the task at hand and his commitment to his patient's well-being necessitated that he should, in Brodie's words, 'be capable of abstracting himself from the consideration of the distress which another endures'.[75] In a similar vein, Charles Bell argued: 'Let no man boast of feelings, until they are of that genuine kind, and amount to that degree, that he can forget himself, in the desire to give aid to another'.[76] It is important to recognise how this differs from conventional understandings of surgical dispassion or detachment. Neither Brodie nor Bell suggest that this is a normative emotional state, nor is it a permanent one. On the contrary, it requires effort and is specific to the moment of the operation. Moreover, emotions of pity and sympathy for another's suffering are not absent here. They are not even 'blunted' by repetition and habituation into a kind of 'insensibility', as Adam Smith might suggest. Rather they are sublimated, through training and moral self-discipline, into a higher form of expression. Hence, situating this emotional transfiguration within the culture of sensibility, Brodie argued that such forms of self-control 'ought to form anything rather than a matter of reproach':

The Surgeon, whose delicate sympathy makes him shrink within himself at every strike of his scalpel, would be ill fitted to perform an operation. He ought not to be characterised as a man of superior sensibility but as one whose zeal in the science of his

[73] See Brown, 'Wounds'.   [74] RCSE, MS0470/1/2/5, ff. 20–1.
[75] RCSE, MS0470/1/2/5, f. 21.   [76] Bell, *Illustrations*, p. vii.

profession, and whose anxiety for his patients welfare, are not sufficiently powerful to suspend for a while feelings of less importance. If present when an operation is tediously and awkwardly performed, I question whether the Surgeon does not feel more severely than an ordinary bystander.[77]

Brodie's comments bring to mind the quotation from *Rab and His Friends* (1859), introduced in Chapter 1, in which John Brown distinguishes between 'pity – as an emotion, ending in itself or at best in tears' and 'pity as a motive'.[78] The *suspension* of 'feelings of less importance' is a professional skill derived from 'zeal' and 'anxiety' for the patient. In the moment of the operation, one particular mode of emotional expression, the active, supersedes another, the passive. What we see at work here is the elaboration of what Barbara Rosenwein calls an 'emotional community'.[79] While recognising the pervasive emotional regime of sensibility, Brodie elaborates a distinctly surgical emotional disposition, which he acknowledges is not always understood by those outside of the professional community of which he is part, and into which his students are being initiated. As such, he suggests that in cases where operations are performed badly, the surgeon feels even 'more severely' than an 'ordinary bystander', not merely because he knows what should be done whereas they do not, but also because, when removed from the act of doing, the surgeon's emotions are no longer held in check to quite the same degree. Brodie's observations on this point resonate with the personal experience of Charles Bell who, in 1805, told his brother that he had 'just returned from an operation' but that 'being bound by certain rules, a *spectator* merely, it was torture to me'.[80]

Everard Home, Brodie's teacher, expressed similar sentiments. He too acknowledged that 'Surgeons have been accused of want of humanity' and suggested that 'The circumstances of their being present so frequently at scenes of distress prevents them from receiving the same shock which others do'. However, like Brodie, he was anxious to exculpate surgeons from the charge of insensibility, claiming that 'an excess of sensibility is of no use & takes away the power of giving relief'. Likewise, he argued that in the moment of the operation, surgeons were required to manage their emotions in order to perform effectively. But to illustrate this point, he chose an intriguing metaphor:

A mother, when the house is on fire will carry her infant through the flames or she may hold her infant to have an operation performed with great firmness & resolution, & afterwards when it is over faint away. During an operation, while he is acting for the relief of another, [the surgeon] is putting a restraint on his own feelings. He does not feel

---

[77] RCSE, MS0470/1/2/5, f. 21.

[78] John Brown, *Rab and His Friends*, 8th ed. (Boston: Colonial Press, 1906), p. 25.

[79] Barbara H. Rosenwein, *Emotional Communities in the Early Middle Ages* (Ithaca, NY: Cornell University Press, 2007).

[80] Charles Bell to George Bell, 23 March 1805, *Letters*, p. 40.

the momentous distress he occasions. As there is nothing in Surgery which can soften an unfeeling man so there is nothing to diminish his benevolence or humanity. Every act which he performs is to relieve distress, to remove temporal evils & to preserve life.[81]

This quotation suggests a number of things, not the least of which is that a surgeon of the early nineteenth century might use maternal metaphors to describe the compassionate, self-sacrificing, and devotional dimensions of his profession. Such analogies complicate Shaw's notion that Romantic surgeons like Charles Bell sought to insulate themselves from 'feminized affects'. In reality, the cultures of sensibility did not necessarily code such emotional expressions as 'feminine'; when Charles wrote of being 'unmanned', this did not equate to feminisation, but rather to a failure of personal and professional duty. Indeed, as in Home's case, the figure of the mother might function as the most obvious motif for selfless devotion, especially if that devotion was conceived in terms of instinctual care. As the century wore on, such analogies, though not necessarily unthinkable, certainly became less common, as medical and surgical metaphors of professional duty and devotion took on more active, intrepid, and warlike forms.[82]

What this quotation also reveals is the limited power of dispassion or detachment to capture the subtleties of the Romantic surgical relationship. After all, as with Brodie's comments, Home's lecture proposes that the emotional restraint of the surgeon is temporary and that, like the mother having rescued her child from the flames, he might afterwards 'faint away'. Moreover, if detachment involves isolating oneself from the suffering and subjectivity of the other, here we have the very opposite, as Home draws parallels between himself and the resolve and fortitude of his patient's mother. Such intersubjectivity was absolutely central to Romantic surgery, for emotional management did not simply involve the surgeon controlling his own feelings, it also necessitated the management of the patient's state of mind, something that could never be achieved through a process of emotional distancing.

The centrality of emotional intersubjectivity to the Romantic surgical relationship was shaped, to a profound degree, by the nature of pre-anaesthetic surgery and by contemporary understandings of the importance of emotional states in the regulation of bodily health. In a period when patients underwent surgery without any significant pain relief and fully conscious of what was happening to them, surgery was an inherently collaborative act that required patient and practitioner to forge an effective (and affective) alliance. A striking case in point took place at Guy's Hospital in January 1824, when Astley Cooper performed the 'formidable operation' of an amputation of the leg at the

---

[81] WL, MS.5604, f. 11.
[82] Michael Brown, '"Like a Devoted Army": Medicine, Heroic Masculinity, and the Military Paradigm in Victorian Britain', *Journal of British Studies* 49:3 (2010), 592–622.

hip joint on a 40-year-old man who was 'rapidly sinking' under the effects of a previous amputation at the knee. The gruelling operation lasted twenty minutes but, according to *The Lancet*, 'the patient bore [it] with extraordinary fortitude'. After it was over, he said to Cooper '"that was the hardest day's work he had ever gone through", to which Sir Astley replied "that it was almost the hardest he ever had"'.[83]

In light of such emotional and physical trials, surgeons of the period were advised to do as much as they could to alleviate the patient's anxiety in advance of a procedure. As we saw in the previous chapter, the public nature of operations in teaching hospitals did not always make this a straightforward task. Nevertheless, the idealised performance of the surgeon as calm and composed did not merely convey moral rectitude and professional self-control, it also helped to put the patient at ease, or as much at ease as circumstances would allow. The same was also true of the surgeon's attire and the arrangement of the operating room. In 1833 James Wardrop told his students that 'the necessary preparations [for an operation] should be made as far as possible, without the knowledge of the patient':

All the instruments ought to be laid on in proper order, and covered over, so that the patient may not witness the preparations which are required. Pains ought also to be taken to avoid all exhibition of blood, as the sight of that never fails to create disquietude in the minds both of the patient and his surrounding friends.[84]

Likewise, 'there is nothing the surgeon should so much avoid, as by his dress, to impress [the patient] with an idea that the operation will be attended by much bloodshed'. Claiming that it 'used to be a very general custom [...] more particularly in public hospitals, that the surgeon attires himself in such a dress as to give rise to the impression that he is about to perform the duties of an executioner rather than those of benefactor', Wardrop advised that it was far better to wear dark clothing so 'that any small quantity of blood which may be spilt shall not be conspicuous', rather than donning a full-length apron, as some surgeons were wont to do.[85] Similar advice was given by John Abernethy. On one occasion, when he was supervising the preparations of a young surgeon, he exclaimed 'No, there is one thing you have forgotten' and laid a napkin over the instruments. 'It is bad enough for the poor patient to have to undergo an operation', he declared, 'without being obliged to see those terrible instruments'.[86] In another instance, he even advised against the use of certain terms

---

[83] *Lancet* 1:16 (18 January 1824), pp. 95–6. This was the very operation that, according to Thomas Wakley, the Scottish journals had unfavourably compared to James Syme's procedure. See Chapter 1, p. 56.
[84] *Lancet* 20:518 (3 August 1833), p. 595.
[85] *Lancet* 20:518 (3 August 1833), p. 595.   [86] Macilwain, *Memoirs*, vol. 2, p. 197.

in theatre. Imagining a surgeon declaring to his assistant during the midst of
a trephination 'Give me the knife Sir', he reflected 'good God, what must the
patients feeling be, blind folded and hearing give me the knife Sir – Had you
not better say give me the Bistoury, a name which not being familiar to the
patient would not alarm him[?]'.[87]

It was not only during an operation that a surgeon's behaviour was important; his demeanour during the clinical encounter might also affect his patient's
emotional state. As we have heard, certain surgeons were perhaps more pol-
ished in their social interactions than others. Nonetheless, Benjamin Brodie
recommended 'guarding against the acquirement of such manners, as may be
apparently rough or really offensive'. At the same time, he also warned against
'the adoption of those courtier like manners, those continued attempts to suit
the inclination and flatter the self-love of others, by means of which mean persons endeavour to make up for their own Ignorance and want of skill'.[88] For
his part, Astley Cooper recommended a 'gentleness of manner', observing that
'patients having a natural dislike to operations, feel still more uneasy if they
discover anything in their practitioner's behaviour that makes them apprehend
rough treatment'. Like Brodie, he was sensitive to the balance between integ-
rity and obsequiousness. Nevertheless, he maintained that 'These qualities forward the interest of professional men, whilst they diminish the sufferings of
human nature'. 'Patients generally form an opinion of a Surgeon's ability by
his manner', he suggested: 'if he be of a dry, morose turn, he is apt to alarm not
only the patient, but his whole family; whereas, he who speaks kindly to them,
and asks for particular information, is supposed to have more knowledge, and
receives more respect'.[89]

In Cooper's configuration, then, manners were not merely social affec-
tations designed to gain an advantage in the competitive world of private
practice, they were a vital tool of therapeutic management. While this might
seem like special pleading, it is important to remember the material effect
that words, deeds, and their emotional correlates were deemed to have on
a patient's health. In making his case for the importance of 'gentleness of
manner', for example, Cooper cited the example of a surgeon who, upon
examining a patient for a compound dislocation of the ankle joint, declared
'Carthage must fall. Thereby implying that amputation must be performed'.
'Indeed', Cooper observed, 'from the rough manner in which he treated his
patient there seemed no other chance for the poor fellow's recovery. In this
case, gentleness might have prevented such an unpleasant circumstance'. In
another instance, meanwhile, a surgical pupil at Guy's asked a man about

[87] RCSE, MS0232/1/5, f. 162.
[88] RCSE, MS0470/1/2/5, ff. 21–2.   [89] *Lancet* 1:1 (5 October 1823), pp. 4–5.

to undergo an operation where he came from, to which the patient replied "'From Cornwall". "'Oh, did you'", the pupil responded, "'I can tell you, you will never see Cornwall again'".[90]

Whatever the pupil's intention here, the effect, unsurprisingly perhaps, was that 'the patient became alarmed' and fled the hospital before the surgeon even had a chance to perform the operation. In other cases, meanwhile, a patient's despondency could have an even more dramatic and unfortunate impact on the outcome of a procedure. 'The mind has great influence over the actions of the body', Cooper wrote in one of his casebooks, 'and it often happens after operations that the least discouraging expression will produce fatal effects'. To support this observation, he cited the case of Mrs Shipley, who had been operated upon by Cooper's mentor, Henry Cline (1750–1827), for a cancerous breast. 'She said she was sure she should die', Cooper wrote, and 'immediately after the operation she became almost lifeless and in three hours she died'. As if to prove the inevitability of her demise, he observed that she had made arrangements to hand over her role as mistress of the household, stating: 'All her keys were found marked that there might be no confusion occasioned by her death'.[91]

Thus, while social graces were doubtless important in the fashioning of an agreeable professional persona, the power accorded to sympathy and imagination within contemporary surgical thought and the intimate connection that was held to subsist between mind and body, mood and health, ensured that emotional sensitivity was no mere ornament. In fact, Romantic surgery demanded a deep emotional communion with one's patient, in order to manage their condition as effectively as possible. According to John Bell, 'the surgeon must be every thing to his patient; watchful, friendly, compassionate, cheerful; for the patient lives upon his good looks; it is when his surgeon becomes careless, or seems to forsake him, that he falls into despair'.[92] Meanwhile, in his *Operative Surgery* (1850), Frederic Skey claimed that 'A man is disqualified [from the duties of surgery] [...] who cannot in imagination place himself in the position of the patient, and reflect on the case in all its bearings and calculate the result as though his own personal health were directly involved'. Skey called this 'the moral relation of the surgeon to his patient' and it was a well-established feature of Romantic surgical culture.[93] In particular, it was a vital tool of surgical decision-making. As we shall see in the next chapter, the performance of an operation almost always involved a process of negotiation between patient

[90] *Lancet* 1:1 (5 October 1823), pp. 4, 9.
[91] RCSE, MS0008/2/1/7, Casebook in the hand of Sir Astley Paston Cooper, 1793–1823, unpaginated.
[92] Bell, *Principles*, p. 15.
[93] Frederic Skey, *Operative Surgery* (London: John Churchill, 1850), p. 3.

and practitioner, but it was nonetheless essential for the surgeon to determine in his own mind whether an operation was in the patient's best interests. As Astley Cooper put it:

> Sorry indeed should I be, to sport with the life of a fellow-creature who might repose a confidence either in my surgical knowledge or in my humanity; and I should be equally disposed to consider myself culpable, if I did not make every possible effort to save a person whose death was rendered inevitable, if a disease were suffered to continue which it was possible for surgery to relieve [...] In the performance of our duty one feeling should direct us; the case we should consider as our own and we should ask ourselves, whether, placed under similar circumstances, we should submit to the pain and danger we are about to inflict.[94]

Not only was it necessary to determine whether an operation was appropriate but, given the gruelling nature of contemporary operative surgery, it was also essential to gauge whether or not the patient had the mental, moral, and physical capacity to withstand a procedure. James Wardrop, for example, gave extensive advice to his students as to the kinds of patients who generally made for better or worse operative subjects. The obese, the gouty, and the scrofulous all presented their challenges but, above all, it was 'Persons of *nervous temperament*' who were 'by no means eligible subjects for operations'. According to Wardrop, fear played a particularly malign role in determining operative outcomes, and he urged his students to 'make a nice distinction between those patients whose nervous system is strongly developed, and those who have little moral courage, or are easily impressed with fear'. 'The physical frame of the former', he alleged, might suffer severely, 'but if they be of a cheerful disposition they soon recover; whereas, when a person has an impression that the operation to which he is to submit is one of great danger, you should consider his recovery doubtful'.[95] Needless to say, almost all patients suffered from some form of apprehension in advance of an operation, which was why it was vital for a surgeon to be able to read his patient's emotions and distinguish normative anxiety from the baleful influence of what he called 'moral depression':

> When [...] you find the patient greatly under the influence of fear, there is one important point to consider, as it ought materially to guide your judgement, and that is, to discover whether the patient's fear arises from the dread of the temporary pain of the operation, or its consequences. If he merely dread the pain, then may you with confidence adopt the measure [...] On the other hand, if he entertain an impression that the operation will cause his death, you ought then only to undertake it with the full conviction and precaution of this additional source of danger before you.[96]

---

[94] Astley Cooper and Benjamin Travers, *Surgical Essays*, Part 1 (London: Cox and Son, 1818), pp. 101–2.
[95] *Lancet* 20:516 (20 July 1833), p. 520.   [96] *Lancet* 20:516 (20 July 1833), p. 522.

As with Henry Cline's patient, the fear of death could very easily become a self-fulfilling prophecy. But even here the surgeon was not helpless, for as well as reading a patient's emotions, he was also expected to be able to influence them through his own manner and emotional countenance. Thus, Frederic Skey maintained that 'the larger the share of confidence entertained by the patient in the skill and resources of the surgeon, the more fully will he be able to divest his mind of apprehension' concerning an operation. 'At such a time', he claimed, the patient was 'an object of just and natural sympathy', and it was 'rare that sympathy does not tell beneficially upon his mind [...] A peculiar kindness, and in the example of a female or child, even tenderness of manner, begets a confidence, which without betraying weakness or uncertainty, fortifies the patient's mind, and reconciles it to the effort'.[97]

For all his evident emotional sensitivity, Skey's caveat alluding to the potential 'weakness' attendant upon emotional expression anticipates a shift in the cultures of surgery that will be the focus of the latter part of this book. Certainly, it was rare for surgeons of the earlier period to express any significant reservations about the rectitude of emotional intersubjectivity in the practitioner–patient relationship. Indeed, as with many other aspects of the emotional cultures of Romantic surgery that we have discussed so far, it was John Bell, at the beginning of our period, who was perhaps the most expressive and eloquent commentator on the value of an emotional and affective engagement with one's patient. In perhaps the most powerful evocation of surgical emotion committed to the page, he wrote:

To become skilled [in surgery], a man must live among the sick: he must have lively feelings, and a sympathizing nature; his mind and senses must be deeply impressed with the character of every kind of suffering; he must have that inward sympathy with the distresses of his fellow-creature [*sic*], which fills the mind with sincere and affectionate interest. What can more aggravate sickness, than to tell the long tale of misery to one who merely listens, who betrays no touch of compassion, whose cold and formal inquiries imply no interest, and end with a prescription in form. Such a man never learnt his profession, will never learn it: he has no feelings towards his individual patients, and can have no enthusiasm towards his general duty [...] To be initiated into our profession, is not merely to be taught the principles of Chemistry, and the Anatomy of the human body; but it is [...] to feel an interest in the fate of each patient; to form apprehensions for his safety which perhaps he himself does not feel [...] to be alarmed by changes of voice, pulse, and countenance, which make no impression even on a patient's friends. This is the true initiation in to our profession; and he, who is once full of these sympathies, takes an interest in every case, and studies with unremitting diligence.[98]

---

[97] Skey, *Surgery*, pp. 3–4.   [98] Bell, *Answer*, Section II, pp. 6–7.

For Bell, then, the ideal surgeon was to be a kind of emotional savant, not only capable of sympathy and pity, mitigating sickness through tender compassion, but also able to read his patient for signs so subtle that they might be missed by their closest friends and to know the patient better than they knew themselves. These qualities were not merely ornamental to a surgeon's identity, they were akin to a knowledge of anatomy and chemistry, a vital source of his moral and professional authority. Of course, in order to regulate the patient's emotional state of mind, the surgeon also had to be capable of managing his own. As already shown, the Romantic surgeon was expected to cultivate an intellectual and emotional self-mastery and, hence, the emotional dynamics of the surgical relationship were never simply subjective, they were always intersubjective, requiring self-reflection and imaginative projection. As Benjamin Brodie put it:

You must ever recollect, Gentlemen, that those beings on whom you are destined to practise are endowed with a percipient, thinking mind, and that that mind will become in the highest degree irritable from a variety of causes such as long confinement, sleepless nights, painful days; now it will prove greatly to your advantage and success if you should be capable of regulating your patient morally as well as physically. But it may be asked here, Who can regulate the minds of others, if they are incapable of commanding their own? and I therefore address to you the expressive words of the poet, inscribed on the portico of the temple of Apollo – "Man, know thyself" […] I do not hesitate to say that he who can look with indifference on the agonies of a fellow creature is not the person to practise surgery in the manner that it ought to be practised; without sensibility, there would not be that anxiety which the humane surgeon feels to relieve pain […] nothing distinguishes the scholar and the gentleman from the barbarian and the ruffian more than this.[99]

For the most part, the expressions of emotional intersubjectivity that we have encountered so far have been idealised and rhetorical. True, the letters of Charles Bell provide an insight into the operations of surgical emotion in the 'real' world, but much of the rest of our evidence has been drawn from textbooks, lectures, and other didactic materials. This is not to say that such expressions are of lesser value; far from it. After all, it is essential to establish the norms of any particular emotional community and there can be no greater testimony to the cultural resonance of an idea than its presentation as an *ideal*, and its inculcation into that community's initiates. Nevertheless, in order to fully appreciate the role played by emotions in the Romantic surgical relationship, it is important to consider how they shaped the everyday dynamics of the clinical encounter and so, in the last section of this chapter, we shall consider the place of emotion in Astley Cooper's casebooks and its relationship to gender identities and ideologies.

[99] *Lancet* 3:54 (9 October 1824), p. 23.

Astley Cooper's Casebooks: Emotions, Gender, and Intersubjectivity in Practice

We began this chapter with Astley Cooper's lively representation of the emotions inherent in the clinical encounter. As we suggested, Cooper's act of literary imagination was based on extensive experience, experience that is, at least in part, preserved in his personal archive, held by the Royal College of Surgeons of England. This material constitutes a particularly rich resource, not only because of its sheer extent, but also because Cooper was one of the preeminent surgeons of the Romantic era, perhaps even its leading light. In Chapter 3, we shall explore the many letters from his patients that are held in Cooper's archive. For the moment, however, our focus is primarily on the casebooks that he kept from his first entry into practice as a pupil of his uncle, William Cooper (1724–c.1800), at Guy's Hospital in 1784, to his retirement from hospital practice in the later 1820s.

Astley Cooper treated a vast range of conditions in the course of his professional career, and many of these are recorded in his casebooks. Above all, however, it is afflictions of the female breast, most especially cancer, that stand out, not only in terms of the frequency of their appearance, but also by virtue of his deep engagement with this particular disease. Cooper became one of Britain's leading experts on breast cancer and, as a result, a large number of women sought his advice. As Erin O'Connor has observed, breast cancer gave rise to a complex set of gendered emotions. For one thing, since at least the eighteenth century, the breast had come to function as a synecdoche for an essentialised femininity. Its destruction by an often virulent and disfiguring disease was therefore deeply troubling to established gender ideologies.[100] Moreover, the fact that the disease was regarded as largely incurable seriously undermined conventional expectations of male guardianship. It is perhaps for this reason that Cooper chose to begin his work on non-malignant growths with a tale of female salvation, even though such instances were comparatively rare. Indeed, as we have already heard, surgeons such as John Abernethy despaired of cure in cases of breast cancer and greatly feared their appearance.

This complex melding of horror and pathos, abjection and fascination, is given powerful expression in a watercolour held in Astley Cooper's archive (Figure 2.2). Its initial creation and subsequent transference to Cooper's collection derived from a collaboration between three professional men: the Cheltenham surgeon Charles Averill (d. 1830), a former pupil of Cooper's whose case it was; the clergyman the Rev. William Brown, who painted it; and 'Mr Turner', probably Charles W. Turner (b. 1804), Averill's own pupil, then

---

[100] Erin O'Connor, *Raw Material: Producing Pathology in Victorian Culture* (Durham, NC: Duke University Press, 2000), ch. 2.

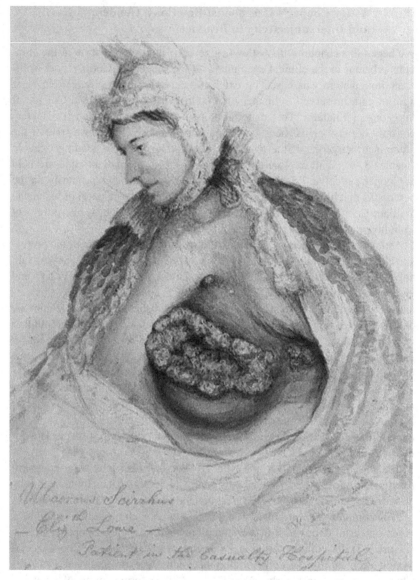

Figure 2.2 Elizabeth Lowe, painted by the Rev William Brown (1828). From the Archives of the Royal College of Surgeons of England

studying at Guy's Hospital, who brought it to Cooper. The woman featured in the image is Elizabeth Lowe, a 29-year-old admitted to the Casualty Hospital in Cheltenham on 26 August 1828. In the accompanying letter, Averill wrote that her case might be of interest to Cooper as 'you are about publishing on

Cancer'. Also, when Averill was a student, Cooper 'had used to state that you had never seen but two cases of schirrous [sic] breast under the age of thirty'. Lowe was therefore remarkable. Not only was she unusually young to be suffering from breast cancer, but her ulceration was particularly pronounced, 'the edges of the sore being very irregularly thickened [...] the middle deeply excavated and partly covered with small yellow sloughs and discharging a bloody sanious fluid'. But she was clearly regarded as extraordinary in other respects too, for, despite the horrific nature of her condition, she held a deep fascination for the men who attended her. This is evident in Brown's portrait, which presents her with humanity, compassion, and not a little tenderness, her downcast look reminiscent of the sublime suffering evoked by Charles Bell's watercolours of the wounded of Waterloo (Figure 2.3).[101] And it is also present in Averill's case history, for he concluded it by noting that, after she died on 16 October, 'her skeleton which is remarkable for the beauty of its symmetry [was] preserved in the Museum attached to the Hospital'.[102]

If Elizabeth Lowe was remarkable, then, in other respects she was eminently typical of the breast cancer patient of this period. Her disease was said to have been caused by a blow to her breast, a commonly cited cause for the development of a tumour. Even more significant, for our purposes at least, was the role played by the trials of motherhood in her condition and treatment. Lowe had borne six children, 'of whom one only is living', and was pregnant again when she developed cancer. Some three and a half weeks before her death, she was delivered of a boy 'who was not permitted to take the breast' and after that point 'she sunk faster' and 'the ulceration extended more rapidly'.[103]

Breast cancer (and female cancers more generally) have attracted a good deal of recent attention from historians of gender and medicine. For the most part, this literature has focused either on the early modern period, up to the end of the eighteenth century, such as with the work of Alana Skuse and Marjo Kaartinen, or on the period from the mid-nineteenth century onwards, such as that of Illana Löwy and Ornella Mosucci.[104] The first half of the nineteenth

---

[101] For an interesting account of the emotionalised gaze of medical illustration, see Mechtild Fend, 'Portraying Skin Disease: Robert Carswell's Dermatological Watercolours', in Jonathan Reinarz and Kevin Siena (eds), A Medical History of Skin: Scratching the Surface (London: Pickering and Chatto, 2013), 147–164. For more on the specifics of Charles Bell, see Brown, 'Wounds'; Shaw, Suffering, ch. 5.

[102] RCSE, MS0008/4/5/6, Letter from Charles Averill to Astley Cooper, 3 March 1829, unpaginated.

[103] RCSE, MS0008/4/5/6, Letter from Charles Averill to Astley Cooper, 3 March 1829, unpaginated.

[104] Illana Löwy, A Woman's Disease: The History of Cervical Cancer (Oxford: Oxford University Press, 2011); Marjo Kaartinen, Breast Cancer in the Eighteenth Century (London: Pickering and Chatto, 2013); Alana Skuse, Constructions of Cancer in Early Modern England (London: Palgrave Macmillan, 2015); Ornella Mosucci, Gender and Cancer in England, 1860–1948 (London: Palgrave Macmillan, 2016).

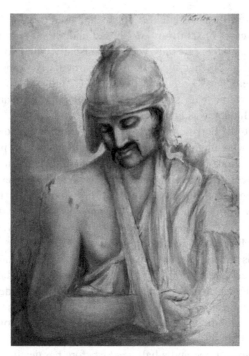

Figure 2.3 Charles Bell, Gunshot wound of the left shoulder (1815). Wellcome Collection. Attribution 4.0 International (CC BY 4.0)

century has, by contrast, been comparatively neglected.[105] Moreover, while Kaartinen dedicates an entire chapter of her book to the subject of 'pain, emotions and cancer in the breast', her analysis is largely concerned, perhaps understandably, with the patient's experience of the disease; she pays comparatively little attention to the intersubjective dimensions of the clinical relationship and the surgeon remains a relatively shadowy figure in her analysis. She briefly considers the qualities of 'empathy and pity' and refers to Frances Burney's mastectomy and the emotional expressiveness of Dominique Larrey. She even acknowledges that Burney's account is embedded in 'early nineteenth[-]century Romanticism and its "sensibility"', but suggests that, as such, 'we cannot [...] extrapolate anything from it'. Indeed, while she speculates that 'most surgeons felt for their patients, and some of them had to struggle to remain sufficiently detached', she does not explore what this might mean, either for surgeons like Larrey or for patients like Burney, and, ultimately,

---

[105] A notable exception to this is Agnes Arnold-Forster, *The Cancer Problem: Malignancy in Nineteenth-Century Britain* (Oxford: Oxford University Press, 2021).

falls back on the familiar narrative of detachment, supporting her point with a secondhand quotation from a book published nearly seventy years prior to Burney's operation.[106]

A more considered exploration of the emotionally intersubjective dimensions of breast cancer is therefore necessary, not simply because surgeons were required to 'read off' emotions from their patients in their treatment and management of the disease, but also because these emotional 'readings' were central to the very conceptualisation of breast cancer in this period. Early nineteenth-century ideas about what caused breast cancer (or any cancer, for that matter) were varied and complex, as indeed they still are. Historians such as Mosucci and Patricia Jansen have identified a general shift in the mid-nineteenth century away from 'constitutional' explanations towards 'local' theories, which emphasised its cellular origins.[107] Most historians of breast cancer acknowledge the role that 'passions' played in 'constitutional' understandings of the disease.[108] For the most part, however, the place of the emotions in the generation of cancer has been given short shrift, with some scholars deferring to generalised arguments about the supposed 'excess emotion' of women.[109] Furthermore, while these scholars point to the importance of the reproductive female body in the aetiology of breast cancer, they have tended to approach such considerations from a purely biological perspective, and none has united such considerations with the emotional dimensions of surgical understanding. As we shall see, however, a contextualised reading of Astley Cooper's casebooks reveals that his understanding of cancer was rooted in what, to co-opt Arlie Russell Hochschild's term, we might call the 'emotion work' of real and idealised femininities. This understanding was forged in the gendered and emotionally intersubjective relationship between the male surgeon and his female patients.[110]

In her essay on breast cancer in the nineteenth century, Erin O'Connor draws attention to what she calls the 'emotional anatomy' of the breast, in other words its profound connectedness to other parts of the body.[111] The basis of this connectedness was the concept of 'sympathy'. As Cooper told his students in 1823:

---

[106] Kaartinen, *Cancer*, pp. 116–17. For a more culturally attuned account, see Wayne Wild, *Medicine by Post: The Changing Voice of Illness in Eighteenth-Century British Consultation Letters and Literature* (Amsterdam: Rodopi, 2006), pp. 256–9.

[107] Mosucci, *Cancer*, ch. 2; Patricia Jansen, 'Breast Cancer and the Language of Risk, 1750–1950', *Social History of Medicine* 15:1 (2002), 17–43.

[108] For example, Kaartinen, *Cancer*, p. 18; Skuse, *Cancer*, pp. 34–5; Jansen, 'Cancer', p. 25.

[109] Mosucci, *Cancer*, p. 24.

[110] Hochschild coined the term 'emotion work' to describe the unpaid work that one undertakes in private life, as opposed to the commodified forms of 'emotional labour' explored in her book *The Managed Heart: Commercialization of Human Feeling* (Berkeley: University of California Press, 1983). See also Arlie Russell Hochschild, 'Emotion Work, Feeling Rules, and Social Structure', *American Journal of Sociology* 85:3 (1979), 551–75.

[111] O'Connor, *Raw*, p. 67.

There exist, among all parts of the body, intimate relations, all corresponding with each other and carrying on a reciprocal intercourse of action. The wonderful and beautiful harmony produced by these concurrent phenomena, is called Sympathy; its real nature is yet unknown but we are acquainted with many of its effects; thus the common and natural sympathy of the uterus and breasts.[112]

The concept of sympathy had been developed from around the mid-eighteenth century by medical men such as Albrecht von Haller (1708–77) and John Hunter, in tandem with its development by moral philosophers such as Adam Smith. The connectedness of the human body and the connectedness of the social body were thus two sides of the same intellectual coin; physiology and philosophy provided equal impetus to the cultures of sensibility.[113]

Unsurprisingly, perhaps, the concept of sympathy could, as in Cooper's example, serve to reify gender ideologies as medical fact. Women were defined by their reproductive capacity and, hence, the two anatomical markers of that function, uterus and breasts, were inseparably linked. Such ideas had ancient origins. The Greek concept of hysteria, after all, rooted women's bodily health in their reproductive system, while the constitutionalism of medieval and early modern medicine was likewise shaped by gender norms.[114] Not by accident did Cooper refer to such connections as 'natural'. It was therefore well recognised by contemporary practitioners that diseases of the breast could be caused by the irregular functioning of the uterus; suspension or retention of menses were regarded as particularly dangerous. But they also ascribed an important role to the operation of the mind and the emotions. Hence, in the Preface to *Illustrations of the Diseases of the Breast*, Cooper said of the breasts that 'malignancy may be lighted up in them by constitutional disease – by anxiety of mind – and the cessation of the menstrual secretion'.[115]

Indeed, for all the talk of mechanical causes, it is anxiety of mind that occupies by far the most prominent place in Cooper's notes on breast cancer. In 1819, for example, he recorded the following case:

---

[112] *Lancet* 1:2 (12 October 1823), p. 37.
[113] G. J. Barker-Benfield, *The Culture of Sensibility: Sex and Society in Eighteenth-Century Britain* (Chicago: Chicago University Press, 1992); Ildiko Csengei, *Sympathy, Sensibility and the Literature of Feeling in the Eighteenth Century* (Basingstoke: Palgrave Macmillan, 2012). For more on the contested social, cultural, and political implications of sympathy, see Mary Fairclough, *The Romantic Crowd: Sympathy, Controversy and Print Culture* (Cambridge, UK: Cambridge University Press, 2013), Part 1.
[114] For example, see Helen King, *Hippocrates' Women: Reading the Female Body in Ancient Greece* (London: Routledge, 1998); Monica H. Green, *Making Women's Medicine Masculine: The Rise of Male Authority in Pre-Modern Gynaecology* (Oxford: Oxford University Press, 2008); Mary E. Fissell, *Vernacular Bodies: The Politics of Reproduction in Early Modern England* (Oxford: Oxford University Press, 2004).
[115] Cooper, *Illustrations*, unpaginated preface.

Mrs Burk: Scirrhous a year and a half ago size of a nutmeg and for half a year there was no pain. Operation by Travers in January. Now June 18th Schirrhous [*sic*] in the same breast and axilla pain and a small lump on the other breast. Age 44 – anxiety the cause – accident and ill health and ill circumstances the cause and nothing has succeeded.[116]

Likewise:

Mrs Webster [...] aged 40 – has had 10/9 children – always healthy except occasionally a cough during pregnancy – bowells [*sic*] rather costive – Menstruation not generally regular = has a swelling in the breast and axilla – its cause is unknown except cold and extreme anxiety of mind.[117]

Even in cases where the disease was not ascribed to anxiety, its relative absence was noted. Hence, another case reads:

Mrs Wilson aged 40 – married but no children has a general enlargement of the breast as if the whole were affected by a sccirhous [*sic*] [...] not regular – bowells [*sic*] irritable no anxiety – cause unknown – unless sympathetic with the Uterus.[118]

It is important to note that breast cancer was not the only disease in Cooper's casebooks for which anxiety was considered as a cause. For example, in the case of a 43-year-old man with 'Fungus Testis' who was described as being of a 'sallow' countenance with 'dark hair and complexion', it was noted that he had 'no anxiety' and was 'not aware of any blow'.[119] Meanwhile, in another case of 'Testis Fungoid', a man similarly described as 'unhealthy', 'wasted', 'sallow', and of 'complexion dark' was said to have 'drank hard and been of late anxious in mind on account of his business going wrong'.[120] However, while there are relatively few instances of testicular cancer in Cooper's casebooks, cases of breast cancer are extremely numerous and the reference to anxiety virtually ubiquitous. Moreover, if the cause of testicular cancer was rooted in men's physical health and appearance, as well as in normatively masculine activities and conventional, albeit excessive, male appetites, in almost every instance of breast cancer reference was made to similarly normative feminine attributes.[121] In part this can be attributed to physiological understandings of disease, such as the role of menses and breast feeding. However, given that the cause was almost always attributed to anxiety of mind, it suggests something quite profound about the place of emotion work in Romantic conceptions of femininity and its pathologies.

[116] RCSE, MS0008/2/1/6, Volume of case notes in the hand of Sir Astley Paston Cooper, 1817–20, unpaginated.
[117] RCSE, MS0008/2/1/6.   [118] RCSE, MS0008/2/1/6.
[119] RCSE, MS0008/2/1/6.   [120] RCSE, MS0008/2/1/7.
[121] For the role of excessive appetites in the propagation of disease in men, see Joanne Begiato, 'Punishing the Unregulated Manly Body and Emotions in Early Victorian England', in Joanne Ella Parsons and Ruth Heholt (eds), *The Victorian Male Body* (Edinburgh: Edinburgh University Press, 2018), 46–64.

The role of women's emotion work in Cooper's breast cancer cases is especially notable in relation to motherhood. As Joanne Begiato has suggested, 'Anxiety was an essential state of parenting', and some in this period even saw it as the natural state of mothers. It was not a shameful emotion, but rather a 'badge of sensitivity and refinement' and 'thus a trait of good parenting'.[122] At the same time, however, Begiato recognises that anxiety could be problematic. This was especially true of pregnancy, which was regarded not only as a joyous occasion but also as a time of great constitutional upheaval, as well as apprehension.[123] This is certainly borne out by the cases in Cooper's archive for, in a number of instances, his patients' tumours either derived from, or coincided with, their confinement. For example, in August 1830, Cooper received several letters from Mary Bradney of Charlton in Somerset and her medical assistant, John Valentine. Mary had a tumour in her right breast and experienced bleeding from the nipple. Valentine wrote that 'She looked forward with great anxiety to her approaching confinement which is expected to be early next month'.[124] Her anxiety was evident from the fact that Valentine followed this statement with the words: 'I know of no good in my writing to you at present, for the purpose of mentioning the above particulars, but it is her will'. And indeed, the very next day Mary wrote herself, ending her letter: 'I cannot expect to trouble you to write both to Mr Valentine and myself but when you write to the former I trust you will give him every advice with regard to my approaching confinement – particularly how to stop the bleeding both now and at the term of labour'.[125]

Another cause of anxiety for mothers that was strongly associated with breast cancer was the ill-health of a child. Mrs Palmer of Wellingborough came to see Astley Cooper in 1836, bearing a note from her surgeon recording that she had received a blow on the breast from 'an intoxicated man'. Furthermore, 'About the time of receiving the blow she was in painful anxiety of mind from the continued illness of her son, which I should suppose so operated upon the constitution as to dispose it to schirrous [sic] inflammation'.[126]

---

[122] Joanne Bailey, *Parenting in England, 1760–1830: Emotion, Identity and Generation* (Oxford: Oxford University Press, 2012), pp. 37–9.

[123] Joanne Begiato, '"Breeding" a "Little Stranger": Managing Uncertainty in Pregnancy in Later Georgian England', in Jennifer Evans and Ciara Meehan (eds), *Perceptions of Pregnancy from the Seventeenth to the Twentieth Century* (Basingstoke: Palgrave Macmillan, 2017), 13–33.

[124] RCSE, MS0008/2/2/4, File of letters and notes of cases sent to Sir Astley Cooper, 1807–36, Letter from John Valentine to Astley Cooper, 23 August 1830.

[125] RCSE, MS0008/2/2/5, Letter from Mary Bradney to Astley Cooper, 24 August 1830.

[126] RCSE, MS0008/2/2/3 pt. 3, File of letters and notes on cases sent to Sir Astley Cooper, Letter from Benjamin Dulley to Astley Cooper, 28 April 1836.

Given the remarkably high levels of infant mortality in this period, it is no surprise that grief was a common experience of motherhood and that it also exerted a powerful influence over mind and body. In the case of a 53-year-old woman named Mrs Bull, for example, Cooper noted that she 'had been very anxious in mind from the loss of a child', while in another, he observed that the patient had 'anxiety of mind from the loss of a daughter 2 years ago'. Most poignant of all, perhaps, is the case of Laetitia Kelly of Carrickfergus in Ireland, who replied to Cooper's inquiry after her health in September 1824. Referring to her recent confinement she wrote:

I had an excellent time and to all appearances a healthful (tho small) Infant – but the Almighty saw fit to take her from us on the third day – the event was so sudden – you will most particularly oblige me by informing me do you or not think the complaint I had in my Breast could have had any influence on the state [...] [of] my dear Infant?[127]

In this particular case it was not that the death of a child had caused cancer, but rather that the patient feared her disease had precipitated her child's untimely demise. Such examples as this attest to the emotion work of motherhood and its role in shaping bodily health. In some cases these emotional demands were unsustainable. In the handwritten notes to his *Illustrations of the Diseases of the Breast*, for example, Cooper recorded the case of an unnamed woman. 'She has been since her last child in ill health', it reads. 'She has been a good nurse – She is defeated and has lost all her feelings of love and affection for [her] children and has lost her appetite'.[128]

It was not only motherhood that was imagined to test women's emotional capacities to the point of physical illness. Other caring roles took their toll, such as in the case of a woman whose cancer was thought to have been 'brought on by anxiety and watching a consumptive sister'.[129] Indeed, all the emotional ties of family life might produce illness, particularly when broken by bereavement. In the case of one woman, for example, her 'anxious state of mind' derived 'from the loss of Brother some time before'.[130] Meanwhile, for Mrs Turner, a 38-year-old with an 'irritable left breast', the cause of her anxiety was a combination of grief and fear, for her 'Mother died of Cancer'.[131] The loss of a husband was a particularly trying circumstance, not only emotionally but also because of the social and economic vulnerabilities of widowhood. Thus, the cause of Mrs le Roux's cancer was given as 'Anxiety of mind – She is a widow', while more specific circumstances were recorded for another Mrs

---

[127] RCSE, MS0008/2/2/4, Letter from Laetitia Kelly to Astley Cooper, 8 September 1824.
[128] RCSE, MS0008/2/1/9, 'Illustrations of the Diseases of the Breast, Part 1', annotation opposite p. 7.
[129] RCSE, MS0008/2/1/6.   [130] RCSE, MS0008/2/1/9, annotation opposite p. 3.
[131] RCSE, MS0008/2/1/9, annotation opposite p. 12.

Turner, 'who has had an anxious state of mind from the loss of her husband and from a Chancery Suit'.[132]

As these last two examples suggest, women's identities as wives were as important in such cases, as were their roles as mothers. Indeed, in almost every instance, Cooper's casebooks make note of both the maternal and marital status of these women. In a number of cases, the anxiety they experienced derived not merely from bereavement, but from husbands who were either abusive or irresponsible. In 1819, for example, the cause of one unnamed 48-year-old woman's tumour was listed as 'anxiety of mind from a drunken husband'.[133] Meanwhile, in the 1830s Cooper was given an account of the case of Elizabeth Sawyer, who had received a blow from a boy in play, but whose notes concluded:

This person was married at twenty eight, the husband died five years afterwards, he being a seafaring man was absent the greatest part of the time they were married and did not pass more than one year with her at home he was very gay and unsteady which caused her much trouble and anxiety. They had no children.[134]

The reason why it is important to consider the emotionally intersubjective qualities of these diagnostic and therapeutic encounters is because, while it is likely that the patient recounted their own case history and may even have provided their own causal explanation for their condition, it is certain that Cooper, like other surgeons in his position, interpreted their testimony and made his own particular determination about the role of emotional experience in the propagation of their disease. Indeed, despite the terse, notational nature of his casebooks, one can find instances therein of Cooper exercising a kind of moral and emotional judgement, such as in the case of an unnamed 30-year-old woman for whom he imagined that a stay in hospital might provide refuge from the rigours of her domestic life, including the burdens of sexual intercourse: 'She is nervous and weak and can not bear fatigue – Bowells [sic] regular – She has had 4 successive miscarriages – Absence from her husband will be useful'.[135]

What the evidence of these casebooks suggests, therefore, is that emotional relations were central to the elaboration of breast cancer as a condition; its diagnosis and meaning were produced in the space between two subjectivities, those of the patient's experience and the surgeon's interpretation. The latter was shaped not merely by contemporary medical theory, but also by the cultural ideologies that sustained it. Those ideologies were

[132] RCSE, MS0008/2/1/9, annotations opposite pp. 12, 5.   [133] RCSE, MS0008/2/1/6.
[134] RCSE, MS0008/2/2/2, File of letters and notes sent to Sir Astley Cooper, 1807–36, unpaginated note.
[135] RCSE, MS0008/2/1/9, annotation opposite p. 1.

not unique to the surgeon, of course. Indeed, the internal evidence suggests that ideas about the causes of cancer and its relation to gendered identities were often shared by patient and practitioner.[136] Even so, the authoritative position of the surgeon, especially within the hospital, which is the context in which these casebooks were produced, gave his perspective a particular significance. For Cooper, breast cancer did not derive from an excess of emotion, nor from a perversion of established gender norms, but rather from the very state of mind, anxiety, that was considered entirely natural to the role of the wife and mother.

While this could potentially be interpreted as a pathologisation of femininity *per se*, such readings would be a simplification. In her essay 'Breast Reductions', Erin O'Connor explores the complex social, cultural, and emotional contours of breast cancer in the mid to late nineteenth century. She aims to critique a style of Victorian literary criticism, and its reading of medical discourse, that represents the breast as the object of an inherently misogynistic male clinical gaze. The extensive use of analogy that characterised medical and surgical discourse, particularly the use of political economic language, she suggests, did not necessarily function to frame the breast within a patriarchal ideology that saw women's place as removed from the public sphere of urban industrial modernity. Rather, it served to shield these practitioners from the emotionally troubling experience of having to watch their patients suffer and die from a painful, malignant, and disfiguring disease with little hope of relief.[137] Similar, though subtly different, readings are appropriate here. The place of anxiety in the elaboration of breast cancer owed much to the sentimentalisation of femininity, and especially motherhood, in the Romantic era.[138] However, rather than distancing or shielding surgeons from the distressing nature of the disease, these associations actually served to enhance the pathos associated with it. Cooper's patients were victims of an emotional, as much as biological, burden, and while breast cancer was certainly fear inducing for the surgeon (to say nothing of the sufferer), the general emotional tenor of Cooper's archive is one of pity, sympathy, and compassion.

Cooper was certainly not alone in acknowledging the influence of emotions on breast cancer. In his *Thoughts on the Cancer of the Breast* (1787), for example, George Bell writes that a 'foundation may be laid for this disease [...] if the mind is agitated by anger, or depressed by fear, grief, or anxiety'.[139] Nonetheless, the

---

[136] In Chapter 3, for example, we shall see that patients' accounts of their own cancer often closely mirrored the predominant medical and surgical theories of the period.
[137] O'Connor, *Raw*, ch. 2.
[138] Bailey, *Parenting*. See also Julie Kipp, *Romanticism, Maternity, and the Body Politic* (Cambridge, UK: Cambridge University Press, 2003).
[139] George Bell, *Thoughts on the Cancer of the Breast* (London: J. Johnson, 1787), p. 7.

sheer ubiquity of anxiety in his casebooks is perhaps more unusual.[140] How to explain this? Well, we might choose to look to Cooper's identity as the quintessential Romantic man of feeling. A youthful radical and suspected Jacobin who honeymooned in revolutionary Paris only to become a titled grandee in later life, Cooper travelled the same path as many of his Romantic contemporaries, from William Wordsworth (1770–1850) to William Lawrence.[141] However, even if he may have tamed his political convictions for the sake of professional advancement, one aspect of his Romantic persona that never left him was his carefully fashioned gender identity and, in particular, his attachment to women and children. As his nephew, Bransby Cooper, later wrote:

The sensibility of his disposition, which throughout life continued to form one of the most distinguishable and loveable traits of his character, led him in his earliest years, even when delighting in the rough and hazardous sports we have described, to appreciate the charms of female character and court friendship in its society. The evident pleasure he took in contributing to the amusement of his sisters and their friends, the respect and attention he always paid to them, together with his elegant form and handsome features – not omitting the other qualities which had exercised so much influence over the companions of his own sex, – all combined to render him an especial favourite with the softer sex; and in their society he spent a considerable portion of his time.[142]

We have already heard how Cooper was said to have cried at the sight of a smiling child about to undergo an operation, a sentiment that may have been enhanced by the loss of his own daughter in 1794 and his subsequent childlessness.[143] In addition to this, his nephew claims that he had 'such a horror [...] of any symptom of privation from food, especially in children, that he never could [...] suppress a tear, when he witnessed an object of his commiseration in the streets of London'. 'I remember', he continues, 'that when I repeated to him the [workhouse] scene in *Oliver Twist* [...] he was quite overcome, and, crying like a child, would not suffer me to continue my description of the distressing tale'.[144]

This compassionate and sensitive demeanour was said to have carried over into Cooper's clinical work. According to John Flint South:

His manner with the patients was always encouraging and kind, and not infrequently he enjoyed a little joke with them as he went along. I never recollect to have seen him lose his temper or treat a patient with unkind, rough language, but, on the contrary,

---

[140] It is certainly far more frequent than in the works of Everard Home, Charles Bell, or John Abernethy, for example. Everard Home, *Observations on Cancer Connected with Histories of the Disease* (London: J. Johnson, 1805); Charles Bell, *Surgical Observations* (London: Longman, Hurst, Rees, Orme, and Brown, 1816); John Abernethy, *Surgical Observations on Tumours and on Lumbar Abscesses*, 3rd ed. (London: Longman, Hurst, Rees, Orme, and Brown, 1822).

[141] On Cooper's early radicalism and later renunciation, see Cooper, *Life*, vol. 1, chs. 5, 12, 16.

[142] Cooper, *Life*, vol. 1, pp. 82–3.

[143] Cooper, *Life*, vol. 1, pp. 253–4.   [144] Cooper, *Life*, vol. 2, p. 93.

with gentle sympathy, which won for him their immediate confidence and warm attachment [...] With all his boldness in acting out his maxim that a surgeon should have 'an eagle's eye, a lady's hand, and a lion's heart,' I cannot doubt that Cooper did think of the suffering of patients on whom he operated; his kind and encouraging and patient manner with them was very striking, and not exceeded by any operator I have ever seen.[145]

Moreover, most commentators noted his particular affinity with his female patients. Not only was frequent reference made to his handsome features and the 'suavity of his manners', but his servant Charles Balderson was even recorded as having said that, when it came to his private consultations, there was often a throng of women waiting to see him and there was always 'more difficulty in drawing one lady than two gentleman', by which he meant 'withdrawing the lady from Mr Cooper's presence'.[146]

Conclusion

As the example of Astley Cooper's casebooks suggests, our understandings of early nineteenth-century surgery and of the relationships between surgeons and their patients can be significantly enhanced by an attention to the operation of the emotions. The dominant emotional regime of the period, Romantic sensibility, with its veneration of women, children, and the family, shaped surgical discourse surrounding breast cancer. Cooper understood the disease primarily through the lens of domesticity and motherhood and, in his dealings with his female patients, he shaped a persona as a sensible, sensitive, and refined gentleman. Clearly, then, established notions of dispassion and detachment fall far short of capturing the emotional complexity and richness of the Romantic surgical relationship. Surgeons not only conceived of their own work in emotional terms, they were also required to make judgements about the emotional dispositions of their patients, determining what forms of treatment were appropriate or whether they could withstand the physical and emotional rigours of an operation. Cooper's archive is full of such judgements. For example, in a scrawled annotation on the proofs of his *Illustrations of the Diseases of the Breast*, he states concerning an unknown case:

No danger in the Operation and it removes Suspence [*sic*] and anxiety of mind which are worse than the real evil of a moment
    It is impossible to promise it shall not reappear but the proper thing is to remove it and then alter the constitution – the removal alone will surely succeed.[147]

---

[145] South, *Memorials*, pp. 53–5.   [146] Cooper, *Life*, vol. 2, pp. 462, 74.
[147] RCSE, MS0008/2/1/9, annotation between 'Contents' and p. 1.

As this comment demonstrates, emotions were not simply a rhetorical device or a professional performance. Emotional intersubjectivity was central to the experience and practice of surgery, especially when confronted by such a dreadful and fearsome disease as breast cancer. Dealing with such conditions required emotional sensitivity and took an emotional toll, giving rise to sensations of pity, sympathy, grief, and regret. However, if emotions shaped surgical identities and subjectivities, then they were equally important in the patient's experience of illness and surgical care. In Chapter 3, we shall continue to explore the nature of the Romantic surgical relationship by switching our perspective and considering how patients experienced sickness, interacted with surgeons, exerted their agency, and negotiated their treatment, through the language of the emotions.

3   The Patient's Voice
Conscious and Unconscious Agency in Romantic Surgery

Introduction

In the previous chapter, we explored the emotions of the Romantic surgical relationship largely from the perspective of the surgeon. A key aspect of the emotional intersubjectivity that was at the heart of this idealised encounter was the ability of the surgeon to put himself in the place of his patient and consider the case 'as [his] own'.[1] Such imaginative projections were a feature of surgical writing in this period. For example, in his *Discourses on the Nature and Cure of Wounds* (1795), John Bell effects a remarkable literary transportation into a patient suffering from an arterial aneurysm:

> The tumour is large, hard, circumscribed, and beating very strongly; the skin over it begins to inflame, the wound of the knife threatens to open again, the whole limb is feeble and cold; the surface of the tumour is livid, and in a few days the beating from such an Artery as the Femoral Artery is most alarming, and to the patient very awful; he spreads his hand broad over the tumour, feels its beating, like the heart in its strongest palpitations [...] He is laid with tourniquets round the limb; he sees by these precautions, and he feels, as it were, that if the tumour burst during the night, he must lose his life with one gush of blood. Lying in this anxious condition, he is watched from hour to hour, till the time appointed for the operation arrives; and it is only then (however great the surgeon's fears about this operation) that the patient is in any degree safe.[2]

Despite the embodied vitality of this passage, such imaginative projections were inherently rhetorical, a testament to the surgeon's sensibility rather than an expression of patient experience. Indeed, even in such a compelling description as this, Bell's subjectivity hovers awkwardly between the surgeon and the imagined other. Thus, his own haptic expertise ('he spreads his hand [...] feels it beating, like the heart in its strongest palpitations') stands in for the embodied consciousness of the patient, while he cannot help but slip from the patient's fear of bleeding to death in the night to the more familiar anxiety of the surgeon anticipating an operation. In order to recover the patient's

---

[1] Astley Cooper and Benjamin Travers, *Surgical Essays*, Part 1 (London: Cox and Son, 1818), p. 102.
[2] John Bell, *Discourses on the Nature and Cure of Wounds* (Edinburgh: Bell and Bradfute, 1795), pp. 68–9.

emotional experience of surgical care, or at least their emotional articulation of that experience, we must, then, look to a different body of material, or at least read the sources in a different way.

The search for the patient's voice has been one of the signal projects of the social history of medicine ever since Roy Porter sought to write a 'medical history from below' in the mid-1980s.[3] In surgery, as in medicine more generally, one of the greatest impediments to that project has been the nature of the source material. Aside from the famous example of Frances Burney's letter to her sister, or retrospective accounts such as that of George Wilson that opened this book, first-hand patient accounts of the experience of pre-anaesthetic surgery are relatively hard to come by. This is not to say that they do not exist. Doubtless there are similar accounts, potentially uncatalogued, in local archives somewhere. But the difficulty of recovering such material has meant that, for the most part, historians have relied on published, or at least well-known, patient testimonies in order to balance their accounts of surgical practice. In his history of early nineteenth-century British surgery, Peter Stanley grapples with precisely this predicament. The patient's voice is 'faint and elusive', he claims. While acknowledging that it is 'possible to devise a "celebrity ward", assembling operations from the great figures of the period' including Lord Nelson (1758–1805), the Earl of Uxbridge (1768–1854), and Sir Walter Scott (1771–1832), Stanley proposes to move 'beyond these well-known figures'.[4] He does this, firstly, by searching for patient voices in the reports of *The Lancet* and, secondly, by using a number of case studies of lesser-known figures taken from published sources or archival collections. The first approach is a reasonable one. This book also mines *The Lancet* for material, especially in Chapter 4. As we shall see, however, *The Lancet* is not a source that can necessarily be taken at face value, and it is important to consider the politics that inform its representation of operative practice, particularly where it concerns the sufferings of patients. The second approach is also appropriate. And yet, while illuminating, Stanley's case studies are presented largely in narrative form and are subject to relatively little analysis, leaving the reader to either flinch at their agonies or marvel at their 'courage in the face of an incurable disease and intense suffering'.[5]

This approach is not uncommon. Patient voices from this period are often allowed to speak for themselves, if only because their relative scarcity, and the fact that we are separated by the phenomenological gulf of modernity, means that their words have an intrinsic power to move us. That power is impossible to deny

---

[3] Roy Porter, 'The Patient's View: Doing Medical History from Below', *Theory and Society* 14:2 (1985), 175–98.

[4] Peter Stanley, *For Fear of Pain: British Surgery, 1790–1850* (Amsterdam: Rodopi, 2003), p. 261.

[5] Stanley, *Pain*, p. 279.

and many of the experiences recorded in this chapter are certainly affecting. But beyond the ghoulish frisson characteristic of much popular history of surgery, or the humanist impulse to feel for our fellow beings, even if removed in time, such accounts serve little *historical* purpose unless they are subject to analysis and read for meaning. In this regard, there is an exemplary model to follow in Stuart Hogarth's essay 'Joseph Townend and the Manchester Infirmary: A Plebeian Patient in the Industrial Revolution'. Townend, a Methodist missionary, wrote a biography of his life, including his 1827 stay in Manchester Infirmary when he was a 21-year-old textile worker. Using this account, Hogarth draws attention to the importance of emotional relationships between patients and practitioners in negotiating treatment. He also demonstrates that being a patient in hospital did not simply involve being a supplicatory recipient of paternalistic largesse, but could also be a profoundly emotional, even spiritual, experience.[6]

Hogarth is exceptionally fortunate in having access to a source as rich as Townend's diary. He describes this as 'possibly the most detailed description of hospital life by a working-class patient in the nineteenth century' and he is almost certainly right, at least for the period prior to the introduction of anaesthesia.[7] Even so, his sensitivity to the emotional relationships between patient and practitioner and the role of emotions in shaping experience, as well as in the exercise of patient agency, are concerns that are applicable to a range of sources from this period, including those examined here. The twin poles of experience and agency are central to the project of recovering the patient's voice, and it is perhaps easier to approach these through manuscript sources, produced by patients themselves, than through printed sources or formal records. This chapter therefore looks to a particularly rich body of archival material that has to date been almost entirely unexplored. In Chapter 2, we used the archives of Astley Cooper to analyse his emotional relationships with the women he treated for breast cancer, drawing primarily on his hospital casebooks. But we also got a glimpse into another dimension of this archive, namely the letters that Cooper received from his patients, their relatives, and medical assistants. These letters are particularly numerous in regard to his breast cancer patients. In her work on breast cancer in the eighteenth century, Marjo Kaartinen explores the agency and experience of women suffering from this disease. But her sources, apart from some manuscript receipt books, are almost entirely printed, and in many cases medical texts.[8] By contrast, the

---

[6] Stuart Hogarth, 'Joseph Townend and the Manchester Infirmary. A Plebeian Patient in the Industrial Revolution', in Anne Borsay and Peter Shapely (eds), *Medicine, Charity and Mutual Aid: The Consumption of Health and Welfare in Britain, c.1550–1950* (Aldershot: Ashgate, 2007), 91–110.

[7] Hogarth, 'Joseph Townend', p. 97.

[8] Marjo Kaartinen, *Breast Cancer in the Eighteenth Century* (London: Pickering and Chatto, 2013), ch. 4.

letters that Cooper received from his patients allow for a greater degree of insight, not just into the experience of disease, or rather its articulation and representation, but also into the ways in which emotions were deployed in corresponding with surgeons and in negotiating treatment.

Cooper's archive is by no means restricted to breast cancer, even if it is an especially prominent presence. Indeed, this chapter includes a range of patients with different afflictions and supplements Cooper's archive with evidence from other sources. Nonetheless, despite the extraordinary richness of this resource, a word or two of caution is necessary. For one thing, while this book pays particular attention to the operative aspects of Romantic surgery, these sources do not contain particularly full descriptions of going under the knife. Many refer to the fear of such procedures, while in other cases we can gain a brief glimpse into the pain and suffering they caused. But the fact remains that Frances Burney's visceral account of surgery remains something of a rarity. In most cases these sources testify to more chronic forms of suffering, and to the anxiety and dread that accompanied serious illness and non-operative forms of surgical treatment. For another, while many of these letters were penned by patients themselves, others were written by family members or by their medical attendants. Mediation is therefore an issue to be reckoned with. There has been much historical debate about the role of mediation in the articulation of non-elite subjectivities in this period. For example, historians of the Poor Law have explored the cultures of pauper correspondence, and have shown the ways in which these letters, even if generic in form or written by amanuenses, often described real circumstances and conveyed authentic sentiments.[9] Others have pointed out the ways in which the cultures of sensibility and an appeal to the emotions were deployed in the pursuit of relief.[10] Likewise, legal historians have considered the extent to which the voices of litigants and other parties were mediated by the lawyers, clerks, and other officials who shaped the public record.[11] In the case of medicine and surgery, it is clear, as we have

---

[9] Thomas Sokoll (ed.), *Essex Pauper Letters, 1731–1837* (Oxford: Oxford University Press, 2001); Steven King, Thomas Nutt, and Alannah Tomkins (eds), *Narratives of the Poor in Eighteenth-Century Britain, Volume 1. Voices of the Poor: Poor Law Letters and Depositions* (London: Pickering and Chatto, 2006); Steven King, 'Pauper Letters as a Source', *Family and Community History* 10:2 (2007), 167–70; Peter Jones and Steven King, 'From Petition to Pauper Letter: The Development of an Epistolary Form', in Peter Jones and Steven King (eds), *Obligation, Entitlement and Dispute under the English Poor Laws* (Cambridge, UK: Cambridge Scholars Publishing, 2015), 53–77; Jones and King, 'Testifying for the Poor: Epistolary Advocates and the Negotiation of Parochial Relief in England, 1800–1834', *Journal of Social History* 49:4 (2016), 784–807.

[10] Joanne Bailey, '"Think Wot a Mother Must Feel": Parenting in English Pauper Letters c. 1760–1834', *Family and Community History* 13:1 (2010), 5–19. See also Bailey, *Parenting In England, 1760–1830: Emotion, Identity and Generation* (Oxford: Oxford University Press, 2012), pp. 42–7.

[11] For example, see Joanne Bailey, 'Voices in Court: Lawyers or Litigants?', *Historical Research* 74:186 (2011), 392–408.

already seen, that practitioners interpreted the patient's narrative in forming their diagnosis. At the same time, however, given the importance ascribed to emotions in the generation, management, and treatment of disease, it seems likely that medical attendants and other interested parties would be concerned to communicate as accurate an account of the patient's state of mind as possible. Therefore, while undoubtedly mediated and imperfect, such sources do allow us to make tentative observations, if not necessarily about the subjective experience of disease, then certainly about the representation and communication of suffering.[12]

The significance, or otherwise, of the patient's narrative in the conceptualisation and treatment of disease has been an underlying concern of much scholarship on pre-modern medicine. If social historians of the early modern period, such as Roy Porter, sought to recover the patient's voice, assert the agency of patients in determining their care, and demonstrate their knowledge of medical theory, historians of the nineteenth century have, for the most part, held to the notion that the patient's narrative was effaced by the rise of 'clinical' or 'hospital' medicine.[13] This idea can be traced to the mid-1970s, more specifically 1976, the year in which Nicholas Jewson published his influential article on 'The Disappearance of the Sick Man from Medical Cosmology' and in which the English translation of Michel Foucault's *The Birth of the Clinic* (1963) was first published in the United Kingdom.[14] Although approaching the issue from very different disciplinary and intellectual perspectives, Jewson and Foucault jointly established the idea that the patient disappeared from the perceptual and conceptual apparatus of nineteenth-century medicine, that subjective testimony was superseded by the medical 'gaze' of clinical investigation and objective measurement, and that the patient became, in Foucault's words, a mere 'accident' of their disease.[15] Though often taken as read, relatively few historians have sought to expound on this phenomenon. A notable exception to this is Mary Fissell, who, in her 1991 essay 'The Disappearance of the Patient's Narrative and the Invention of Hospital Medicine', argues that, by the turn of the nineteenth century, 'the patient's narrative of disease was made utterly redundant' as hospital doctors came to focus on 'symptoms and

---

[12] For a good account of the communication of suffering within the context of eighteenth-century medical epistolarity, see Wayne Wild, *Medicine by Post: The Changing Voice of Illness in Eighteenth-Century British Consultation Letters and Literature* (Amsterdam: Rodopi, 2006).

[13] For example, see Roy Porter, 'Laymen, Doctors and Medical Knowledge in the Eighteenth Century: The Evidence of the *Gentleman's Magazine*', in Roy Porter (ed.), *Patients and Practitioners: Lay Perceptions of Medicine in Pre-Industrial Society* (Cambridge, UK: Cambridge University Press, 1985), 283–314.

[14] Michel Foucault, *The Birth of the Clinic: An Archaeology of Medical Perception*, trans A. M. Sheridan (London: Tavistock, 1976); Nicholas D. Jewson, 'The Disappearance of the Sick Man from Medical Cosmology, 1770–1870', *Sociology* 10 (1976), 225–44.

[15] Foucault, *Birth*, p. 14.

signs' discernible by 'physical diagnosis and post-mortem dissection'.[16] Fissell only makes a brief reference to Foucault, and her essay perhaps owes more to Jewson's developmental model of change than to Foucault's revolutionary one.[17] Nonetheless, it is in keeping with a post-Foucauldian approach to the hospital that unites a social historical concern with institutional discipline to a more epistemic conception of social control.

In 2007, Flurin Condrau observed that 'a full debate between these two positions – that the patient's view can be unearthed from the sources, against the statement that the patient is a construct of the medical gaze – has, to my knowledge, never taken place'.[18] Fifteen years later, this remains broadly true.[19] In many ways, however, the political context for these positions has changed markedly. As Condrau recognises, Porter's co-opting of a Thompsonian rhetoric of 'history from below' linked his work to a political project with which it was only ambivalently aligned. The patient, though often poor, was not necessarily so, and in their case the 'condescension of posterity' was less clearly the product of political oppression than of 'medicalisation', a prominent bugbear for those at either end of the political spectrum in the 1970s.[20] By the 1980s, this focus on the agency of the individual lent itself, however inadvertently, to a neo-liberal Thatcherite agenda.[21] At the same time, not dissimilar observations have been made of the poststructuralist approaches of Foucault, in that they make the individual, rather than social class, the locus of power.[22] It is perhaps of little surprise, therefore, in our post-postmodern era when medical authority is increasingly tenuous and when internet expertise, anti-vaccination movements, and 'patient choice' abound, that the literature has sought to assert the agency of the individual in the face of clinical medicine, or at least to nuance established ideas about the hegemony of the medical gaze. Thus, even if Hogarth is wary of substituting power for the emotions in his account of Townend's stay in hospital, the effect of his argument is

[16] Mary E. Fissell, 'The Disappearance of the Patient's Narrative and the Invention of Hospital Medicine', in Roger French and Andrew Wear (eds), *British Medicine in an Age of Reform* (London: Routledge, 1992), 92–109, at pp. 93, 100.

[17] Fissell, 'Disappearance', p. 108, n. 28.

[18] Flurin Condrau, 'The Patient's View Meets the Clinical Gaze', *Social History of Medicine* 20:3 (2007), 525–40, at p. 529.

[19] For a response to Condrau's challenge, see Anne Hanley and Jessica Meyer, 'Introduction', in Anne Hanley and Jessica Meyer (eds), *Patient Voices in Britain, 1840–1948* (Manchester: Manchester University Press, 2021), 1–30.

[20] Condrau, 'Patient's View', pp. 530–5. For example, leading critics of 'medicalisation', particularly in the field of psychiatry, included the Roman Catholic priest Ivan Illich, the conservative libertarian Thomas Szasz, and the New Left thinker R. D. Laing.

[21] Condrau, 'Patient's View', p. 535.

[22] Roger Cooter, '"Framing" the End of the Social History of Medicine', in Frank Huisman and John Harley Warner (eds), *Locating Medical History: The Stories and Their Meanings* (Baltimore: Johns Hopkins University Press, 2004), 309–37.

to emphasise intersubjectivity over alienation, agency over subjugation, and complexity over oppositional binaries.[23] This chapter follows a similar path in that it demonstrates the continued resonance of the patient's narrative, as well the instrumentality of emotions, within the Romantic surgical relationship.

One of the characteristics of the literature on the patient's narrative has been to conflate Jewson's model of 'Hospital Medicine' with all aspects of the nineteenth-century clinical encounter, when in fact the private consultation continued to exemplify many of the features of his 'Bedside' model.[24] Even so, it is still important to acknowledge the different contexts of hospital medicine and private practice. We cannot be sure that Cooper's hospital patients were treated in a radically different way from his fee-paying ones, although the political dynamics pertaining to a dependent hospital patient and a (largely) autonomous patron were clearly distinct. Indeed, the very fact that commentators alluded to Cooper's sympathetic handling of hospital patients suggests that such practices were not necessarily taken for granted (though equally, as we have seen, 'rough treatment' was not unknown in private practice). What is certainly true is that, within Cooper's archive, these patients are represented and 'heard' very differently. Whereas his private patients can be read through letters written by them, their family members, or their medical attendants, his hospital patients are only glimpsed through his case notes. At the same time, however, this might give us pause to think about the nature of agency and how we conceptualise it. Ever since the 1990s, historians of early modern poverty have traced the agency of the poor through similar institutional records.[25] Like them, we might see agency in such acts of resistance as drunkenness on the ward or leaving the hospital under treatment. We might go one step further. If pre-anaesthetic surgery was a collaborative process, then patients might not collaborate as effectively as their surgeons desired. Indeed, this resistance, as we shall see, might even take on 'unconscious' forms, a revolt of the body and nervous system against violation and pain.

This chapter opens by considering the emotional experiences of patients in Romantic surgery, using the letters they sent to Cooper to explore their thoughts, feelings, and the ways in which they negotiated their treatment. Through a close reading of Cooper's hospital casebooks and other sources, it

[23] Hogarth, 'Joseph Townend', p. 108. See also Mary Wilson Carpenter, 'The Patient's Pain in Her Own Words: Margaret Mathewson's "Sketch of Eight Months a Patient in the Royal Infirmary of Edinburgh AD 1877"', *19: Interdisciplinary Studies in the Long Nineteenth Century* 15 (2012), http://doi.org/10.16995/ntn.636 (accessed 12/04/19).

[24] Jewson himself took the scheme from Erwin Ackerknecht, *Medicine at the Paris Hospital, 1794–1848* (Baltimore: Johns Hopkins University Press, 1967), though with scant acknowledgement; Jewson, 'Disappearance', p. 227, n. 7.

[25] For example, Tim Hitchcock, Peter King, and Pamela Sharpe (eds), *Chronicling Poverty: The Voices and Strategies of the English Poor, 1640–1840* (New York: St Martin's Press, 1997).

then proceeds to consider the various ways in which poorer patients asserted their agency and resisted forms of surgical authority and treatment. The final section considers forms of unconscious resistance to surgical treatment, notably the phenomenon of the 'obstreperous' patient and the failure of the individual, or their nervous system, to confirm to the idealised trope of operative fortitude.

'A Sensation of Half Dying': The Patient's Account of Surgical Illness

In October 1832, Astley Cooper was visited by a woman bearing a note from Roger Nunn of Colchester (1783–1844), which read:

Mrs Ekins the Bearer of this is a Widow Lady with a Large Family and very very small means. This I know will be a sufficient passport to your heart and lay claim to your judgement without a fee – Do her and me the favour to look at her breast and say whether you think it malignant or otherwise, for myself I hope and believe that it is not. Any plan you may suggest for her benefit I shall have pleasure in following up, upon the same feeling and principle, with which I have taken the liberty of sending her to you.[26]

So began one of Cooper's many relationships with his patients. His archive is full of such letters of introduction, in which provincial medical practitioners, often exploiting some personal connection, referred their patients to his expert insight. These are particularly prevalent in cases of afflictions of the breast. Indeed, just a few days after Mrs Ekins' visit, Cooper received another patient from Essex, this time a woman by the name of Mrs Durrant, who bore the following note from her surgeon, Thomas King of Chelmsford:

You will oblige me by giving me your candid opinion as to the Bearer Mrs Durrant's case 1st Whether you consider the disease affecting her Breast scirrhous and likely to become cancerous 2nd Whether it is that kind of case in which extirpation will be likely to prove availing and whether you would recommend it. It would afford me very great pleasure to find that you are of opinion anything can be done effectually to relieve this Patient a Widow with 5 Children whose life is of great consequence to her Family.[27]

Both of these letters are couched in a language of feeling. While Nunn expresses his hope that Ekins' growth is not malignant, King tells Cooper that it would give him 'great pleasure' should he think himself capable of treating Durrant. What is more, the women themselves are presented as objects of pity, deserving, in the first case at least, of *pro bono* treatment. In keeping with Cooper's identity as a man of feeling with a particular attachment

[26] RCSE, MS0008/2/1/9, 'Illustrations of the Diseases of the Breast, Part 1', Letter from Roger Nunn to Astley Cooper, 17 October 1832.
[27] RCSE MS0008/2/1/9, Letter from Thomas King to Astley Cooper, 24 October 1832.

to women and children, these women's medical attendants appeal directly to his 'heart', highlighting their patients' status as poor widows and the mothers of large families. As we saw at the beginning of the previous chapter, Cooper himself imagined the idealised female patient in this way, as the 'mother of a large family dependent on her for protection'.[28] Joanne Bailey has argued that parents and children 'were "good to think with" and "to feel with" in the culture of sensibility'; they 'stimulated the sympathetic identification required for feeling and benevolent behaviour'. Importantly, however, 'the need had to be genuine and the recipient deserving'.[29] Thus, notions of familial 'distress', including the financial burdens of widowhood and dependence, were especially important to the poor, who invoked this language themselves or, as in these examples, had it deployed on their behalf by others. According to Bailey, 'The language of distress was familiar to the elite who read literature and donated to charity. Parental distress stimulated especial sympathy and consideration', in part because it 'signalled that the poor possessed sensibility which made them all the more deserving of relief or charity'.[30]

At one level, then, these expressions of, and appeals to, emotion were generic, having close parallels with other supplicatory relationships. However, Cooper's archive also reveals a more active emotional expressiveness and agency. Perhaps understandably, among the emotions given most prominent expression in this archive are those of apprehension, anxiety, and dread. A particularly powerful example of this can be found in the case of Mrs Sheath of Lincolnshire. Unlike many of the patients in Cooper's archive, Sheath's case appears more than once and provides a sustained insight into the emotional relationship between a patient and her surgeon, albeit one mediated by third parties. The first letter relating to her case was written by her husband in February 1832, revealing that she had already undergone an operation to remove a breast tumour:

About three years ago Mrs Martin Sheath of Wyberton near Boston, my dear Wife, was in Regent Street with her Sister [...] under your Care having a lump in her right breast, and which was skilfully extracted by you; since that time Mrs S has had the misfortune to lose an affectionate Brother and not many months have elapsed since her only Sister, who was her nurse and Companion, departed this life after a very short illness, which

[28] Astley Cooper, *Illustrations of the Diseases of the Breast*, vol. 1 (London: Longman, Rees, Orme, Brown, and Green, 1829), p. 3.
[29] Bailey, *Parenting*, pp. 122–3.
[30] Bailey, *Parenting*, p. 43. See also Donna Andrew, '*Noblesse Oblige*: Female Charity in an Age of Sentiment', in John Brewer and Susan Staves (eds), *Early Modern Conceptions of Property* (London: Routledge, 1995), 275–300; Andrew, '"To the Charitable and Humane": Appeals for Assistance in the Eighteenth-Century London Press', in Hugh Cunningham and Joanna Innes (eds), *Charity, Philanthropy and Reform: From the 1690s to 1850* (Basingstoke: Macmillan, 1998), 87–107.

circumstances have left her in great grief and affliction and I fear have contributed a great deal to a return of the complaint. There is a small lump by the side of the same breast which now and then gives her pain but she dislikes to mention it to Mr Snaith, her apothecary, I therefore cannot allow it to proceed any further without acquainting you of the circumstance and requesting you to give me your excellent advice in what manner we ought to pursue. It has not been of so long standing as the former nor near so large, and it would be a great comfort to us both, if it could possibly be dispersed in preference to another operation, the thoughts of which make her as you may suppose very uneasy and dejected. I shall wait anxiously for your opinion.[31]

Martin Sheath's identification of 'great grief' as a cause of his wife's renewed affliction was, as we have seen, in keeping with Cooper's own views on the aetiology of cancer. Evidently, Cooper took on the case and recommended topical treatments, perhaps given the patient's fear of another operation. Clearly, too, he advised the Sheaths to trust to their local surgeon-apothecary, Frank Snaith, given that the next letter relating to her case, dated September 1834, is written by him and addressed to Cooper's manservant, Charles Balderson:[32]

I address this to you by desire of Mrs Sheath, who supposes Sir Astley has not returned to Town. Mrs S begs me to inform you that there is a sore in that part of the Breast [...] formed from the healing of the sore in the first operation; she said she had the same when in Town and that Sir Astley soon healed it principally by the application of a white powder, but Mrs Sheath does not know whether it be the same she is using at present [...] She has considerable pain in the fresh Ulceration [...] afore mentioned [...] Do suggest something if Sir Astley has not returned. Mrs Sheath is miserable about this new Ulceration and the adhesion of the lint, to [...] which [...] she attributes the new ulceration.[33]

Sheath's profound misery concerning the progress of her complaint and her anxiety to receive Cooper's advice are clearly communicated in this letter and only amplified by the next message from Snaith, some two months later. 'Mrs Sheath is so anxious to hear from you respecting the excoriations I mentioned in my last letter', it reads, 'that she would have me to write again today from Wyberton. She is alarmed lest the excoriations should spread under the arm, which is not improbable they will do if their progress cannot be arrested'.[34] Meanwhile, in one of the last letters in the archive, dated June 1835, Snaith records the alarming state of Sheath's condition and conveys her desperation:

---

[31] RCSE, MS0008/2/2/4, File of letters and notes of cases sent to Sir Astley Cooper, 1807–36, Letter from Martin Sheath to Astley Cooper, 7 February 1832.

[32] His actual surname was Osbalderson, but he was given this 'cognomen which offered a greater facility of pronunciation'; Bransby Blake Cooper, *The Life of Sir Astley Cooper, Bart.*, vol. 1 (London: John W. Parker, 1843), p. 329.

[33] RCSE, MS0008/2/2/4, Letter from Frank Snaith to Charles Balderson, 23 September 1834.

[34] RCSE, MS0008/2/2/4, Letter from Frank Snaith to Astley Cooper, 11 November 1834.

Our poor patient Mrs Sheath, has again requested me to trouble you with a statement of her present condition; the original sore is much the same it is a little more filled up from the bottom so that it does not look so much like a scooped out cavity, but the small ulceration, which she calls excoriations have spread since I last addressed you. They have extended from the Breast across the axilla to the back part of the arm, but they have extended much further downward along the abdomen, & on the Breast which has never been affected before [...] We apply the lotion to the Ulcerations [...] but it appears to make no alteration to the parts, she is anxious you should order something else, as she says, that if one thing does not answer, you always try another, now do my Dear Sir, write immediately, she is so anxious, and I was to have written to you two days ago, but was prevented.[35]

It is not known what happened to Mrs Sheath; given the nature of her symptoms, it seems likely that she succumbed to her condition. These letters therefore give voice to the profound anxiety of living with a painful, disfiguring, and almost certainly terminal disease.[36] But they also point to the importance of emotions in soliciting advice and treatment. Clearly Snaith was taking direct instruction from Mrs Sheath in his communications with Cooper. His role was not simply to report his clinical observations, but also to pass on her feelings and to leverage changes in treatment based, to a significant degree, on her state of mind. Perhaps unsurprisingly, given the widespread apprehension of its incurability, such expressions of anxiety and fear on the parts of patients were particularly common in cases of breast cancer. But they were also evident in other conditions too, especially other instances of cancer. Thus, a note delivered to Cooper by one of his male patients states:

Our Patient Mr Stayner the Bearer, has requested us to give you the outline of his Case [...] He has during the last two years suffered a considerable pain in the Lumbar Region and the urine has deposited a lateritious sediment. But latterly he has been apprehensive of some Scirrhous affection of the rectum we have not discovered such disease existing but our patient's mind has been strongly impressed with this idea in consequence of his Father and Mother both having died from Cancer of the Rectum and the latter sloughing Mamma [breast cancer].[37]

Sheath's case thus illustrates the apprehension and anxiety that attached to the experience of disease in general, as well as the ways in which those fears were instrumental in shaping therapeutic decision-making. For example, her initial wariness of revealing her condition to her surgeon-apothecary was not uncommon. Whether from fear of an unfavourable diagnosis or from a belief that nothing could be done to alleviate their condition, patients often concealed

[35] RCSE, MS0008/2/2/4, Letter from Frank Snaith to Astley Cooper, 10 June 1835.
[36] On the experience of pain and cancer, see Kaartinen, *Cancer*, pp. 94–101; Javier Moscoso, 'Exquisite and Lingering Pains: Facing Cancer in Early Modern Europe', in Rob Boddice (ed.), *Pain and Emotion in Modern History* (Palgrave: Palgrave Macmillan, 2014), 16–35.
[37] RCSE, MS0008/2/2/3 pt. 1, File of letters and notes on cases sent to Sir Astley Cooper, unpaginated note dated 11 October.

their symptoms, even from loved ones.[38] In 1836, for instance, Frances White of
Thatcham in Berkshire wrote to Cooper with a history of her case, which began,
aged 28, when she 'discovered a small lump forming about the size of a nutmeg
on the top of my left Breast near my duct'. White 'took little notice of it for a year
or more', as it gave her little pain. However, she later 'began to have shooting
pains in my Breast and the lump gradually increased'. It was only aged 36, when
the tumour started to discharge 'something like clear water', that she went to see
Cooper, 'something I very much regret not having done in the first beginning of
the Disease'. As she explained, 'I never let any Medical Gentleman see it before
Sir Astley for as I resided in the country I had not sufficient confidence to think
they could do me any good, the doctors in Berkshire having but little experience
in such cases'.[39] Meanwhile, in December 1833, Cooper received a letter from
the Lancaster physician Edward Denis De Vitré (1806–78) asking his advice
in the case of Mrs Mackreth, the 62-year-old wife of a local clergyman who
had already undergone a previous operation. 'Unfortunately', De Vitré wrote,
'she has all along observed the strictest secrecy regarding her complaint, and
only informed her husband of it a week ago'. As such, her condition was quite
advanced and De Vitré told Cooper that 'I have not flattered Mr Mackreth's
expectations'.[40] Practitioners were well aware of this inclination to conceal, and
another Lancastrian correspondent, the Blackburn surgeon James Barlow, wrote:

It is lamentable to recount the numerous cases of tumours which I have witnessed and
which have either been neglected on the one hand by the supinity of the Patient, or from
ignorance and timidity of the surgeon on the other insomuch that the disease has ultimately become exasperated [sic] beyond the aid of the scientific surgeon.[41]

In other cases, however, it was the surgeon who might conceal the full reality of a patient's condition from them. This was a matter of some contention
within Romantic surgery. As we have heard, surgeons of the period spoke of
the necessity of putting the patient's needs and desires at the centre of decision-making. And indeed, at a time when operative surgery required active
resolve on the part of the patient, consent and collaboration were absolute
necessities. Thus, Frederic Skey proclaimed that 'However, desirable it may
be, that the mind of the patient be animated by a full share of hope and confidence in the issue, this desideratum cannot justify his withholding the honest,
and unreserved declaration of his thoughts and opinions'.[42] Skey's reference

[38] Kaartinen, *Cancer*, pp. 64–7.
[39] RCSE, MS0008/2/2/4, Letter from Frances White to Astley Cooper, 22 May 1836.
[40] RCSE, MS0008/2/2/3 pt. 3, Letter from Edward D. de Vitré to Astley Cooper, 14 December 1833.
[41] RCSE, MS008/2/2/12, Notebook of notes on a case of the removal of a tumour from the cheek,
    unpaginated. The notion that women were particularly inclined to conceal their condition was
    widespread in this period; Kaartinen, *Cancer*, p. 66.
[42] Frederic Skey, *Operative Surgery* (London: John Churchill, 1850), p. 12.

to the patient's state of mind hints at the delicate balancing act inherent to the clinical consultation. In the early part of our period in particular, when, as we have seen, emotions such as anxiety and grief were thought to have a powerful influence on the propagation and exacerbation of physical complaints, presenting the patient with a full account of their predicament might only serve to compound it. Certainly, patients occasionally feared they were not being told the whole truth. For example, in 1832 Maria Wigg of Honiton in Devon wrote to Cooper, stating:

Could you, Sir think of any thing to afford me relief I should for ever feel extremely thankful, for I must acknowledge that I still feel apprehension of a cancer, and when most troubled with pain am fearful you did not tell me exactly what it really was, therefore dear Sir your candid answer will be very very acceptable to me and greatly ease my mind.[43]

Neither were such fears unfounded, for in 1822 John Rosewarne, a surgeon of Wadebridge in Cornwall, wrote relative to his patient:

As Miss Best is extremely anxious and agitated on the subject I have endeavoured as much as possible to keep the real nature of the complaint from her until imperious [sic] changes in it should oblige me to be more explicit, and I still think that the most cautious manner of proposing an operation would be necessary; I have as yet only ventured to hint at it.[44]

Evidently, the patient's fear of the operation could be as profound as that of the condition itself and had a material effect on their treatment.[45] In 1835 Dr Bowen of Carmarthen wrote to Cooper concerning his patient, Mrs Hughes, from whom Cooper had already removed a tumour and the whole left breast the previous year. Subsequent shooting pains in the region produced 'great despondency' and 'She now has a great drea[d of being] obliged to submit to another [operation]'. 'I have therefore said nothing to her on the [subject]', he wrote, 'but recommended her to consult you personally and thereby have her mind made easy'.[46] As we have seen in the case of Mrs Sheath, her husband's desire that her tumour be 'dispersed' through the use of caustics derived from the fact that the prospect of another operation made her 'very uneasy and dejected'.[47] Likewise, Mrs Mackreth doubtless kept the return of her cancer secret from her husband in part because 'She dreads the idea of another

---

[43] RCSE MS0008/2/1/9, Letter from Maria Wigg to Astley Cooper, 24 September 1832.
[44] RCSE, MS0008/2/2/3 pt. 1, Copy of a letter from John Rosewarne to Thomas Stewart, 9 July 1822.
[45] Kaartinen, Cancer, pp. 91–4.
[46] RCSE, MS0008 2/2/3 pt. 3, Letter from Dr Bowen to Astley Cooper, 26 November 1835. This page of the letter is badly damaged and the words in square brackets are conjecture.
[47] RCSE, MS0008/2/2/4, Letter from Martin Sheath to Astley Cooper, 7 February 1832.

operation'.[48] All three of these women had endured the agony of surgical excision, and had no desire to repeat the experience, even if that came at the cost of their life. But in any case, surgical removal was well known to be a most uncertain 'cure' and many women were understandably cautious of undergoing the ordeal unless there was a real chance of success. In Chapter 2, we encountered Mrs Palmer of Wellingborough who visited Cooper in 1836 for a tumour of her left breast, caused by the combination of a physical blow and the ill-health of her son. In the accompanying note from her surgeon, Benjamin Dulley (c.1807–88), he observed:

There does not seem to be any great enlargement of the glands in the axilla but there is a kind of chain of communication from them to the tumour which has deterred me from submitting to her the prospects of an operation until I had had your opinion thereon – for in the few cases in which I have operated there has been the usual tendency to reproduction of the disease which precludes giving so favourable a prospect of real ease as Patients generally require before submitting to a painful operation.[49]

In 1815, Mrs Etchley of Hereford attended Cooper with similar questions as to the efficacy of an operation. The note she bore from her surgeon, Mr Griffiths, stated: 'The principle questions we wish to submit to your decision are [...] Whether you think it advisable to remove the Tumour by excision? and in the next, how far you think this Lady a good subject to undergo such an operation, looking forward to permanent advantages?'[50]

As it turned out, Cooper did not think Etchley's case to be a 'true scirrhous', and hence she did not require an operation. Meanwhile, in other instances patients had to be convinced of the imminent risk to their health in order to go under the knife. For example, a note in Cooper's archive gives an account of the case of Mrs Davis of 'Old St Pancras Church', a 34-year-old woman who developed a tumour of the right breast weighing five pounds (her breast as a whole weighed fifteen). 'This immense enlargement was not attended with much pain', the note observes, the main issue being its weight, 'and this inconvenience, added to the apprehension that the patient's health must soon give way under the influence of such a disease, induced her to consent to its removal with the knife in the judicious hands of Sir A Cooper'.[51] However, perhaps the most striking example of a patient being persuaded to consider an operation, by dint of their own experience as much as by surgical advice, is that of Jane Watson, a Quaker from Waterford in Ireland. She began her letter by asking 'perhaps Astley Cooper may recollect being applied to for advice by Jane

---

[48] RCSE, MS0008/2/2/3 pt. 3, Letter from Edward D. de Vitré to Astley Cooper, 14 December 1833.
[49] RCSE, MS0008/2/2/3 pt. 3, Letter from Benjamin Dulley to Astley Cooper, 28 April 1836.
[50] RCSE, MS0008/2/2/4, Letter from J Griffiths to Astley Cooper, 14 April 1815.
[51] RCSE, MS0008/2/2/3 pt. 1, unpaginated note dated 19 September 1822.

Watson, respecting a tumour in her breast on the 29th of the 5th month (May) in the present year'. '[H]e rather approved an immediate removal', she notes, 'but as she could not at that time submit, he prescribed a plaister, daily aperient pills, and occasional application of leeches'. There follows a detailed account of her complaint, complete with emphatic underlining. She observes that in the 'last three [months], there has been evidently a considerable encrease [*sic*] of size, as well as of pain' in her tumour. She had followed Cooper's instructions, including in the application of the 'plaister' and the daily 'aperient pills', and while the pills operated 'moderately', the leeches did not produce 'the inflam- mation she feared'. 'Still', she adds, 'she has not been sensible of deriving much, if any benefit from them'. Watson maintained that 'she has not had any medical advice since seeing Sir A C – considering herself his patient, and acting according to his directions'. She therefore 'solicits Sir Astley Cooper's candid opinion, whether from what she has now communicated he thinks there is still a prospect of her being relieved by an opperation [*sic*]'. '[C]rossing the waters at such a late season of the year with the journey to London appears a formidable addition', she concluded, 'but still she might be induced to under- take it, if there appears a probability of success and begs Sir Astley Cooper will kindly favour her with a reply at the earliest period that finds his convenience as she waits it, with considerable anxiety'.[52]

Jane Watson's letter is remarkable in many ways. Here is evidence, if ever it were needed, that the patient's voice was by no means entirely effaced by the advent of clinical medicine. Like many others in her position, she uses the language of emotion, particularly anxiety, to leverage a response. But what is particularly striking about her letter is the fact that it is couched in the third person. While this might be a quirk of Quaker prose, it also served to give her observations a greater degree of clinical authority, as if they had been written by a medical attendant. Indeed, at one point in the letter she acknowledges the oddity of her address, stating that 'if he [Cooper] thinks he could understand her situation better by having it stated by a Surgeon she will have it done'.[53] Watson was clearly an assertive and capable woman, managing her illness to the best of her abilities. Sadly, the records suggest that she died, aged 62, some six years after penning this letter.[54]

If some patients required persuasion about the need for an operation, oth- ers were far more readily disposed to submit. In August 1835, for example, Cooper received a letter from his former pupil Henry James Prince (1811–99), surgeon to the General Infirmary at Bath, who would later become notorious

---

[52] RCSE, MS0008/2/2/3 pt. 1, Letter from Jane Watson to Astley Cooper, 10 July 1839.
[53] RCSE, MS0008/2/2/3 pt. 1, Letter from Jane Watson to Astley Cooper, 10 July 1839.
[54] www.igp-web.com/IGPArchives/ire/waterford/churches/quaker-deaths-w3.html (accessed 01/05/22).

as the founder of the Agapemonite religious sect.[55] Prince wrote that during his medical studies in London, which were attended with 'some degree of mental anxiety, my attention was attracted to a gradual decline of general health by the Enlargement of two or three glands in the right groin', a condition that was exacerbated by his contracting gonorrhoea in 1833. At the time of writing, his right testis had swelled to the 'size of a large hen's egg', which 'acts as a mechanical impediment to my taking exercise so successfully that I am crippled by it'. He therefore requested Cooper to remove it in its entirety, stating:

The impression upon my own mind is that the presence of the diseased Testis is the only prevention to recovery and that my health will never be restored without the extirpation of the gland. I am 24 years of age, of a nervous and irritable temperament, and extremely susceptible to external impressions of every kind.[56]

The idea that the mental anxiety produced by a tumour could only be remedied by its excision, regardless of its pathological status, can also be found in one of Cooper's casebooks, wherein the entry for a 20-year-old patient by the name of Mrs Hole ends with the resolution: 'To be removed on the ground of anxiety as it prays upon the mind'.[57] For others, however, no amount of persuasion could overcome the fear of an operation. Thus, one of Cooper's patients, who was herself being treated for breast cancer, wrote that she 'had a Sister that was afflicted with a Cancer for many years who had not courage to undergo an operation and had Causticks applied'. She broke out in ulcers, which were healed with 'the juice of Clivers, or Goose Grass, but she Dyed [sic] in 2 years apparently of consumption at the age of 47'.[58]

As this correspondent's reference to her sister reminds us, relations between patients and surgeons were often mediated, not only by medical attendants, but also by friends and family. Benjamin Brodie told his students that the 'Medical practitioner necessarily sees more of the interior of the families whom he visits than other persons', while Frederic Skey maintained that family members could play a vital role in the surgical consultation, allowing the surgeon to 'speak more freely and unreservedly to persons only secondarily concerned' and enabling the 'exercise of the calmer and more disinterested judgement of one [...] more competent to meet the occasional idiosyncrasies of a patient's mind'.[59] Skey's somewhat idealised representation of familial disinterest neglects the fact that friends and family often brought their own

---

[55] Timothy C. F. Strutt, 'Prince, Henry James (1811–1899)', *ODNB*.
[56] RCSE, MS0008/2/2/4, Letter from Henry James Prince to Astley Cooper, 10 April 1835.
[57] RCSE, MS0008/2/1/6, Volume of case notes in the hand of Sir Astley Paston Cooper, 1817–20, unpaginated.
[58] RCSE, MS0008/2/2/4, Letter from E. Wood to Astley Cooper, 22 November [no year].
[59] RCSE, MS0470/1/2/5, Benjamin Brodie, 'Introductory lecture of anatomy and physiology' (October 1820), f. 5; Skey, *Surgery*, p. 13.

emotions into the bargain. As we shall see, parents could exert considerable agency in refusing surgical treatment for their children, whereas others were anxious to procure it. In February 1835, for example, the surgeon John Dalton (1771–1844) of Bury St Edmunds sent his daughter Hannah to see Cooper in the company of his son and fellow surgeon John Dalton junior (1803–59). The accompanying letter reveals that she had a 'Serious stricture' in her rectum and a 'malformation of Parts' that had prevented the consummation of her marriage. Dalton apologised to Cooper for having 'troubled you with what all eminent consulting Surgeons hate, a long prosing and to you perhaps ignorant, stupid story', but he begged Cooper's forgiveness and hoped he would 'attribute it to the anxiety I feel as a Parent'.[60] In other instances, family members played a mediating role that was closer to Skey's ideal. Thus, in 1832, the surgeon Caleb Woodyer (1766–1849) of Guildford wrote to Cooper about a patient of his named Miss Hayden, a 70-year-old 'maiden lady' suffering from 'a diseased Breast'. Woodyer noted that 'Her niece, Miss Sophia Hayden will now likely accompany her, who has a strong mind'. This was probably just as well, he claimed, as her aunt 'has the high nervous sensibility, which requires caution in your observations'.[61]

As we have heard, first-hand accounts of operations written by patients themselves are relatively rare. The closest we have to such a thing in Cooper's archive is a letter sent to him in 1823 by the former East India Company surgeon John Cairnie (1769–1842) of Largs. In October 1816, a canister of gunpowder exploded in Cairnie's left hand, 'whereby the muscles of the thumb and palm of the hand were much lacerated, and the bone of the first phalanx of the thumb was broken'. He appeared to be recovering well, but some days later he began to haemorrhage and 'we were unable after repeated attempts and much suffering to me to find from whence it proceeded'. As a result:

the palmar arch was cut down upon and tied, but to no purpose the bleeding returning at intervals without any warning reduced me extremely – The radial artery was next cut down upon and tied[.] [I]n doing a sheath [of] the nerve had been included, as when the Ligature was tightened, I started involuntarily from my back to my legs and a severe pain struck me from the occiput to the forehead over the right eye.[62]

This operation 'proved also unsuccessful and the thumb was next removed at its junction with the Carpal bones'. Still, the source of the bleeding could not be found and so Cairnie had to undergo an amputation between the elbow and the wrist. However:

[60] RCSE, MS0008/2/2/6, Letter from John Dalton to Astley Cooper, 22 February 1835.
[61] RCSE, MS0008/2/2/4, Letter from Caleb Woodyer to Astley Cooper, 7 February 1832.
[62] RCSE, MS0008/2/2/3 pt. 1, Letter from John Cairnie to Astley Cooper, 8 April 1823.

The assistant in charge of the Retractors let them slip during the sawing of the bone and some of the soft parts got into the teeth of the saw when the pain was most excruciating I could compare it to nothing but boiling lead running into a fresh wound, happily it was but momentary or I must have died under it.[63]

In another, not dissimilar instance, William Dann, a 34-year-old shipwright, was admitted to Guy's Hospital in May 1816 and found to have an aneurysm of the popliteal artery. During the operation, which appears to have been performed by the notoriously incompetent William Lucas junior, the femoral sheath was tied up with the ligature and 'as this was done the Patient's cries were deplorable [and] he seemed to suffer in an extreme degree'.[64] Evidently curious about the pain he had caused, the surgeon asked Dann after the operation to describe what he had felt:

He says the first incision into the integuments was a sharp smarting pain, but that produced from the application of the ligature round the sheath was of an exquisite burning nature; he describes it as if the limb was sliced down with an [sic] hot lance – the pain shot down to the knee, and was described as tho [sic] a lance had passed into the part – then it went down in like manner to the ankle where the same feeling occurred as in the knee – When the artery was properly separated from the sheath he felt it raised distinctly, and was relieved of a stretching pain when it was divided and retracted, he felt it go in, on his word.[65]

These two instances provide a fleeting, yet intensely visceral, insight into the embodied experience of pre-anaesthetic surgery. In her pioneering study, Elaine Scarry argues that the experience of pain ultimately destroys language, rendering it inexpressible.[66] This is because she treats pain as a thing in itself, which stands outside of language. By contrast, scholars such as Javier Moscoso and Joanna Bourke have sought to understand pain as a cultural and linguistic phenomenon, an 'event' that only achieves 'significance' (or meaning) through its expression.[67] Certainly, Carnie and Dann's use of simile and metaphor suggests something of the ineffability of such intense embodied experiences, as does George Wilson's account of his operation in 1842, in which he claims that 'suffering so great as I underwent cannot be expressed in words, and thus fortunately cannot be recalled'.[68] And yet, if Wilson's account supports Adam

[63] RCSE, MS0008/2/2/3 pt. 1, Letter from John Cairnie to Astley Cooper, 8 April 1823.
[64] On Lucas' incompetence, see Cooper, *Life*, vol. 1, p. 302; John Flint South, *Memorials of John Flint South* (London: John Murray, 1884), pp 52–3.
[65] RCSE, MS0008/2/2/3 pt. 1, unpaginated case of 'Popliteal aneurism'.
[66] Elaine Scarry, *The Body in Pain: The Making and the Unmaking of the World* (Oxford: Oxford University Press, 1985), pp. 3–11.
[67] Joanna Bourke, *The Story of Pain: From Prayers to Painkillers* (Oxford: Oxford University Press, 2014), pp. 1–19; Javier Moscoso, *Pain: A Cultural History* (Basingstoke: Palgrave Macmillan, 2014).
[68] James Young Simpson, *Acupressure: A New Method of Arresting Surgical Haemorrhage* (Edinburgh: Adam and Charles Black, 1864), p. 568.

Smith's assertion that 'Nothing is so soon forgot as pain', Carnie's memory of that sensation was clearly alive and well some seven years after the event.[69] In the relative absence of such first-person testimony, we find that the language used to describe the experience of patients in the operating theatre was often more generic. As we shall see in Chapter 4, where operations went wrong, or where it suited the reformist agenda of journals like *The Lancet* to highlight the sufferings of the patient, that language used could be emotive and expressive. For the most part, however, descriptions of successful operations either make little reference to the bearing of the patient or, if the operation was particularly gruelling, highlight the 'fortitude' of the sufferer. Thus, in the case of Mrs David, noted above, it was said that the operation to remove the tumour from her breast lasted 'about eighteen minutes, without the patients [*sic*] hands (at her own desire) being confined or her eyes darkened and without her uttering one word of complaint'.[70]

Within Cooper's archive, first-hand descriptions of pain most commonly relate to the chronic sensations of illness, or the acute agonies of therapeutic treatment, rather than the experience of operative surgery. In part, this may have something to do with the clinical value of such testimony. Except in such cases as Dann's, where the surgeon's curiosity was piqued, the pain of undergoing an operation was ubiquitous and thus of comparatively little clinical interest or relevance. Let us remember, too, that Wilson's account of his operation only assumed meaning through its contrast with the relative *painlessness* of anaesthetic surgery. By contrast, patients' descriptions of the pain of disease, or of treatment, could serve a diagnostic, prognostic, or therapeutic purpose. Hence, at various points in his casebooks, Cooper records the subjective sensations of his patients, such those of Mrs Smith, a 59-year-old woman with a tumour in her left breast, who described her condition thus: 'The pain is by fits – like a Cork Screw – like a Knife at others – sometimes like [illegible] – sometimes like an aching'.[71] Moreover, for patients themselves, such descriptions had a moral and emotional force. They might generate pathos and encourage a favourable response from their surgeon, or they might leverage a change in treatment. In the case of 'W Davy' from Marlborough, they testified to his diligence in following Cooper's instructions, and provided information by which to determine his future treatment. Davy suffered from a tumour on his cheek and in May 1831 he supplied Cooper with 'a statement of the progress and success of the application of arsenic to my face', in 'compliance with your request'. He describes a pain that the modern reader can hardly begin to imagine:

[69] Adam Smith, *The Theory of Moral Sentiments* (London: A. Miller, 1759), p. 56. On the use of metaphor in descriptions of pain, see Bourke, *Pain*, ch. 3.
[70] RCSE, MS0008/2/2/3 pt. 1, unpaginated note dated 19 September 1822.
[71] RCSE, MS0008/2/1/9, annotation opposite p. 1.

I applied the Pulv: arsenic to the face. The pain was very severe and <u>incessant</u> for the <u>first day and night</u> – The <u>second</u> day the pain was at times, <u>great</u> but not <u>unremitting</u>, During the day, from weakness induced by want of rest and continual pain, I fainted – The <u>third</u> and <u>fourth</u> days were days of suffering, but <u>not excessive</u>. I had but little rest at night. The <u>fourth</u> night was more painful than any, except the <u>first</u>. I conclude, that was occasioned by a disposition to separate, the dead from the live flesh, as after this, it became more easy [...] From this time, both pain and swelling gradually subsided. I should observe that the <u>enflamed</u> state and <u>swelling</u> of the cheek were very great. One eye was <u>nearly</u> closed, and the mouth <u>almost</u> shut up by the swelling [...] At the end of <u>one month</u> the past portion of the dead flesh sloughed off [...] the wound gradually contracting, till at the end of one week, May 10th, it healed completely –

The pain, for the <u>two first days</u>, after the application to the face, was like violent pricking of needles, the thrusting of knives, and often as if something were gnawing the flesh, at times there was a sensation of numbness.[72]

Given such suffering, even in an ostensibly successful case, it is perhaps unsurprising that patients frequently expressed deep despondency about their condition. As we have heard, this was a state of mind that was regarded with grave concern by surgeons, for dejection, especially after an operation, could prove fatal. Thus, in Cooper's casebooks, accounts of patients' aftercare make frequent reference to their mood. In one instance, for example, a 'Stout healthy man was brought into Guys Hospital who had a compound fracture of his leg'. Amputation was immediately performed but, after two days, it was noted that 'his countenance is desponding' and just under a week later he died, 'apparently of weakness'.[73] Occasionally it is possible to hear the patient give voice to feelings of despair or resignation. For example, in 1804, the surgeon John Leadam (1780–1845) of Tooley Street, Southwark, told Cooper of the case of a woman under his care who suffered from a severe stomach complaint and exhibited 'the most distressing symptoms', including vomiting and twitching. Two or three times a day she felt '(to use her own expression) "a Sensation of Half Dying" for which she considered Fainting away would be the happiest relief'. According to Leadam, she had frequent recourse to opium, 'more from her particular watchfulness, than pain [and] ... in her latter moments, she loudly called for it, to ease the pangs of death'.[74] Similarly, a description of a woman who suffered from erysipelas following an operation on her face recounts that she was in such pain that she 'could not swallow the bark which was poured gently into her mouth'. Soon afterwards she 'said "she wished the Lord would free her from pain" in a manner scarcely intelligible' and 'at 2 o'clock on the morning of the 22 Dec she died'.[75]

[72] RCSE, MS0008/2/2/3 pt. 1, Letter and case report from W. Davy to Astley Cooper, 30 May 1831.
[73] RCSE, MS0008/2/1/4, Cases in Surgery, Volume 4 (1788), 'Case 28th', ff. 70–2.
[74] RCSE, MS0008/2/2/4, Letter from John Leadam to Astley Cooper, November 1804.
[75] RCSE MS0008/2/2/7, File of letters and notes on cases sent to Sir Astley Cooper, 1813–38, Letter from 'RB' to Astley Cooper, undated.

Even in less acute cases, patients could experience profound despair. One of the most notable examples of this in Cooper's archive concerns the Reverend Dr Michael Burke (1789–1866), Catholic Rector of the Parish of St Peter and Paul in Clonmel, Ireland. Burke fractured his left thigh in a fall from a coach travelling from Boulogne to Paris. According to the case report:

Dr Burke was to all appearance a very healthy man, but suffered intense anxiety of mind owing principally to an apprehension of the result of his accident being fatal, an idea which seemed to occupy his mind incessantly, almost to the exclusion of every other thought, and partly to his absence from home in a foreign country away from his friends and his parish.[76]

The celebrated surgeon Philibert Joseph Roux (1780–1854) declared that it 'required only time for nature' to heal the fracture, but Burke expressed 'the utmost desire to get home'. Indeed, another surgeon, M. Durand, 'attributed the tardiness of the union to the patient's state of mind which he alleged to be [...] distracted by nostalgia, and apprehension of a fatal result'. As Thomas Dodman has shown, Romantic conceptions of nostalgia were intimately tied to absence from home, and the 1820s and 1830s constituted its 'golden age' as a clinical condition, especially in its spiritual homeland of France.[77] Even after his return to Clonmel, however, Burke's mind was 'still in a state of the greatest despondency [...] his fears of a fatal result have continued' and 'his depression of spirits is such that he is often affected even to tears'. Indeed, his despondency was so persistent and unyielding that his attendants began to lose their patience, for his case concludes with the observation that due to 'his peculiar temperament [...] his complaints are supposed to be often much greater than in proportion to any actual pain or annoyance suffered'.[78]

In a number of instances, despondent patients contacted Cooper because they believed him to be their last hope of relief. In March 1817, for example, Charles Jamieson of Inverness wrote to Alex Mackenzie in London, repeating his 'earnest wish that you would once more lay my case before Dr [sic] Cooper' for 'if he will or cannot do any thing for me there is no help'. Included with the letter was an account of his 'long distressing state', which involved a sore on his penis that prevented him from urinating without intense pain and putting his 'whole frame [...] in a kind of stupefied state'. 'The medical men here when they call

[76] RCSE, MS0008/2/2/3 pt. 1, unsigned, undated case notes.
[77] Thomas Dodman, *What Nostalgia Was: War, Empire, and the Time of a Deadly Emotion* (Chicago: University of Chicago Press, 2018), pp. 128–30. See also Philip Shaw, 'Longing for Home: Robert Hamilton, Nostalgia and the Emotional Life of the Eighteenth-Century Soldier', *Journal for Eighteenth-Century Studies* 39:1 (2016), 25–40; Joanne Begiato, 'Selfhood and "Nostalgia": Sensory and Material Memories of the Childhood Home in Late Georgian Britain', *Journal for Eighteenth-Century Studies* 42:2 (2019), 229–46.
[78] RCSE, MS0008/2/2/3 pt. 1, unsigned, undated case notes.

say "how do you do" and promise to call [again] in the evening', he wrote, but while 'they are my real friends and would do me good if they could', they availed him nothing. As such, he sought to procure Cooper's advice, 'as may either relieve me or that I may conclude nothing can be done for me' and that 'I must struggle with my distress and meet the consequences'.[79]

Jamieson's letter brings us to the final set of emotions that are given expression by patients in Cooper's archive. Perhaps unsurprisingly, given the limited power of early nineteenth-century surgery to cure many of the most serious conditions that came under its purview, expressions of relief, joy, and gratitude are somewhat less common than those of anxiety, fear, and despondency. Nevertheless, there are a number of instances in which patients either wrote to Cooper themselves, or had their recovery communicated to him by third parties. Cooper's breast cancer patients were especially expressive on this point, and particularly indebted to him as an individual. Thus, in reply to Cooper's enquiry after her health, a woman from West Burton in the Yorkshire Dales, signing herself 'E Wood', wrote 'You tell me you have not forgot me, I should be a most ungrateful person if I ever forget my obligation to you, as, under providence, you were the means of saving my life when Mr Hay of Leeds told my Son that I could not survive 6 weeks, and that all the Surgeons in England could not save my life'.[80] Meanwhile, Frances White, whom we encountered earlier, claimed that 'I must always consider my life has been prolonged owing to my going to Sir Astley and the kind attentions of his worthy assistant Mr Balderson'.[81] As we saw at the beginning of Chapter 2, in the introduction to his *Illustrations of the Diseases of the Breast* (1829) Cooper imagined telling one of his patients that her breast was not cancerous and seeing her face brightened 'with the smile of gratitude'. These letters clearly show that such imaginings were grounded in reality and, indeed, in his casebooks Cooper recounts an even more powerful, affective response on the part of 'Mrs Stuart', who 'consulted a medical gentleman respecting a tumour which she had in her breast and immediately as he told her it was not cancerous or ever would be she fainted'.[82] However, as Hannah Newton's work has shown, recovery from illness was not simply an occasion for joy and gratitude, or even overwhelming relief, but also for religious reflection and praise.[83] Hence,

---

[79] RCSE, MS0008/2/2/4, Letter from Charles Jamieson to Alex Mackenzie, 24 March 1817.
[80] RCSE, MS0008/2/2/4, Letter from E. Wood to Astley Cooper, 22 November [no year].
[81] RCSE, MS0008/2/2/4, Letter from Frances White to Astley Cooper, 22 May 1836.
[82] RCSE, MS0008/2/1/7, Casebook in the hand of Sir Astley Paston Cooper, 1793–1823, unpaginated.
[83] Hannah Newton, *From Misery to Mirth: Recovery from Illness in Early Modern England* (Oxford: Oxford University Press, 2018), ch. 4.

while Wood referred to Cooper as a tool of providence, in 1837 George Chamberlaine, the Rector of Wyke Regis and Weymouth in Dorset, told him that 'By the blessing of God, I have every reason to believe that the whole of the stone which tormented me for four years is dissolved' and that 'my heart is filled with gratitude to the almighty disposer of all events; I consider myself a most fortunate Man for being in mercy, reprieved for a short period, and for being permitted at my advanced age to enjoy my life, free from pain and disease'.[84] Sadly for Chamberlaine this reprieve was indeed short, for records suggest that he died four months later.[85]

Thus far in this chapter we have mostly heard from Cooper's private patients. Even if their interactions with him were mediated by others, the letters sent on their behalf nonetheless suggest a certain intimacy. This quality of intimacy was, no doubt, dependent upon an equivalence of social status, combined with the security and confidence of the patron. However, it also had complex emotional dimensions. This was especially pronounced in the case of Cooper's female patients, notably those undergoing treatment for breast cancer. As we have just seen, these women were particularly expressive of their gratitude to Cooper and often projected onto him the identity of a saviour. This derived, in part, from the severity of their condition, and the relatively low chances of a successful cure, which made the joy of deliverance all the more intense. But it also stemmed, as we suggested in Chapter 2, from Cooper's identity as a man of feeling with an especial attachment to the opposite sex. This emotional dynamic is clearly evident in his correspondence. For example, in reporting on the satisfactory state of his patient Mrs Barratt, the surgeon Thomas Plum of Bath wrote that 'she bids me say (with her best Compliments) that if you would address the other side of the letter a few lines to herself, she should feel most happy'.[86] Cooper's other patients, namely those whom he treated in his capacity as surgeon to Guy's Hospital, no doubt had somewhat less latitude in their dealings with him. Moreover, those dealings have left far fainter traces in the historical register. In the next section we shall therefore turn our focus to the relationships between Romantic surgeons and their poorer patients, demonstrating that, while the latter's voices are certainly less distinct than those of wealthy clients, we can nonetheless unearth evidence of an emotional agency and, even, of a resistance to clinical authority.

---

[84] RCSE, MS0008/2/2/7, Letter from George Chamberlaine to Astley Cooper, 27 June 1837.
[85] NA, PROB 11/1885/81, Will of Reverend George Chamberlaine, Clerk, Rector of Wyke Regis and Weymouth, Dorset (31 October 1837).
[86] RCSE, MS0008/2/1/9, Letter from Thomas Plum to Astley Cooper, 10 June 1832.

'Wilful and Bad to Manage': Agency and Resistance in the Hospital

Historians have long been conscious of the links between the growth of the hospital system in the eighteenth century and that of contemporary disciplinary institutions, such as the workhouse and prison.[87] Traditionally, they have characterised the relationship between hospital patient and practitioner as one of dependence and subordination. At the same time, however, they have been sensitive to the reciprocity of medical charity and to the fact that patients had something to gain from admittance to a hospital, even if it came at the price of obedience and gratitude.[88] Indeed, in keeping with the historiography on the Poor Law, historians of medicine have increasingly recognised that such institutions might be 'resources strategically deployed by the poor, rather than oppressive regimes imposed on them'.[89] These ambivalences are neatly encapsulated in a quote from John Abernethy, who told his students that 'I am certain that people are saved in a Hospital who would have died in a palace from the fear of having recourse to [a] decisive plan of treatment'.[90] For Abernethy, therapeutic efficacy was, in part, the consequence of an abnegation of autonomy. This is not to say that hospital patients could be operated on without their consent. Rather, it implied that clinical *decisiveness* was a function of clinical *authority*, and that the patient who could be more easily persuaded might also be more easily saved.

Of course, we might see in Abernethy's remarks a kind of wry commentary on exactly the forms of emotional autonomy and agency that we have seen at work with Cooper's private patients. But this is not to say that hospital patients, and poorer patients generally, did not exercise their own agency when it came to negotiating surgical authority. For one thing, while admittance to a hospital like Guy's generally required the personal recommendation of a governor (except, that is, in the case of accidents, when patients were brought in off the street), many patients came into the hospital with a very distinct sense of what they wanted and expected from their treatment.[91] When Joseph Townend arrived at the Manchester Infirmary, for example, he managed to convince the

---

[87] Lee Davison, Tim Hitchcock, Tim Keirn, and Robert Shoemaker (eds), *Stilling the Grumbling Hive: The Response to Social and Economic Problems in England, 1689–1750* (New York: St Martin's Press, 1992); Donna Andrew, *Philanthropy and Police: London Charity in the Eighteenth Century* (Princeton: Princeton University Press, 1989).

[88] For example, see Roy Porter, 'The Gift Relation: Philanthropy and Provincial Hospitals in Eighteenth-Century England', in Roy Porter and Lindsay Granshaw (eds), *The Hospital in History* (London: Routledge, 1989), 149–78.

[89] Hogarth, 'Joseph Townend', p. 96. See Hitchcock, King, and Sharpe (eds), *Chronicling Poverty*.

[90] RCSE, MS0232/1/5, John Flint South, 'Lectures on Natural and Morbid Anatomy and Physiology, delivered by John Abernethy Esq. FRS in the Anatomical Theatre at St Bartholomew's Hospital in the years 1819 & 1820, Vol. 4th', f. 211.

[91] Roy Porter, 'Accidents in the Eighteenth Century', in Roger Cooter and Bill Luckin (eds), *Accidents in History: Injuries, Fatalities and Social Relations* (Amsterdam: Rodopi, 1997), 90–106.

surgeons to attend to his injured wrist, as well as attempt a 'risky and untested surgical procedure' to remedy the consequences of a childhood accident and sever the web of skin that attached his right arm to his side.[92] Astley Cooper's archive reveals similar examples of patient assertiveness. Thus, one of his casebooks notes that 'Mr Dixon of Newington Butts sent a young woman into the Hospital with a tumour in her breast which was unaccompanied with any signs of ill health and altho [sic] she was anxious for an operation I refused to perform it and she quitted the Hospital'. However, the woman returned a few months later 'with the swelling increased and I then made an opening into it and discharged several ounces of clear serum'.[93]

Leaving the hospital, either under treatment or in the face of an unsatisfactory response, constituted the most basic, and most extreme, exercise of patient agency. In 1819, for example, Cooper received an extensive report from the York surgeon James Atkinson (1759–1839) on the case of a young man with aneurysmal varix whose arm had to be amputated. Atkinson reported that his patient was 'detained rather longer in York than he would have wished, to keep him under subjection (being a sort of sailor) and to insure the firm cicatrisation of the wound'. The man had spent nearly two weeks in York County Hospital and, while his identity as free-roaming, free-living Jack Tar evidently required him to be kept under especially close observation, it also militated against him staying put. Hence, he 'was very desirous (in his own terms) "to slip his cable" some days before he was permitted' and he 'left York in good plight on the 27th of the month'.[94]

Atkinson remarked that this patient left hospital 'with more grateful feelings upon the occasion, than might have been expected from the discipline he had received from his doctors'.[95] As such comments suggest, this case provides a revealing insight into the dynamics of patient agency. This young man had fallen 'near twenty feet from the top of a Vessel that was going to be launched, and injured his head and back'. After the accident he was bled by a surgeon but 'in a very inconvenient situation, in a bad light, and with the left hand'.[96] Thereafter his arm began to swell and he was taken to the County Hospital, where it was determined that he had developed an aneurysm and that 'an operation appeared to be the only recourse'. As Atkinson explained:

It became necessary now, as a crisis drew nigh, to enter into some explanation with the patient and his mother, as to the nature, consequence and relief of the complaint. They had been taught to apprehend that it was possible an operation might be required.

---

[92] Hogarth, 'Joseph Townend', pp. 97–8.   [93] RCSE, MS0008/2/1/7, unpaginated.
[94] RCSE, MS0008/2/2/3 pt. 2, James Atkinson, 'Case of Aneurysmal Varix, operation and subsequent amputation', f. 25.
[95] RCSE, MS0008/2/2/3 pt. 2, Atkinson, 'Aneurysmal Varix', f. 26.
[96] RCSE, MS0008/2/2/3 pt. 2, Atkinson, 'Aneurysmal Varix', f. 1.

And to this expedient, they were not much averse; but they had somehow attached the idea, that it could be performed on one day, and entire recovery take place on the next. Our prospects however were by no means so flattering. And Mr Saunders and myself endeavoured to set them right in this particular. A very sensible and a very firm question was put to us, whether, after the operation, there might not possibly be still a necessity for amputation. We replied that it was an event intended to be prevented, but that we could not pledge ourselves to answer for the success.[97]

Clearly, then, even within the context of hospital treatment, such procedures were subject to serious negotiation, with the patient and his mother making 'very firm', yet also 'very sensible', inquiries as to the nature of the operation and its chance of success. It was, as Atkinson explained, 'On these grounds [that] we started'. Unfortunately, the operation proved problematic. 'Those parts under the skin were very irritable' and the pain was such that it was 'scarcely supportable by the patient', even though he was 'a hardy man and bred up in pitch and tar'. After the operation, he suffered restless nights and was 'flushed, hot and feverish, with a pulse above one hundred'. Subsequently, ecchymosis appeared on his elbow and gangrene began to set in. During this time, Atkinson notes:

We had frequent occasion to chide him, for removing the arm out of the favourable position, in which we left it after the dressing. He was ill nursed by his mother, and was wilful and bad to manage, and would suffer his arm to get laid under him or in a descending posture, notwithstanding he was requested to avoid it.[98]

Eventually it was decided that, because of the spread of gangrene, 'all chance of saving his limb was over', and 'with his consent it was agreed to amputate'. His recovery, however, was good; his arm 'healed very well' and he was eventually able to leave the hospital, albeit somewhat earlier than his attendants would have liked.[99] Atkinson's patient was evidently a 'wilful' man and, on occasion, 'bad to manage'. He entered hospital as an object of charity, but was by no means entirely submissive to surgical 'discipline'. Indeed, he appears to have given full expression to his feelings, including irritation, despondency, and impatience. Having said that, even if he was a less compliant and agreeable patient than Townend, he likewise left hospital in accordance with the social expectation of gratitude for his treatment.

This case provides a point of entry into a number of issues relating to the agency of poorer patients, both within and without the walls of the hospital. For one thing, the involvement of the patient's mother (by whom he was apparently 'ill-nursed') suggests that parents and other relatives could exert as much

[97] RCSE, MS0008/2/2/3 pt. 2, Atkinson, 'Aneurysmal Varix', ff. 6–7.
[98] RCSE, MS0008/2/2/3 pt. 2, Atkinson, 'Aneurysmal Varix', ff. 7, 11, 12, 15.
[99] RCSE, MS0008/2/2/3 pt. 2, Atkinson, 'Aneurysmal Varix', ff. 16, 23, 25.

influence in these cases as in those of wealthier, fee-paying patients. Henry
Robert Oswald's diary records his interaction with the 'poor father' of a 'boy
with a Diseased Leg'. '[W]hen I told him the probability of its being necessary
to amputate the leg', Oswald recounts, 'he was very averse to such a thing and
said it was shocking to do so and that he would rather see the boy go to the
grave'. In response, Oswald told him it was 'more shocking to see a fine boy
die for want of assistance and that many a man and these great men were alive
and well after the operation useful to themselves and Society'. However, while
he apparently 'saw the force of Reason [...] prejudice prevailed' and the father,
who claimed that 'he had never used a dose of medicine in his life', refused the
operation, leaving the boy to an uncertain fate.[100]

Relatives could also resist surgical authority in other ways. For example,
Abernethy told his students about one of his former hospital patients at St
Bartholomew's who had a sore on his leg and whose 'nervous system was
extremely wrong'. When the patient eventually died, Abernethy was 'very
anxious to examine the body'. As we shall see in Chapter 5, at the time of this
lecture (1818), British surgeons had no legal right to the bodies of those who
died under their care, and yet they were acutely aware of the system that had
been established in France, whereby pathological anatomy had become rou-
tinised in hospitals, something that, they argued, had enabled Paris to become
the leading centre for clinical education in the world.[101] By contrast, men
like Abernethy were reliant upon the compliance of relatives in order to gain
access to such bodies for the purpose of post-mortem dissection. In this case,
he claimed 'a little turn against who called herself his relation would not allow
me', adding 'A very wrath I was in with her'.[102] Abernethy's frustration was
shared by Thomas Paget junior (1796–1875), Honorary Surgeon to Leicester
Royal Infirmary, who, in October 1832, wrote to Cooper to provide an 'unsatisfactory account of the late Mrs Slater' who 'sank rapidly on her return to
Leicester and died suddenly' of breast cancer. '[O]f the internal appearances I
could not prevail upon the friends to allow me examination', he lamented, for
'there is much contradict [sic] feeling and of course obstinacy in these parts'.[103]

[100] NLS, MS9003, Diary of H. R. Oswald Snr, describing his first six months as surgeon to the
4th Duke of Atholl, Governor General of the Isle of Man (1812–13), ff. 65v–66r.
[101] John Harley Warner, 'The Idea of Science in English Medicine: The "Decline of Science" and
the Rhetoric of Reform, 1815–45', in French and Wear (eds), British Medicine, 136–64.
[102] RCSE, MS0232/1/1, John Flint South, 'Lectures on the Principles of Surgery delivered by
John Abernethy Esq. FRS in the Anatomical Theatre at St Bartholomew's Hospital in the
years 1818 and 1819', ff. 153–5.
[103] RCSE, MS0008/2/19, Letter from Thomas Paget junior to Astley Cooper, 25 October 1832.
This was just after the passage of the Anatomy Act, but even so the relatives still had the right
to retain the body. It may, however, have contributed to public 'obstinacy' on the subject of
anatomical dissection. See Chapter 5.

In addition to demanding treatment or leaving the hospital, another form of patient agency was to refuse particular forms of treatment. This was not an uncommon occurrence. As we have heard, the disciplinary cultures of the hospital, as well as the paucity of other options available to them, may have encouraged poor patients to acquiesce to an operation that, had they more money and more autonomy, they might have declined. Nonetheless, as we have also heard, therapeutic treatment within the hospital still required a degree of negotiation, and patients were at liberty to determine their treatment, albeit within more limited parameters than were available to private patrons within the 'medical marketplace'.[104] Thus, one of Cooper's casebooks records that a man named 'Goodfellow was admitted into Guys with a bad compound fracture of the Elbow Joint [...] He was strongly urged to submit to the Operation of Amputation but positively refused'. In this case the patient's decision seems to have paid off, as 'The most simple treatment was pursued [...] The wound healed kindly and the man recovered'.[105] In another instance, the patient's reticence to submit met with a more ambivalent response. The surgeon Robert Cook of Gainsborough, Lincolnshire, wrote to Cooper in May 1831 informing him that 'At length I [will] send you the Tumour from Miss Davenport's breast – it is a good deal shrivelled from having become dry before it was put in spirit'. Its excision, he observed, 'left a large Chasm which it was impossible to bring together either by sutures or straps'. However, he did not specify how Davenport was persuaded to agree to the procedure, saying only that 'she would not have it removed' and that 'she bore the operation very ill although it was of short duration not 2 minutes'.[106]

Even if patients did not directly refuse treatment, they might nonetheless prove challenging to surgical authority, particularly by means of their behaviour on the wards. In Cooper's casebooks this seems to have been an especial problem for those patients who were brought into the hospital having suffered an accident, many of whom were drunk, disruptive, or otherwise 'bad to manage'. Early in his career, for example, he attended a 'young man' who was admitted to St Thomas' Hospital having 'received a violent blow from another on the left side of his head'. 'There was a wildness & irrationality about the Patient', Cooper notes, 'wh[ich] Mr C[line] suspected arose from his having been intoxicated & wh[ich] was proved to have been the case afterwards for

---

[104] On the concept of medical patronage, see Nicholas D. Jewson, 'Medical Knowledge and the Patronage System in 18th Century England', *Sociology* 8:3 (1974), 369–85. For its ambivalent relation to the social historical concept of the 'medical marketplace', see Mark S. R. Jenner and Patrick Wallis, 'Introduction', in Jenner and Wallis (eds), *Medicine and the Market in England and Its Colonies, c.1450–c.1850* (Basingstoke: Palgrave Macmillan, 2007), 1–23.

[105] RCSE, MS0008/2/1/7, unpaginated.

[106] RCSE, MS0008/2/2/3 pt. 3, Letter from Robert Cook to Astley Cooper, 28 May 1831.

soon after he became sick & vomited up a considerable quantity of superfluous liquor of some kind'.[107] As this example suggests, cases of intoxication
were particularly problematic when accompanied by injuries to the head, as
the symptoms were often hard to distinguish from delirium. John Abernethy
told his students of the case of a woman who had her 'skull knocked in with a
cane on Blackfriars Bridge'. 'I closed the scalp as well as I could', he claimed,
'and laid on a compress to give support to the Dura Mater – but I could not
make out whether the symptoms were those of Concussion, Compression or
Drunkenness'. '[S]he was stupid enough', he continued, 'but did not appear
insensible for she howled at the operation very much'. The next day she
refused to let the dresser touch her head, but did consent to Abernethy inspect-
ing her wound. Thus, he concluded, she 'had been nothing more than drunk
for she had a perfect recollection of my having performed the operation upon
her'.[108] If this patient's drunkenness made her more expressive in the operating
theatre, Cooper gives an account where the opposite was the case. 'A Woman
was brought into Guys Hospital completely intoxicated', he notes, 'and with
much injury done to her leg by a compound fracture [so] that an amputation
was deemed necessary and was performed':

She was totally insensible to pain during its performance – but the following day when
she was expected to be recovered from her intoxication her senses seemed imperfect
her memory had failed her and it was with great difficulty she could be made to believe
that her Leg was removed – She continued in a sort of Stupor for several weeks – her
stump looked well yet her wit was disturbed – she had much pain & at length death
ensued.[109]

This case raises the question of how much consent was involved in the decision to amputate her leg. Clearly, Cooper determined that her injuries were life
threatening and that an operation could not wait for her to regain her sobriety.
Such issues of consent and coercion were especially difficult to navigate in
the case of patients who, through either illness or injury, were deemed to be
'deranged'. In one case, for example, Cooper attended a man who was injured
in the collapse of a house, which had fractured his leg and left him disordered
in his senses. 'When I saw him […] he was extremely restless and talked incessantly, yet he knew his Wife', Cooper noted: 'He layed [sic] for 4 or 5 minutes
as if dead and would then suddenly start and commit the greatest violence'.[110]
In another instance, a 37-year-old patient called John Smith was admitted to
Guy's Hospital with a tumour in his elbow. He 'suffered great pain' after the
operation, Cooper recorded, and at six in the evening he 'suddenly rose from

---

[107] RCSE, MS0008/2/1/1, Cases in Surgery, Volume 1 (1788), 'Case 4th', ff. 6–7.
[108] RCSE, MS0232/1/5, f. 107.   [109] RCSE, MS0008/2/1/4, 'Case 24th', f. 63.
[110] RCSE, MS0008/2/1/3, Cases in Surgery, Volume 3 (1790–1), 'Case 4th', f. 6.

his bed, to quit as he said the hospital, and return home. He earnestly desired the removal of the ligatures, convinced that the blood was obstructed in its course, talked in an unconnected manner about his family and appeared to labour under mental aberration'. Four hours later he was 'much the same' and refused a request 'to remove to another ward'. Eventually he 'was removed by force to Isaac's [ward] and an opiate draft given by Compulsion'. According to 'The person who accompanied him to Town', he was deranged, and thus required 'Coercion'. For the next few days he continued to be as 'bad as ever, calling aloud, sitting up in bed, and using the arm used [sic] in the operation roughly'. However, his mind was soon 'reconciled' by a visit from his brother and he remained in Guy's for another month, until he 'Went away, his Intentions being unknown'.[111]

Lest it appear that patient agency and subjectivity on the wards of the hospital merely involved resistance to surgical authority, or disruptive and challenging forms of behaviour, it is important to note that the archive also provides evidence of emotional communion and tenderness between hospital patients and their attendants. Although less evident than in the extensive and often expressive correspondence between surgeons and their private patients, such feelings were also an important aspect of the dynamic of institutional care. In Stuart Hogarth's account of Joseph Townend's stay at the Manchester Infirmary, for example, he points out the deep affection that Townend had for a number of the practitioners and students who attended him and 'whose unmistakable tokens of real kindness I shall never forget'.[112] Meanwhile, in reference to the St Bartholomew's patient whose body he was 'anxious' to examine, Abernethy remarked that he was 'a very good hearted and good tempered man, for when I had done dressing him, I used to sit down and we told one another stories'.[113] Moreover, in an especially poignant instance, the young Astley Cooper recorded the case of a 13- or 14-year-old boy who fell from a scaffold, fracturing his skull and driving pieces of bone 'into the substance of the brain'. He lost all sense and movement in his right side, accompanied by 'very painful sensations'. In his distress, 'He was often supplicating the nurse to rub his arm with her hand'. Sadly, he was to die less than five weeks after the accident.[114]

Resistance to surgical authority was not always a conscious or calculated act. Even in those instances where patients acquiesced to the surgeon's directions and were, to all intents and purposes, a model of good behaviour, the nature of pre-anaesthetic surgery meant that willpower alone did not necessarily make

[111] RCSE, MS0008/2/2/3 pt. 1, unpaginated case, 'Aneurism from Bleeding'.
[112] Hogarth, 'Joseph Townend', p. 99.   [113] RCSE, MS0232/1/1, f. 154.
[114] RCSE, MS0008/2/1/1, 'Case 8th', ff. 15–17.

one a good operative subject. In the final section of this chapter, we shall therefore explore the issue of nervous irritability and its role in shaping the concept of the 'obstreperous' surgical patient.

'Obstreperous' Patients and 'Bad Stumps': Irritability and Unconscious Resistance

The title of this chapter makes a distinction between conscious and unconscious forms of patient agency. It is important to acknowledge, however, that Romantic conceptions of the unconscious differed somewhat from modern ones. The notion of the unconscious as a constituent of the psyche that is inaccessible to the conscious mind and is the seat of various mental processes, including phobias, desires, and drives, is largely, though not exclusively, the product of Sigmund Freud (1856–1939).[115] However, in the Romantic period, idealist philosophers such as Friedrich Schelling (1775–1854) and Samuel Taylor Coleridge were developing notions of the transcendent mind that would shape later concepts of the unconscious, while by the 1830s and 1840s, physiologists such as Marshall Hall (1790–1857) and Thomas Laycock (1812–76) had established the basis for the autonomic nervous system, whereby bodily processes, even bodily actions, might take place without wilful intent.[116] For the earlier part of the Romantic period, namely 1790–1830, the term unconscious, though often used in the same manner as 'insensible' (and implying a *loss* of consciousness), is less frequently used to describe actions outside of conscious volition. Nonetheless, such meanings were clearly inchoate, for one of the earliest uses of the term in *The Lancet* concerns a man suffering from a severe injury to the head who is described as having 'unconsciously pass[ed] his evacuations'.[117]

Moreover, by invoking the concept of unconscious agency (or resistance), I want to suggest more than merely unwilled actions; I want to approach something closer to Bruno Latour's reading of object agency. For Latour, everything within the network of relations has agency, including non-humans and inanimate objects. These objects have agency because they interact with humans

---

[115] For a classic account of the 'discovery' of the modern unconscious, and of the contribution of individuals other than Freud, see Henri F. Ellenberger, *The Discovery of the Unconscious: The History and Evolution of Dynamic Psychiatry* (New York: Basic Books, 1970).

[116] Sean J. McGrath, *The Dark Ground of Spirit: Schelling and the Unconscious* (London: Routledge, 2013); Alan Richardson, *British Romanticism and the Science of the Mind* (Cambridge, UK: Cambridge University Press, 2001); Edwin Clarke and L. S. Jacyna, *Nineteenth-Century Origins of Neuroscientific Concepts* (Berkeley: University of California Press, 1987). Laycock was himself heavily influenced by German idealist philosophy, particularly that of Johann Gottlieb Fichte (1762–1814). See Michael Brown, *Performing Medicine: Medical Culture and Identity in Provincial England, c.1760–1850* (Manchester: Manchester University Press, 2011), pp. 193–4.

[117] *Lancet* 6:137 (15 April 1826), p. 93.

and can often frustrate, obstruct, or otherwise shape their actions.[118] While, of course, surgical patients were not merely objects, their agency did transcend the level of conscious action and wilful intent. Surgical bodies are always, in a sense, sites of resistance, in that they can defy cure, or 'behave' in ways that confound the wishes of both the surgeon and the patient. In the pre-modern and pre-anaesthetic period, these tendencies were all the more marked, and surgical bodies frequently proved extremely difficult to manage, both inside and outside of the operating theatre.

In this regard, one of the most important concepts in early nineteenth-century surgical thought was that of 'irritability'. This idea originated in the mid-eighteenth-century work of the vitalist physician Albrecht von Haller, who regarded irritability in reaction to stimuli to be one of the defining characteristics of muscular fibres (as opposed to nervous fibres, whose key characteristic was sensibility). Haller's conception of irritability thus provided a rationale (prior to the autonomic nervous system) for why the muscles of the heart functioned without direct conscious input.[119] But for surgeons of the early nineteenth century, the language of irritability expanded to encompass a range of other concepts, notably *irritation*, characterised by inflammation and caused by disease or operative intervention, as well as the influence of the nervous system and the patient's state of mind.[120] As we saw in Chapter 2, these concepts were linked by another of Haller's ideas, namely sympathy, so that each could affect the other. Thus, Astley Cooper spoke of irritability (mediated by sympathy) in terms of a 'stone in the bladder' causing 'pain in the extremity of the penis', or a 'disease of the liver' causing 'pain the shoulder'.[121] Likewise, he claimed that 'Persons affected by cancerous or fungous complaints are of exceedingly anxious minds (at least nine times in ten)' and that 'this anxiety occasions a sort of irritable fever, that invariably proves detrimental'.[122] In this way, irritability shaped the patient as a deeply unstable entity, composed of complex and interdependent bodily and mental relations that always threatened to confound the best efforts of the surgeon. At the same time, however, and as Cooper's reference to cancer patients suggests, irritability (or irritation) also came to describe a kind of constitutional state or personal idiosyncrasy. Thus, as he told his students, 'Constitutional irritation will be very different; that is, much greater in some persons than in others, so that a wound, which in

[118] Bruno Latour, *Reassembling the Social: An Introduction to Actor-Network Theory* (Oxford: Oxford University Press, 2005), pp. 63–86.
[119] Hubert Steinke, *Irritating Experiments: Haller's Concept and the European Controversy on Irritability and Sensibility, 1750–90* (Amsterdam: Rodopi, 2005).
[120] For example, see Benjamin Travers, *An Inquiry Concerning That Disturbed State of the Vital Functions Usually Denominated Constitutional Irritation* (London: Longman, Rees, Orme, Brown, and Green, 1827).
[121] *Lancet* 1:2 (12 October 1823), p. 37.   [122] *Lancet* 1:3 (19 October 1823), p. 75.

one man would be attended by the most dangerous consequences, would not probably in another [...] diminish a single ordinary function'.[123]

In this way, patients, through no fault of their own, could be denominated as more or less easy to manage in terms of treatment and operative intervention. Cooper's archive provides an insight into this process, as well as into the complex relationship between concepts. In his notes, for example, he opined that 'Irritability is greatest in the young' before adding that 'it is the power of being excited to action – Irritation is the effect of Irritants on the Irritability'.[124] Elsewhere we can see the ways in which the concept of irritability shaped perceptions of patients. For example, concerning one of his male hospital patients he wrote that '32 hours after his admission he became extremely irritable, restless and quick in all his motions'.[125] In reference to a female patient, he observed that 'She keeps her bed generally. The least noise or talking excites pain, so does agitation of mind. She is very irritable'.[126] Likewise, in the case of another female patient, Cooper recorded that one of his colleagues 'amputated the Leg of a Girl who possessed wonderful Irritability both of body and mind particularly the latter'.[127]

It would be a mistake to infer from these examples that there was a starkly gendered aspect to the concept of irritability, for men were just as likely to be regarded as irritable as women. What is clear, however, is the link between irritability, mental states, and occasionally obstreperous behaviour. When taken together, the concepts of irritability and anxiety can be said to have provided the fundamental logic for the ontological and epistemological 'messiness' of the pre-anaesthetic operative subject, accounting for the uncertainties that surrounded the success or failure of a procedure. But irritability also took on a kind of moral aspect, determining the forms of treatment a patient might receive and defining certain individuals as difficult or troublesome. This is particularly evident in descriptions of operative practice. For example, in 1824, *The Lancet* reported on the case of William Rose, an 18-year-old man of 'scrophulous [sic] habit' with 'dark hair, dark grey eyes and a saturnine complexion'. Since childhood, he had been afflicted with a disease of the knee joint, which had ultimately required amputation. However, the procedure had not been a total success and, even after the passage of eight years, 'the patient [...] loudly complains of the result of the operation'. The stump was extremely irritable and 'the least touch, however slight, [was] sufficient to excite the most excruciating sensation'. A second operation was therefore carried out, but not, according to the report,

[123] *Lancet* 1:2 (12 October 1823), p. 40.   [124] RCSE, MS0008/2/1/7, unpaginated.
[125] RCSE, MS0008/2/1/3, 'Case 5th', f. 9.
[126] RCSE, MS0008/2/2/3 pt. 1, unpaginated case of 'Internal Aneurism'.
[127] RCSE, MS0008/2/1/3, unpaginated case notes.

without some difficulty, in consequence of the extreme irritability of the stump [...] and partly from the obstreperous conduct of the patient [...] that fortitude which induced him to solicit an operation, and which supported him when placed on the table, forsook him in an instant, on the first touch of the knife. His motions, which were almost convulsive at this period, seriously endangered the fingers of the operator.[128]

In this case, the author of the report stated that the patient's conduct in the operating theatre 'may be readily excused', perhaps because of the extreme constitutional upheaval occasioned by his previous amputation.[129] Even so, his irritability still served to construct him as difficult, the kind of patient to 'loudly complain'. Moreover, in other instances, the links between obstreperous conduct and moral judgement were even more explicit. For example, in 1829 *The Lancet* reported on the case of Michael Graeme, a 31-year-old man who had injured himself falling from scaffolding and who was brought into Westminster Hospital. Drawing on a set of established ethnic stereotypes about over-emotionality and ungovernability, the report noted that 'The patient was an Irishman, obstreperous in his complaints, and very much impeded by his cries and struggles, the diagnostic examination'.[130]

It is within the context of such *misbehaviour* that we might gain a greater understanding of the concept of operative fortitude that we highlighted earlier in this chapter. As we suggested, the language of fortitude was positively ubiquitous in those cases reported in *The Lancet* where the severity of the procedure was matched by the stoicism of the patient. This language not only served as a shorthand for myriad instances of personal resolve, it also shaped a vision of the idealised operative patient, one who was both bodily acquiescent and emotionally self-controlled, the opposite of William Rose, or John Abernethy's patient who, when undergoing a lithotomy, 'exhibited great degrees of nervous irritation crying out "damn my hearties, now you have pull away my hearties"'.[131] In a mirroring of the expectation of calm resolve to which the surgeon himself was beholden, the patient who displayed the requisite degree of fortitude not only set a moral example, they also stood a better chance of recovery. Appearances could be deceptive, of course. In 1832, the surgeon John Scott (1799–1846) of the London Hospital excised a tumour from the face of a 45-year-old man, removing the whole superior maxillary bone. According to the report, 'The patient throughout behaved with the most stoical fortitude'. On being asked by the surgeon 'whether he suffered much during the operation', he smiled, saying that he would 'tell [him] another time', before 'cheerfully' walking to his bed unaided, a display of sangfroid that was 'greeted with the hearty plaudits of all the spectators'. Despite such

[128] *Lancet* 1:19 (8 February 1824), pp. 190–1.   [129] *Lancet* 1:19 (8 February 1824), p. 191.
[130] *Lancet* 11:283 (31 January 1829), p. 575.   [131] RCSE, MS0232/1/5, f. 226.

positive indications, the author of the report noted that 'the patient is dead, having expired in convulsions'.[132] Such cases notwithstanding, the display of fortitude continued to be seen as both a moral and a practical good, with clear, though not unambiguous, links to gender and racial ideologies. Thus, an 1830 report from the Glasgow Royal Infirmary, published in *The Lancet*, warned against using 'the patient's feelings or manifestations of pain' as a measure for the appropriate amount of force necessary to reduce dislocations, observing:

In this hospital we often see hardy mountaineers, whether exposed to the lacerating extension by pulleys, or to the agonizing march of the knife through the living fibre, display a fortitude and composure, from a confidence in the surgeon and a command over their feelings, that, to a unreflecting spectator, would seem to augur deficient sensation […] But it is equally true, that another and a numerous class of patients, yell with apparent agony, on the slightest interference, even sometimes before it has commenced, or after it has terminated, clearly proving it to be the result of mental trepidation, or a deficiency of that animal *forte* or *bottom*, that so conspicuously characterises the former class of individuals.[133]

While this author clearly associated fortitude with the rugged masculinity of the Scottish Highlander, and while terms such as 'bottom' were often used to describe hyper-masculine figures like boxers, such gender associations were not uncomplicated, for just as men might prove as irritable as women, so too might women display as much resolve as men.[134] Indeed, according to some commentators, fortitude was a positively feminine trait; in 1834, the report of an operation undertaken at Guy's Hospital to remove the greater portion of the lower jaw of a 25-year-old servant named Maria Laler commented that the 'fortitude displayed by the patient was very great, and tended further to confirm the impression that females nearly always bear painful operations with greater courage and patience than men'.[135] And yet, as the century wore on, the discourse surrounding fortitude increasingly emphasised masculine values above all others. In 1843, for example, just three years before the first use of inhalation anaesthesia in Britain, the naval surgeon Richard Dobson (1773–1847) wrote to *The Lancet* stating that 'the fortitude of mind which is necessary to enable a patient to bear a surgical operation without making any exclamations of suffering can be produced through the mind only, without having recourse to either mesmerism or opium'. He then proceeded to provide examples of what James Kennaway has shown to be the cult of operative nonchalance

---

[132] *Lancet* 17:438 (21 January 1832), p. 604.   [133] *Lancet* 13:343 (27 March 1830), p. 927.
[134] David Day, '"Science", "Wind" and "Bottom": Eighteenth-Century Boxing Manuals', *International Journal of the History of Sport* 29:10 (2012), 1446–1465.
[135] *Lancet* 22:559 (17 May 1834), p. 285. For more on women and pain, see Bourke, *Pain*, pp. 206–14.

that attached to military personnel in this period.[136] As Kennaway argues, this military conception of fortitude had a significant racial dimension, with commentators establishing a moral hierarchy that placed either Anglo-Saxons or Highland Scots at the top, with the Irish below and non-white races occupying the lower tiers of the scale.[137] As the examples cited here suggest, such hierarchies also seem to have informed the perceptions of civilian surgeons.

For some commentators of this period, the moral force of emotional self-control was such that it was held to suppress symptoms that might otherwise be regarded as innate to a particular condition. In one remarkable instance, the Worcester physician and later founder of the Provincial Medical and Surgical Association (1832), Charles Hastings (1794–1866), told his colleagues of a case of rabies 'without parallel' in which 'the manly bearing and fortitude' of the patient 'raised his mind above fear and excluded the influence of prejudice'. According to Hastings, the case 'exhibits the action of the rabid poison on *a man* in its true colours, without the mimicry of feigned symptoms, or those aggravations of terror which too often lash and goad the unhappy patient into frenzy and madness'.[138]

Though by no means as extreme, the language surrounding the limbs of amputees likewise exhibits a somewhat moralistic tone. For the most part, patients were not held personally responsible for the irritability of their stumps. Certainly, there is little evidence of a discourse similar to that identified by Erin O'Connor in the aftermath of the American Civil War (1861–5), wherein the 'hysterical' irritability of the stump or the 'neurotic' delusions of the phantom limb actively feminised the male amputee.[139] Indeed, in his lecture on 'Bad and Irritable Stump[s]' delivered to the students of the North London Hospital in 1836, Robert Liston, like many of his contemporaries, expressed pity and sympathy for those patients whose stumps were the source of extreme pain and irritation. Liston was quite clear that the responsibility for this state of affairs lay with the surgeon, for it was his duty to 'proceed in a manner as to do away with all chance of these painful and distressing circumstances'. In particular, he urged his students to ensure that the bone was properly bisected and that the nerves did not 'become entangled in the scar'.[140] At the same time, however, the language of the 'bad stump' still served to cast some patients'

[136] *Lancet* 39:1012 (21 January 1843), p. 623; James Kennaway, 'Military Surgery as National Romance: The Memory of British Heroic Fortitude at Waterloo', *War & Society* 39:2 (2020), 77–92.
[137] James Kennaway, 'Celts under the Knife: Surgical Fortitude, Racial Theory and the British Army, 1800–1914', *Cultural and Social History* 17:2 (2020), 227–44.
[138] *Lancet* 14:363 (14 August 1830), p. 783.
[139] Erin O'Connor, *Raw Material: Producing Pathology in Victorian Culture* (Durham, NC: Duke University Press, 2000), pp. 106–11.
[140] *Lancet* 26:660 (23 April 1836), pp. 133–5.

bodies as obstructive and difficult. This was especially so because an irritable or 'bad' stump was often accompanied by mental despondency, so that the patient became complicit in their own decline. In one case this was almost literally true. Abernethy told his students of a patient who broke his leg while riding in Hyde Park and had to have it amputated. '[S]oon after the operation', he remarked, 'his Stomach and Bowels got wrong – his head became affected and he was delirious':

[O]n the third day, whilst the nurse was gone down stairs, she heard something go thump thump thump about the drawing room which was on the same floor, with that in which he slept, and in running up stairs found that he had got out of bed and was hopping about, and she was just in time to catch him by his shirt to prevent his jumping out of [the] window.[141]

According to Abernethy, such delirium was not uncommon because hectic fever was a marked feature of this condition, for which 'nothing can be done because the cause cannot be removed'; the fever was 'but a violent exertion of the Constitution' itself. Abernethy informed his students that 'Mr [John] Hunter [...] called this "a state of dissolution" [...] implying that all hope of relief is at an end'.[142] Indeed, while he maintained that patients could, in principle, recover, the prognosis was generally not good. This was particularly true of those who had suffered from a compound fracture. 'There have been a number of cases of compound fracture since I have been in this Hospital', he claimed, 'but they have all done well except where amputation has been performed, not a single case had a good stump and many died but God knows why'.[143]

Abernethy's confusion is suggestive. With no concept of post-operative infection in which the extruded bone of the compound fracture might introduce microbes into the body, surgeons like Abernethy were only able to account for the success or failure of such amputations by reference to constitutional irritability and mental anxiety. But we must not frame our explanations in such presentist terms. Rather, we must have recourse to what we have called the ontological 'messiness' of the pre-modern operative subject, in which a complex melding of constitutional, nervous, and emotional factors combined to determine a patient's fate. Within this framework, the concept of irritability provided a powerful way of thinking about the patient's capacities and susceptibilities and served to distinguish difficult patients from easier ones. While the discourse surrounding the notion of fortitude suggests that such ideas had a strong moral component, the patient could not always be held fully responsible for their failure to conform to the ideal. Sometimes their bodies simply resisted all attempts to save them. After all, even a 'good' patient might have a 'bad' stump.

---

[141] RCSE, MS0232/1/1, f. 242.
[142] RCSE, MS0232/1/1, f. 11.   [143] RCSE, MS0232/1/1, f. 241.

Conclusion

This chapter has been concerned to recover the patient's voice in the articulation of experience, demonstrating how emotions played a vital role in their dealings with surgeons. At the same time, it has shown how patients, like surgeons, were often expected to conform to certain idealised forms of behaviour, be that the gratitude of the hospital patient or the stoic fortitude of the operative subject. While manuscript archives such as those of Astley Cooper provide an extremely valuable insight into the patient's account of their own condition, the fact remains that their experience of disease, injury, and operative surgery was often mediated by the representations of others, be that medical attendants, family members, medical journalists, or surgeons themselves. In this sense, it is often difficult, not to say futile, to attempt to disentangle lived experience from cultural and representational conventions. This ambiguity is powerfully evident in the case of a Chinese labourer by the name of Hoo Loo, who came to London in 1831 to have a large tumour removed from his groin (Figure 3.1). As Peter Stanley observes, Hoo Loo's case is 'unusually well-documented'.[144] This was in large part because of his exotic appeal at a time of heightened Orientalist interest in China, as well as the sheer size of his growth. The operation to remove Hoo Loo's tumour was undertaken by Charles Aston Key (1793–1849), Astley Cooper, and Thomas Callaway (1791–1848) at Guy's Hospital in front of some 680 spectators, and was reported in *The Lancet*. Initially, the surgical team had proposed to retain the patient's genitals but, after complications arising from the length of the procedure (it lasted over an hour and three-quarters), it was decided that they should be 'sacrificed'. By this time, however, it was too late and 'the depressing effects of the operation' had begun to 'exhibit themselves'. Hoo Loo experienced serious blood loss and syncope, dying shortly after being removed from the table.[145]

What is remarkable about *The Lancet*'s description of Hoo Loo is the way in which it cast him as a model patient and an object of great pity and sympathy. It consistently described him as a man of 'amiable' character, his countenance occasionally melancholic but mostly 'very cheerful and good-tempered'. It reported that he had become a 'great favourite' with the Guy's Hospital nurses and that his death 'elicited the utmost commiseration' and 'perhaps a few tears'. Moreover, in its description of the operation itself, Hoo Loo was cast as a model of moral fortitude and, ultimately, Romantic sublimity:

The fortitude with which this great operation was approached, and throughout undergone, by Hoo Loo, was, if not unexampled, at all events never exceeded in the annals of surgery. A groan now and then escaped him, and now and then a slight exclamation, and

---

[144] Stanley, *Pain*, pp. 262–3.   [145] *Lancet* 16:398 (16 April 1831), pp. 86–8.

POOR HOO LOO AND HIS TUMOUR.   89

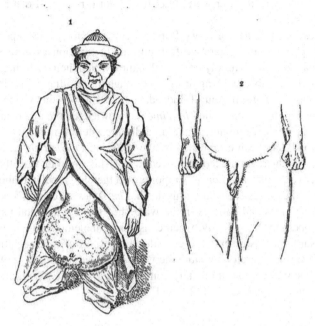

Figure 3.1 'Poor Hoo Loo and His Tumour', *The Lancet* 16:398 (16 April 1831), p. 89. Public Domain Mark

we thought we could trace in his tones a plaintive acknowledgement of the hopelessness of his case. Expression of regret too, that he had not rather borne with his affliction than suffered the operation, seemed softly but rapidly to vibrate from his lips as he closed his eyes, firmly set his teeth and resignedly strung every nerve in obedience to the determination with which he had first submitted to the knife.[146]

There is only one problem with this account. Hoo Loo did not speak any English; neither did *The Lancet*'s reporter, nor any of the surgical attendants, understand a word of his native Cantonese. In the absence of an intelligible voice, *The Lancet* therefore created one for him. The reality of his situation was, however, somewhat more complex, and certainly less picturesque, than *The Lancet*'s report suggested. As Stanley points out, nearly two weeks after the operation *The Times* carried a report from an eyewitness to the event who understood 'the Chinese language' and claimed that what Ho Loo had actually said during the course of the procedure was '"Unloose me,

---

[146] *Lancet* 16:398 (16 April 1831), pp. 86–8.

unloose me! Water! Help! Water! Let me go!"', and that the 'last articulate sounds he was heard to utter were, "Let it be – let it remain! I can bear no more! Unloose me!"'[147]

The Times therefore gave a very different account of Hoo Loo's experience, suggesting, perhaps, that operative fortitude might function as a means by which the patient was culturally contained and by which their sufferings were rendered more palatable by being refracted through the familiar cultural tropes of pathos and personal self-control. Indeed, so powerful was this vision of the Romantic patient that even while *The Times* acknowledged the agony and terror of Hoo Loo's final minutes, it could hardly present him in any other way than that which had been established by the reporting of *The Lancet*. Hence, it concluded its distressing account by reaffirming his 'mild and gentle manners'. Moreover, while *The Lancet*'s reporter had merely speculated about the possibility of the nurses crying after his death, *The Times* stated it as a positive fact that the 'nurses and patients in the ward shed tears at the fatal termination of the operation'.[148] Clearly, when considering the emotional cultures of Romantic surgery, it is essential to consider the politics of representation. In Chapter 4, we shall therefore explore the ways in which the language of emotion shaped, sustained, and ultimately complicated *The Lancet*'s reporting of London hospital surgery in the 1820s and 1830s.

---

[147] *Times* 19 April 1831, p. 3.   [148] *Times* 19 April 1831, p. 3.

4   'Scenes of Cruelty and Blood'
Emotion, Melodrama, and the Politics of Romantic
Surgical Reform

Introduction

In July 1824, an anonymous correspondent wrote to *The Lancet* to express his concern about the manner in which operations were being conducted at the Borough hospitals of Guy's and St Thomas' in London. 'When the fiat of an hospital surgeon has determined a patient to an operation', he began, 'the space of time from that moment to the moment of his conveyance to the theatre must be a time of increasing anxiety and distress'. As we have seen, the ordeal of surgery in this period often required considerable mental preparation, and this delay could therefore range from hours to days, even weeks. However, as this correspondent observed, 'such anxious expectation, such painful agitation, must [...] disturb [the body's] functions and render it more unfit for the operation'. Hence it was the duty of the surgeon to 'make this anxious interval as short as possible'. Yet if the period of waiting was fraught, it was of only 'minor importance' when compared to the emotional trials of the operation itself:

Feverishly heated, and frequently very much exhausted by his previous sufferings, every additional moment, at this dreadful crisis, becomes to him an hour, and every additional moment that he continues under the torture of the different instruments, diminishes the chance of success and, of course, encreases [*sic*] the danger of his life.[1]

With this in mind, the correspondent was pained to recount an operation he had witnessed for the removal of a stone from the bladder of a young boy of about 8–10 years of age. Patients undergoing lithotomy, which was one of the most invasive and dangerous of pre-anaesthetic surgical procedures, first had to be 'sounded'. This involved the insertion of a metal probe through the urethra into the bladder in order to determine the presence and location of the stone (or 'calculus'). This was normally done well in advance, but for some reason the surgeon in this case, whose name the author thought it 'improper to mention', chose the 'dreadful moment' immediately prior to the operation to re-examine the boy. 'Unfortunately he could not feel the stone', he recalled, 'till after

[1] *Lancet* 2:42 (17 July 1824), p. 91.

149

trying in all directions, and putting the boy in excruciating pain for several minutes, he, at last, satisfied himself and gave the instrument into the hand of another surgeon, for further testimony'. This surgeon likewise had great difficulty in locating the calculus and so handed the sound to a third colleague. According to the correspondent:

These examinations occupied a full twenty minutes, during the whole of which time the boy continued screaming and was nearly exhausted before the operation commenced [...] Now a great part of this painful process might be, or ought to be, avoided. It is woeful to the patient, it is disgraceful to the surgeon.[2]

This letter was only one of many similar accounts of botched and bungled surgical procedures to appear in the pages of *The Lancet* in the first two decades of its existence. As we have seen in the opening chapters of this book, operations in this period were a carefully calibrated performance, frequently subject to quasi-public scrutiny from students and fellow practitioners. Surgeons were not only expected to operate effectively and competently, but also, through a display of calm resolve, to exert a moral influence over their anxious patients. Failure to perform any of these tasks adequately could critically undermine one's reputation as an operative surgeon. However, while operative competence had long been subject to professional scrutiny, the 1820s witnessed a radical transformation, not only in the extent of this oversight, but also in its forms and functions. Shortly after its foundation in 1823 by the radical surgeon-turned-journalist (and later coroner and Member of Parliament) Thomas Wakley, *The Lancet* embarked on a campaign to 'expose' and 'censure' what it considered to be instances of surgical incompetence, particularly among those holding 'public office' at London's teaching hospitals. We shall explore the politics of this campaign in due course, but for our immediate purposes, what was perhaps most remarkable about it was the extent to which it was couched in a language of the emotions, characterised by frequent and vociferous expressions of anger, outrage, sympathy, and pity. The author of the letter with which we opened this chapter was clearly aware that he was participating in a wider radical and reformist discourse. He began by stating that 'As the principal object of the LANCET is to improve the medical and chirurgical practice, and [...] to ameliorate the condition, and to diminish the distress of the subjects of its operation; you may not, perhaps, think the following observations unworthy of insertion'.[3] And indeed, emotions played a vital role in his narrative. Drawing upon that intersubjectivity that, as we have seen, was a prominent feature of Romantic surgical culture, he effected a sympathetic engagement with the agonies of this child-patient, claiming that 'the

---

[2] *Lancet* 2:42 (17 July 1824), p. 92.   [3] *Lancet* 2:42 (17 July 1824), p. 91.

operation [...] was tedious and the effect of the whole upon my mind was distressing – What must it have been to the young sufferer?'[4]

Historians have long been aware of the importance of the early nineteenth-century movement for medical and surgical reform in the making of the modern medical profession.[5] They have likewise been alert to the role played by periodical publications, especially *The Lancet*, in shaping the ideologies and agendas of that movement.[6] For example, they have shown how *The Lancet* functioned as an intertextual space for the elaboration of the medical profession as an 'imagined community'.[7] By combining agenda-setting editorials with letters from practitioners, *The Lancet* allowed its contributors and readers to imagine themselves as participants in a collective endeavour, existing in a deep and extensive communion with others of whom they had little or no direct knowledge. Indeed, so powerful was its function in this respect that it encouraged the idea of a reforming consensus and unity of purpose where none existed.[8] As various scholars have shown, the movement for medical reform drew heavily on the broader cultures of early nineteenth-century political reform, echoing its appeals to meritocracy and attacks on institutional 'corruption' and 'tyranny'.[9] Moreover, recent work has drawn particular attention to

---

[4] *Lancet* 2:42 (17 July 1824), p. 92. The word 'tedious' is used here in its meaning of 'Wearisome by continuance; troublesome; irksome [...] Slow', rather than as a synonym for dull; Samuel Johnson, *A Dictionary of the English Language*, 4th ed., vol. 2 (1777), p. 1493.

[5] For example, Ivan Waddington, *The Medical Profession in the Industrial Revolution* (Dublin: Gill and Macmillan, 1984); Irvine Loudon, *Medical Care and the General Practitioner, 1750–1850* (Oxford: Clarendon, 1987); John Harley Warner, 'The Idea of Science in English Medicine: The 'Decline' of Science and the Rhetoric of Reform, 1815–45', in Roger French and Andrew Wear (eds), *British Medicine in an Age of Reform* (London: Routledge, 1991), 136–64; Ian Burney, 'Medicine in the Age of Reform', in A. Burns and J. Innes (eds), *Rethinking the Age of Reform: Britain, 1780–1850* (Cambridge, UK: Cambridge University Press, 2003), 163–81; Michael Brown, *Performing Medicine: Medical Culture and Identity in Provincial England, c. 1760–1850* (Manchester: Manchester University Press, 2011); Brown, 'Medicine, Reform and the "End" of Charity in Early Nineteenth-Century England', *English Historical Review* 124: 511 (2009), 1353–88.

[6] Mary Bostetter, 'The Journalism of Thomas Wakley', in Joel Howard Wiener (ed.), *Innovators and Preachers: The Role of the Editor in Victorian England* (London: Greenwood Press, 1985), 275–92; William F. Bynum and J. C. Wilson, 'Periodical Knowledge: Medical Journals and Their Editors in Nineteenth-Century Britain', in William F. Bynum, Stephen Lock, and Roy Porter (eds), *Medical Journals and Medical Knowledge: Historical Essays* (London: Routledge, 1992), 29–48; Jean Loudon and Irvine Loudon, 'Medicine, Politics and the Medical Periodical, 1800–50', in Bynum, Lock, and Porter (eds), *Medical Journals*, 49–69; Debbie Harrison, 'All the *Lancet*'s Men: Reactionary Gentleman Physicians vs. Radical General Practitioners in the *Lancet*, 1823–1832', *Nineteenth-Century Gender Studies* 5:2 (Summer 2009), www.ncgsjournal .com/issue52/harrison.html (accessed 15/10/21).

[7] Brown, 'Medicine'. See also Brown, *Performing Medicine*, pp. 159–60.

[8] Brown, 'Medicine', pp. 1379–80, 1382–3.

[9] Burney, 'Medicine'; Brown, 'Medicine'; Brown, '"Bats, Rats and Barristers": *The Lancet*, Libel and the Radical Stylistics of Early Nineteenth-Century English Medicine', *Social History* 39:2 (2014), 182–209.

the importance of literary style and discursive form in the articulation of this reforming agenda. Brittany Pladek, for example, has highlighted *The Lancet*'s links to the wider world of publishing, its early combination of miscellany and political invective resembling such journals as *Blackwood's Magazine*.[10] Meanwhile, other work has analysed *The Lancet*'s stylistic associations with radical publications such as the *Black Dwarf* and *Political Register*, the latter of whose editor, William Cobbett (1763–1835), was a profound early influence on Wakley. Like Cobbett, Wakley deployed literary devices such as ridicule and epithet, positively inviting the charge of libel, in an effort to 'align himself with the cultures of popular radicalism'.[11]

This account of the stylistics of *The Lancet* is grounded in a rich interdisciplinary literature on Romantic radicalism that has paid close attention to the importance of symbolism and language in political discourse.[12] This literature has shown how what James Epstein called 'radical expression' could be expressed through such forms as clothing and material culture, as well as through ritualised and embodied performances in courtrooms, taverns, or other public spaces.[13] The performative aspects of Romantic radicalism have highlighted the particularly strong interconnections between the theatrical and political cultures of the era. In the words of Boyd Hilton, 'if the theatre was political, it is equally true that politics was theatrical'.[14] Indeed, so deeply entwined were politics and the theatre in this period that, as Mike Sanders suggests, we might best think of them together 'in terms of both a "culture of politics" as well as a

---

[10] Brittany Pladek, '"A Variety of Tastes": *The Lancet* in the Early Nineteenth-Century Periodical Press', *Bulletin of the History of Medicine* 85:4 (2011), 560–586.

[11] Brown, '"Bats, Rats"', p. 185.

[12] Olivia Smith, *The Politics of Language, 1791–1819* (Oxford: Oxford University Press, 1984); Ian McCalman, *Radical Underworld: Prophets, Revolutionaries and Pornographers, 1795–1840* (Cambridge, UK: Cambridge University Press, 1988); James Epstein, *Radical Expression: Political Language, Ritual and Symbol in England, 1790–1850* (Oxford: Oxford University Press, 1994); Marcus Wood, *Radical Satire and Print Culture, 1790–1822* (Oxford: Oxford University Press, 1994); Kevin Gilmartin, *Print Politics: The Press and Radical Opposition in Early Nineteenth-Century England* (Cambridge, UK: Cambridge University Press, 1996); Peter Spence, *The Birth of Romantic Radicalism: War, Popular Politics and English Radical Reformism, 1800–1815* (Brookfield, VT: Scholar Press, 1996).

[13] Epstein, *Radical Expression*; Robert Poole, 'The March to Peterloo: Politics and Festivity in Late Georgian England', *Past and Present* 192 (2006), 109–53; Katrina Navickas, '"That Sash Will Hang You": Political Clothing and Adornment in England, 1780–1840', *Journal of British Studies* 49:3 (2010), 540–65; Navickas, *Protest and the Politics of Space and Place 1789–1848* (Manchester: Manchester University Press, 2016); Mary Fairclough, *The Romantic Crowd: Sympathy, Controversy and Print Culture* (Cambridge, UK: Cambridge University Press, 2013); Katie Barclay, *Men on Trial: Performing Emotion, Embodiment and Identity in Ireland, 1800–45* (Manchester: Manchester University Press, 2019); Ian Newman, *The Romantic Tavern: Literature and Conviviality in the Age of Revolution* (Cambridge, UK: Cambridge University Press, 2019).

[14] Boyd Hilton, *A Mad, Bad and Dangerous People? England, 1783–1846* (Oxford: Oxford University Press, 2006), p 33.

"politics of culture"'.[15] The theatrical mode that has received the greatest attention from historians and literary scholars of the Romantic era is melodrama, and the appeal of melodramatic forms to Romantic radicals has long been recognised. Patrick Joyce observes that 'the plot structure of melodrama concerned virtue extant, virtue eclipsed and expelled, virtue tested (in struggle), virtue apparently fallen, and virtue restored and triumphant', a narrative trajectory that resonated with 'the moral drama of an unequal society'.[16] Indeed, in her pioneering study *Melodramatic Tactics* (1995), Elaine Hadley proposes that melodrama 'seems to have served as a behavioural and expressive model for several generations of English people' throughout the nineteenth century.[17] These observations on the appeal of the 'melodramatic mode' have been developed and extended by scholars such as Robert Poole and Katherine Newey, so that we now have a rich understanding of the implications of melodramatic theatricality for late Georgian and early Victorian political discourse.[18]

Work on the radical stylistics of *The Lancet* makes brief mention of its melodramatic aspects, notably in relation to its affinities with the *Black Dwarf*.[19] However, this chapter takes the analysis of *The Lancet* and melodrama much further. As scholars have recognised, one of the characteristics of Romantic melodrama was its use of powerful emotions and its appeals to feeling; it was 'a mode of high emotionalism and stark ethical conflict' in which 'eyes were opened, hearts moved, conspiracy exposed and tyranny dissolved'.[20] Melodrama thus provides a revealing lens through which to analyse *The Lancet*'s campaign of radical surgical reform and within which to frame its use of a highly emotionalised discourse in the exposure of alleged surgical incompetence and corruption.

One of the reasons, perhaps, why the melodramatic mode held such appeal for Wakley and *The Lancet* in their campaign to reform the structures and hierarchies of metropolitan surgery was that, as we have seen, surgical practice

---

[15] Mike Sanders, 'The Platform and the Stage: The Primary Aesthetics of Chartism', in Peter Yeandle, Katherine Newey, and Jeffrey Richards (eds), *Politics, Performance and Popular Culture: Theatre and Society in Nineteenth-Century Britain* (Manchester: Manchester University Press, 2016), 44–58, at p. 44.

[16] Patrick Joyce, *Democratic Subjects: The Self and the Social in Nineteenth-Century England* (Cambridge, UK: Cambridge University Press, 1994), pp. 178, 189, quoted in Robert Poole, '"To the Last Drop of My Blood": Melodrama and Politics in Late Georgian England', in Yeandle, Newey, and Richards (eds), *Politics*, 21–43, at p. 22.

[17] Elaine Hadley, *Melodramatic Tactics: Theatricalized Dissent in the English Marketplace, 1800–1885* (Stanford: Stanford University Press, 1995), p. 3.

[18] Katherine Newey, 'Bubbles of the Day: The Melodramatic and the Pantomimic', in Yeandle, Newey, and Richards (eds), *Politics*, 59–74. Indeed, Rohan McWilliam identifies a 'melodramatic turn' in the scholarship, but warns against such a diffuse application that it risks losing its explanatory power: Rohan McWilliam, 'Melodrama and the Historians', *Radical History Review* 78 (2000), 57–84, at pp. 59–63, cited in Poole, '"Last Drop"', p. 22.

[19] Brown, '"Bats, Rats"', pp. 190–1.   [20] Poole, '"Last Drop"', p. 27.

was often not only highly emotional and intensely dramatic, but also deeply theatrical. As a form of rhetorical emplotment, therefore, melodrama, with its emphasis upon the suffering of the virtuous in the face of tyranny and cruelty, could be literally played out on the stage of the operating theatre, as the innocent object of charity writhed beneath the arrogant and cruel hand of surgical incompetence. By extension, such moral binaries could also serve to describe the professional and political situation of meritorious general practitioners oppressed by a corrupt and tyrannical surgical elite. However, the use of such an emotionally charged language, especially when harnessed to a campaign of radical scrutiny and personal, as well as structural, critique, was not without its discontents. As Sanders suggests of the somewhat later debates around Chartism, there was 'a definite anxiety that the theatrically effective must be politically suspect, precisely because it appeals to the emotions rather than to reason'.[21] This is not to suggest that emotion and reason were always counterposed as simple binary opposites, certainly not within Romantic political discourse. But what is nonetheless true is that *The Lancet*'s highly emotive language was productive of great debate and vociferous opposition concerning its propriety and its implications for surgical identities and reputations.

This chapter opens with an account of London surgery in the 1820s and 1830s, establishing the context for *The Lancet*'s campaign of radical reform. It then proceeds to consider the melodramatic mode in relation to *The Lancet*, exploring its emplotment of medical reform in terms of the moral binaries of tyrannical oppression and virtuous heroism. Meanwhile, the final section explores the particular stratagem of reporting and exposing examples of supposedly bungled operations performed at London's teaching hospitals. As well as demonstrating the rhetorical force of such melodramatic representations, it also considers the anxieties and complexities surrounding the use of emotive forms of radical critique within a conflictual world of inchoate professional norms.

The Politics of London Surgery

Before we turn to the issue of melodrama and radical style, it is necessary to provide some context as to the professional and political landscape of early nineteenth-century metropolitan surgery. It is important to note, from the beginning, that *The Lancet* considered itself to be a journal of national, even international, scope. It included regular reports on medical and surgical events in Scotland and Ireland, as well as communications from the Continent and beyond. It also had a broad readership (far larger than for any

---

[21] Sanders, 'Platform', p. 52.

other contemporary British medical journal) and, as argued elsewhere, was instrumental in shaping an imagined community of medicine that was, in many cases, deeply provincial.[22] And yet, in other respects *The Lancet* remained a resolutely metrocentric publication. Wakley was decidedly hostile to most things Scottish and Irish, claiming that there were 'few people under the sun, or the clouds, who have more exalted notions of their own physical, moral and intellectual pre-eminence than the Scotch' and asserting that his was 'the only English medical journal free from Scotch influence, and not subject to Scotch control'.[23] Wakley was equally disdainful of any initiative for reform that came from outside of London. In 1836, for example, he dismissed what he incorrectly, though probably not unintentionally, called the 'Provincial Medical Association' as a 'little knot of M.D.'s [*sic*]' composed of 'insignificant personages' whose demise 'cannot be protracted to a distant period'.[24] In this prediction he was mistaken, for the Provincial Medical and *Surgical* Association (to give it its full title) would, in 1856, change its name to the British Medical Association (BMA), under which designation it continues to serve as the principal professional association for British medicine. But in 1836 all this was far off and the failure of a small provincial venture seemed, in Wakley's eyes at least, to be inevitable. When it came to mass meetings of the profession, meetings that, as in the political realm, performed a powerful symbolic function in manifesting the 'body politic', Wakley claimed that they 'ought undoubtedly to be held *in London*', not only because they 'would secure the attendance of an assembly always four times as numerous as would be found in any other part of England', but also because London was 'the great centre of every important movement and transaction in the empire'.[25]

Such metrocentrism could, of course, be readily justified. Despite the ever-increasing importance of the provinces to the economic life of Britain, and despite the growing significance of provincialism as a distinct form of political (and medical) identity, London remained at the heart of national political and professional governance.[26] In the former case, London's status as capital was unrivalled; with the abolition of the Irish Parliament in 1800 its authority extended throughout the British Isles. In the latter instance, the picture was

---

[22] Brown, 'Medicine'; Brown, *Performing Medicine*, chs. 5 and 6.
[23] *Lancet*, 10:246 (17 May 1828), p. 211. All of this was before Wakley became friends with Robert Liston, as discussed in Chapter 1. Even after that, however, *The Lancet* continued to resist what it called the 'Scotch influence' in English medicine and surgery.
[24] *Lancet*, 27:686 (22 October 1836), p. 173.
[25] *Lancet*, 27:686 (22 October 1836), p. 173. Emphasis in original. For the political significance of mass meetings, see Navickas, *Protest*.
[26] For provincial political identities, see Simon Gunn, *The Public Culture of the Victorian Middle Class: Ritual and Authority in the English Industrial City, 1840–1914* (Manchester: Manchester University Press, 2000). For medical ones, see Brown, *Performing Medicine*.

more complex. Both Edinburgh and Glasgow had their own corporate structures, as did Dublin. Moreover, the capacity of the Royal College of Physicians
of London to regulate anything outside of the city and its immediate environs
was limited, while the Royal College of Surgeons of *London* only became the
Royal College of Surgeons of *England* in 1843.

At the same time, however, changes in medical and surgical training did
much to cement London's professional hegemony. As Susan Lawrence has
shown, the eighteenth and early nineteenth centuries saw the decline of traditional forms of surgical education and the rise of new ones. Since the medieval
period, aspirant surgeons had generally been trained by apprenticeship, a long-
term dyadic relationship in which young men served under a master, often living in his household for up to seven years, in order to learn the 'mysteries' of
their craft. During the eighteenth century this was increasingly supplemented,
and eventually superseded, by a system of 'pupillage', in which students paid
fees to attend surgical lectures and 'walk the wards' of the hospital for the
purposes of practical clinical instruction.[27] For some surgical pupils, especially
the privileged class known as dressers (who paid for the right to participate in
operations), this contractual relationship could very closely resemble apprenticeship, even if it did not require such intimate domestic arrangements.[28] For
others, however, a more ad hoc curriculum could be assembled through a mix-
and-match combination of lectures and practical instruction. This was a system of education that was recognised by the Court of Examiners of the Royal
College of Surgeons and formalised by the Apothecaries Act of 1815, which
stipulated the minimum number, and requisite types, of courses that a licentiate
must attend in order to be judged suitably qualified to practice.

In the absence, before the mid-nineteenth century at least, of suitably large
provincial hospitals, what all of this meant was that a growing number of surgical pupils were required to undertake a significant portion of their training
in the medical metropolises of Edinburgh and London. What it also meant
was that metropolitan hospitals, and their associated practitioners, assumed an
ever more central place within British surgery. According to Lawrence, 11,059
pupils signed up to walk London's hospital wards between 1725 and 1815. As
she argues, this not only 'embedded pupilage into the hospital economy' as
'pupils became sources of income for surgeons [...] and of free labour on the
wards', but it also 'confirmed and strengthened hospital men's prestige and

[27] Susan Lawrence, *Charitable Knowledge: Hospital Patients and Practitioners in Eighteenth-Century London* (Cambridge, UK: Cambridge University Press, 1996), ch. 4.
[28] Indeed, Margaret Pelling has suggested that such forms of training were simply apprentice-ship by another name: 'Managing Uncertainty and Privatising Apprenticeship: Status and Relationships in English Medicine, 1500–1900', *Social History of Medicine* 32:1 (2019), 34–56.

influence as the arbiters of medical knowledge'. 'Well before the eighteenth
century, staff physicians and surgeons had practiced publicly', she acknowledges, yet 'having increasing numbers of pupils on the wards extended hospital men's interpretations of disease and treatment to ever larger circles'.[29]

Other historians, notably Adrian Desmond and Carin Berkowitz, have
shown how the surgical-educational ecosystem of early nineteenth-century
London extended beyond the walls of the hospital to encompass new forms of
private teaching, such as the Great Windmill Street Anatomy School, founded
by William Hunter in 1767, or the Webb Street and Aldersgate Schools,
founded in 1819 and 1825, respectively.[30] Yet the reality was that such private ventures were often relatively short-lived and, while they challenged the
hegemony of the hospital schools, at least for a time, they were, if not exactly
parasitical, then certainly highly dependent on them. For one thing, they were
often geographically proximate, Webb Street being but a short walk from the
Borough hospitals of Guy's and St Thomas', and the Aldersgate School being
adjacent to St Bartholomew's. For another, they were generally established by
disappointed hospital men. Both Edward Grainger (1797–1824) and Frederick
Tyrrell (1793–1843) failed in their attempts to lecture at the United School
of Guy's and St Thomas', leading them to found, or help found, the Webb
Street and Aldersgate Schools.[31] In some cases, private teaching might even
act as a springboard to a hospital post. This was the case for Charles Bell,
whose purchase of a share of the Great Windmill Street School in 1811 was
followed by his appointment as surgeon to Middlesex Hospital in 1814, as
well as for Frederick Tyrrell and William Lawrence, whose short stints at the
Aldersgate School ended with them being appointed lecturers to St Thomas'
and St Bartholomew's, respectively.[32]

The rising importance of hospital teaching concentrated surgical wealth
and power in the hands of a relatively small group of men who, in turn,
wielded authority over the education and careers of a far larger body of students and junior practitioners. In 1828, Astley Cooper estimated that some
700 students studied surgery in the metropolis each year.[33] Most all of these
would, at some point, have been enrolled at one of the hospital schools that,
by the mid-1830s, consisted of St Bartholomew's, St Thomas' and Guy's

[29] Lawrence, *Charitable*, pp. 108, 110.
[30] Adrian Desmond, *The Politics of Evolution: Morphology, Medicine, and Reform in Radical London* (Chicago: Chicago University Press, 1989); Carin Berkowitz, *Charles Bell and the Anatomy of Reform* (Chicago: Chicago University Press, 2015).
[31] Desmond, *Politics*, p. 155; Michael Bevan, 'Grainger, Edward (1797–1824)', *ODNB*; D'Arcy Power and Anita McConnell, 'Tyrrell, Frederick (1793–1843)', *ODNB*.
[32] Berkowitz, *Charles Bell*, ch. 1; L. S. Jacyna, 'Bell, Charles (1774–1842)', *ODNB*; Jacyna, 'Lawrence, Sir William, first baronet (1783–1867)', *ODNB*; Power and McConnell, 'Tyrrell'.
[33] *Report from the Select Committee on Anatomy* (1828), p. 16.

(which had split into two schools in 1825), St George's, Westminster, the London Hospital, the Middlesex, and the North London (later University College) Hospital. The men who taught at these institutions were sometimes referred to as 'pure surgeons', or simply 'pures'. In other words, they were in the relatively unique position of being able to practise primarily as operative surgeons and to gain extensive practical experience of surgical cases of all kinds. It is these men who have featured most prominently in this book so far and many, such as Astley Cooper at Guy's, John Abernethy at St Bartholomew's, Charles Bell at the Middlesex, and Robert Liston at University College Hospital, were among the leading lights of surgery in the early nineteenth century. In most cases, they held office in a pro-bono capacity. However, because the fees received from pupils could be extremely lucrative, these positions were highly sought-after. As a result, their incumbents often sought to hand them on to relatives and favourites. Perhaps the most egregious example of this bias towards what *The Lancet* called 'neveys and noodles' centred on Astley Cooper; during the 1820s and 1830s no fewer than four of his nephews (Edward Cock [1805–92], Frederick Tyrrell, Charles Aston Key, and Bransby Cooper) as well as several of his pupils (including Benjamin Travers [1783–1858], Thomas Callaway, and John Morgan [1797–1847]) held office at either St Thomas' or Guy's.[34]

In contrast to the hospital 'pures', those studying under them were destined, for the most part, to become surgeon-apothecaries or general practitioners. As we have heard, these men were not surgical specialists and it might be possible for them to pass through their entire career without once performing a capital procedure such as an amputation, lithotomy, or trephination. Instead, they were generalists, catering to the broad health requirements of a burgeoning middle class, men who might open veins, dress wounds, and set fractures, as well as prescribe medicines. They were also to be found in lesser public offices, either in the Poor Law system (notably, from 1834 onwards, as District Medical Officers) or in the military and commercial trading companies. Their qualifications consisted not only of the Licence of the Society of Apothecaries (LSA), but also often Membership of the Royal College of Surgeons (MRCS), the so-called 'conjoint' qualifications of 'College and Hall'.[35]

It was in relation to this latter qualification that the 'pures' wielded an authority equal to their role as lecturers, for as well as occupying the most prestigious hospital posts, they also dominated the Council of the Royal College of Surgeons. For example, during its first four decades as a chartered institution, Astley Cooper was elected President on two occasions

---

[34] *Lancet* 11:282 (24 January 1829), p. 535.   [35] Loudon, *Medical Care*, p. 224.

(1827 and 1836), as were Everard Home (1813 and 1822), Henry Cline (1815 and 1823), and Anthony Carlisle (1828 and 1837). Meanwhile, the St George's Hospital surgeon Thomas Keate (1745–1821) served as Master (as the post was known between 1800 and 1821) on no fewer than three occasions (1802, 1809, and 1818).

Even more importantly, perhaps, these men also dominated the Court of Examiners, the body that decided whether a candidate was fit to practise and eligible to be accepted as a member of the College. In this role they had considerable power in determining the careers of aspirant practitioners and a significant degree of latitude in shaping the regulations to fit their own interest; or so it was claimed. In May 1824, for example, *The Lancet* noted that the Court of Examiners, which included Cooper, Cline, Abernethy, and Home, had instigated a change in the bye-laws of the College by which 'Candidates for the diploma will be required to produce, prior to examination, a certificate of having regularly attended three courses at least, of anatomical lectures, *which shall have been delivered during the winter season*'. As Wakley pointed out:

It must be recollected that nearly all the examiners have been, and that five out of the ten are still, hospital surgeons; that the anatomical lectures delivered at the hospitals with which they are connected are only delivered during the winter season, while there are other teachers unconnected with these institutions [i.e. private lecturers] who give lectures on anatomy during the summer – what step do the examiners (two of whom are anatomical lecturers) adopt? Why, endeavour to crush the men who oppose them [...] by passing a bye-law which [...] render[s] an attendance on lectures delivered during the summer [...] of no use as far as regards passing the college.[36]

This quotation highlights the extent of professional rivalry and factionalism within metropolitan anatomical and surgical education. As Desmond has demonstrated, there was a politics of knowledge to this factionalism, as those in the private schools were often more inclined towards radically materialist forms of anatomical knowledge than those in the hospital schools, whose epistemological conservatism generally took the form of a Paleyite natural theology.[37] Berkowitz, meanwhile, has highlighted the role played by moderate Whig reformers such as Charles Bell, who might yet cleave to a natural theological position.[38] However, what is clear is that this intellectual politics mapped onto a broader cultural politics of power, authority, and social identity. Within radical discourse, the supposed intellectual backwardness of the hospital surgical elites was 'made the epistemic corollary of nepotism, of a system of succession and patronage which mirrored

---

[36] *Lancet* 2:35 (29 May 1824), pp. 256–6. Emphasis in original.
[37] Desmond, *Politics*, ch. 4.   [38] Berkowitz, *Charles Bell*.

the corruption of pocket boroughs and aristocratic governance'.[39] In other
words, the intellectual conservatism at the heart of the hospital schools was
held to be a direct product of a wider systemic malaise in which incompetent
placemen were gifted high-status posts by virtue of their wealth and social
connections, rather than their ability, while men of talent and industry were
forced to establish their own private schools outside of the 'family system'.[40]
Worse still, it was alleged that these corrupt placemen used their authority to
protect their sinecures and crush the aspirations and hard-won influence of
the anatomical entrepreneurs. For Wakley and his radical supporters, therefore, the system required wholesale reform, wherein hospital posts would
be opened up to genuine competition. Only in this way, they argued, could
hospitals come to realise their true function as scientific institutions for the
cultivation and dissemination of advanced surgical knowledge.[41] Embedded
in this critique was an assumption that hospitals were not *private* ventures,
nor merely charitable concerns, administered by their patrons and govern-
ing committees, but were instead *public* bodies with a *public* duty, rightfully subject to *public* scrutiny and oversight. In this sense, the campaign
concerning hospital surgery, which lasted from around the mid-1820s to the
mid-1830s, was part of a wider movement in which those 'half-public, half-
private' institutions, such as asylums and prisons, which straddled the line
between civic society and the state, were subject to aggressive intervention
by middle-class reformers.[42]

It should be noted that the reform of hospital surgery was but one aspect of
a wider medical reformist agenda. However, there are particular reasons why
it occupied such a prominent place within the pages of *The Lancet*. For one
thing, among the journal's core constituency were those general practitioners
who were most affected by the standards and structures of hospital teaching. By contrast, the experience of university medical graduates was of less
concern, although this did not prevent *The Lancet* from attacking the Royal
College of Physicians and its perennial President, Henry Halford (1766–
1844), on a regular basis. For another, Wakley had direct personal experience
of this particular system, having been a student at the United School of Guy's
and St Thomas' between 1815 and 1817. Shunning the excesses traditionally associated with medical student life, he allegedly pursued the course of
a 'self-respecting, sturdily independent labourer' who would regularly work

[39] Brown, '"Bats, Rats"', p. 189.
[40] For the use of the term 'family system', see *Lancet*, 15:386 (22 January 1831), pp. 564–8. See
also Desmond, *Politics*, p. 112.
[41] Brown, 'Medicine'.
[42] Michael Brown, 'Rethinking Early Nineteenth-Century Asylum Reform', *Historical Journal*
49:2 (2006), 435–52, at p. 439.

'fifteen hours a day'.[43] This industry was not matched by his teachers, however, and while 'he was allowed to do his part – to pay his fees and attend his classes – the authorities were not prepared to play their part by him'. According to his biographer:

The lectures advertised were not delivered by the eminent people who received the fees, but by their demonstrators [...] the honorary staff from whose lips he was to learn the science of healing were capricious in their visits and were generally dumb upon the occasions when they put in an appearance; the list of operations was not published to the students and only the favoured pupils of the staff knew what was going to be done by the great men and when. And to cap all these injustices, he found that he was relegated to a class in his profession marked out from the beginning to constitute the ranks and file, not in the least through want of personal merit, but because he had not paid exorbitant fees to apprentice himself to a great man.[44]

Wakley was not universally averse to his tutors. On the contrary, he had chosen to attend the United School precisely because Astley Cooper lectured there and, while his attacks on nepotism and the alleged abuse of power by hospital surgeons inevitably brought Cooper within his journalistic sights, Wakley retained a deep and abiding respect for Cooper's abilities, whose reputation he guarded with some jealousy. As his former colleague at *The Lancet*, James Fernandez Clarke (bap. 1812, d. 1875), noted, a clear indication of the esteem in which Wakley held Cooper was the fact that he was one of the very few high-profile London hospital surgeons never to receive one of the sarcastic monikers that, as we shall see, were such a characteristic of *The Lancet's* censorious style.[45] By contrast, Wakley's attitude towards Cooper's acolytes was less favourable, and his apparent disdain for men like Benjamin Travers may well have stemmed not only from Travers' privileged status as Cooper's former pupil, but also from a low estimation of his abilities as a lecturer, for Travers would often deputise for the 'great man' during Wakley's student days.

It should by now be clear how closely the campaign for the reform of hospital surgery paralleled the broader cultures of political reform. Indeed, Wakley often made a direct association between the two movements, even if he appreciated that a medical reformer might yet be a political conservative.[46] In January 1831, for example, he claimed that 'Medical [...] must stand or fall with political reform; for it is because the vices of our professional corporations have formed a part of the system by which we are oppressed, that

[43] Samuel Squire Sprigge, *The Life and Times of Thomas Wakley* (London: Longmans and Green, 1897), p. 21.
[44] Sprigge, *Wakley*, p. 31. For more on the political elaboration of Wakley's biography, see Brown, '"Bats, Rats"', pp. 186–7.
[45] James Fernandez Clarke, *Autobiographical Recollections of the Medical Profession* (London: J. and A. Churchill, 1874), p. 18.
[46] Brown, *Performing Medicine*, p. 203.

they have hitherto escaped correction'.[47] Like political and social reform more generally, medical reform was in many ways both a class conflict and a generational one, with young men from the middling sorts, like Wakley, frustrated by the lack of preferment to which they believed their talent and industry entitled them.[48] Given this fact, and the importance ascribed to educational structures and practices in shaping the politics and cultures of an inchoate profession, it should come as no surprise that *The Lancet* regarded the medical students of the metropolis as one of its principal constituents. Wakley frequently figured himself as a champion of the student interest, calling them 'our beloved but cruelly-plundered friends, the British students in medicine'.[49] It could even be argued that the interests of the student market shaped the very essence of *The Lancet*. Wakley's biographer, Samuel Squire Sprigge (1860–1937), pithily claimed the journal was conceived both to '*in*form' and '*re*form'.[50] In pursuit of the former agenda, it sought, from its very first volume, to publish surgical lectures, beginning with those of Astley Cooper, so that 'the numerous classes of Students, whether here or in distant universities' might have the benefit of knowledge that, by dint of cost or convenience, they could not otherwise obtain.[51] With regard to the latter, meanwhile, *The Lancet* sought, among other things, to expose the 'illiberal' treatment of students and defend their 'rights' in the face of 'oppression' or exploitation by the hospital authorities and surgical elites.[52]

It is important to recognise that in both of these endeavours, the students of the metropolis were not simply avid readers of *The Lancet*, but often also active collaborators. The practice of pirating surgical lectures (they were initially published without the consent of the lecturers concerned) was dependent upon students taking shorthand notes and passing them on to Wakley. In fact, Wakley actively recruited students such as James Lambert (d. 1831) and James Fernandez Clarke to report on hospital matters, while hospital surgeons frequently cautioned their students against supplying information to *The Lancet*, even calling upon those responsible to identify themselves.[53] Indeed, according

---

[47] *Lancet* 15:385 (15 January 1831), p. 529.
[48] On the significance of generational conflict in the cultures of reform, see Heather Ellis, *Generational Conflict and University Reform: Oxford in the Age of Revolution* (Leiden: Brill, 2012). For the importance of age and social status in shaping adherence to radical epistemologies, see Roger Cooter, *The Cultural Meaning of Popular Science: Phrenology and the Organization of Consent in Nineteenth-Century Britain* (Cambridge, UK: Cambridge University Press, 1984), pp. 42–8.
[49] *Lancet* 17:422 (1 October 1831), p. 1. Wakley's opponents were certainly conscious of his courting of the student body. For example, see *London Medical Gazette* 12 April 1828, pp. 571–2.
[50] Sprigge, *Wakley*, p. 80.   [51] *Lancet* 1:1 (5 October 1823), p. 2.
[52] *Lancet* 13:338 (20 February 1830), p. 710.
[53] For example, see Benjamin Travers' warning to his students in *Lancet* 2:38 (19 June 1824), pp. 371–2. John Abernethy called upon the 'hireling' of *The Lancet* to step forward so that he could

to Clarke, after the exclusion of James Lambert from the Borough hospitals in 1828 for his account of Bransby Cooper's botched lithotomy operation (of which more anon), a sign was erected in the hall of Guy's Hospital warning any student against reporting for *The Lancet*, under pain of expulsion.[54]

However, if the unauthorised publishing of surgical lectures angered the hospital 'pures', it was as nothing compared to other forms of reporting that developed during the 1820s. As we shall see in the latter part of this chapter, *The Lancet* did not begin by publishing reports of hospital cases with the express intention of exposing instances of incompetence. Nevertheless, such reports quickly assumed an ever greater importance within the journal's reformatory armamentarium. As with the reporting of surgical lectures, it was students who played a vital role in witnessing and reporting such occurrences. Susan Lawrence observes that the expansion of hospital teaching not only allowed the surgical elites to broaden their influence and increase their income, it also exposed them to a far greater degree of scrutiny, 'allowing more medical men to witness, discuss, and (potentially) praise or criticize the bedside decisions of these elite practitioners'.[55] As in the political realm, then, scrutiny, exposure, and publicity were held to be among the most potent tools for reshaping the *ancien régime* of metropolitan hospital surgery. Likewise, as in the political realm, such radical and reforming ideologies encouraged the drawing of sharp moral polarities between oppressors and victims, heroes and villains, polarities that lent themselves, in turn, to intensely emotional and melodramatic forms of emplotment.

The Lancet and the Melodramatic Mode

In her account of *The Lancet*'s literary style, Brittany Pladek highlights the journal's early engagement with theatricality and extensive use of literary form. She notes the observation, made by Sprigge, that Wakley had 'an extreme love of the stage', that 'he was well-read in dramatic literature and a constant attendant at the play'.[56] As she points out, *The Lancet* ran a regular theatrical review column in its early numbers, although ultimately only for about two months.[57] Pladek considers Wakley's embrace of literature and theatricality, together with what she calls *The Lancet*'s other 'nonmedical' features, such

---

refund his money and have him leave the course. 'Take the substance of what I say, you are perfectly welcome to it – you have paid for it – it is yours', he claimed: 'but I do protest that I think no one has a right to publish it to the world'. *Morning Chronicle* 15 October 1824, p. 1; *Lancet*, 3:56 (23 October 1824), p. 114.

[54] This sign apparently remained there until the late 1840s or early 1850s: Clarke, *Recollections*, p. 65.
[55] Lawrence, *Charitable*, p. 110.
[56] Sprigge, *Wakley*, p. 104; Pladek, '"Variety"', pp. 576–7.
[57] Pladek, '"Variety"', p. 575.

as the chess and gossip columns, to be an attempt to appeal to broader tastes and to chart 'a middle course between the journalistic gravity expected by his medical colleagues and a commercial strategy he was reluctant to abandon'.[58] There is no doubt that Wakley conceived of *The Lancet* as having a broad appeal, although the fact that he gave up this 'miscellaneous fluff' after less than a year of publication suggests a limited aspiration to be a truly inclusive periodical along the lines of *Blackwood's Magazine*.[59] Even so, *The Lancet*'s investment in theatricality and literature went far deeper, and continued for far longer, than the ephemerality of such structural forms might suggest. Where Pladek's otherwise insightful analysis lacks scope is in her separation of the literary and commercial aspects of *The Lancet* from its medical and political ones.[60] It is clear that Wakley had a genuine love of the theatre, and that his near-constant literary references served, in his mind at least, to enliven *The Lancet*'s prose and to distinguish it from the 'uniformly dull' content of rivals such as the *Medico-Chirurgical Review*. But theatricality played a far more vital role in shaping Wakley's public persona, providing the very foundation for his political performances, both figurative and literal.[61] Sprigge even suggests that Wakley's regular play-going was 'a fact upon which his future oratorical successes were largely dependent'.[62]

Furthermore, in order to understand the political cultures of the Romantic period, we must be attentive to the politics of literature; and we do not have to look very hard to find an early instance of literary political engagement within the pages of *The Lancet*. Pladek notes that the very first number of *The Lancet* concludes with an extended extract from an open letter penned by the essayist and poet Charles Lamb (1775–1834). For Pladek, Wakley's re-publication of this letter indicates his assumption that his audience was familiar 'with a wider periodical press, including literary journals like the *Quarterly Review*' and reveals his desire to 'place [*The Lancet*] in dialogue with a broader periodical market, underlining the relevance of its contents beyond the sphere of medical specialization'.[63] There is, however, rather more to it than this. Lamb's letter was originally published in the *London Magazine* and was addressed to the poet laureate, Robert Southey (1774–1843). Southey had recently published a review of Lamb's *Essays of Elia* (1823) in which he claimed that the book 'wants only a sounder religious feeling, to be as delightful as it is original'. In response, Lamb wrote 'with unusual anger [...] impunging both Southey's judgement and his character'.[64] Wakley confessed himself 'at a loss to conceive

[58] Pladek, "'Variety'", pp. 574, 586.   [59] Pladek, "'Variety'", p. 574.
[60] Pladek, "'Variety'", p. 576, n. 69.   [61] *Lancet* 1:10 (7 December 1823), p. 333.
[62] Sprigge, *Wakley*, p. 104.   [63] Pladek, "'Variety'", p. 576.
[64] Peter Swaab, 'Lamb, Charles (1775–1834)', *ODNB*.

what Southey can have done, to thus arouse the feelings of Elia [Lamb], whose spirit has ever appeared to us as gentle as the "summer air"'. Clearly, however, the reason Wakley chose to include this letter was because of his fierce political opposition to Southey, a man whose transition from radical republicanism to ultra Toryism, and consequent royal preferment, warranted his description as a 'sack-hunting, hypocritical rhymer' and who, according to Wakley, 'cannot yet have recovered from the lashing that Lord Byron gave him' after he had referred to the young, radical Romantic poets as a 'Satanic school'.[65] For Wakley, literature and politics were not discrete entities: they were co-constitutive aspects of the same social and cultural sphere.

As can be seen from Southey's comments about Byron and his circle, radical reformers did not have a monopoly on emotive and censorious language. Nonetheless, *The Lancet*, in common with its radical political equivalents, evinced a particularly pronounced desire to arouse and sustain powerful emotions, so much so, in fact, that the *Medico-Chirurgical Review* decried what it called its 'mock-heroic bombast, and sentimental lachrymation'.[66] *The Lancet*'s investment in dramatic sentiment is clearly evident in its early theatrical reviews, which exhibit an attachment to emotional authenticity, to the elision of artifice and the expression of true, honest feeling. In its second number, for example, it commented on the performance of Lionel Benjamin Rayner (1787–1855) as 'Tyke' in Thomas Morton's (1764–1838) *School of Reform* (1805), especially the scene 'where the old affection quivers on his lips and dissolves him in welcome tears', tears that 'were so powerful and true, that we almost hesitate to call them *acting*'. 'The audience', it claimed, 'not only testified their sense of his excellence [...] by loud applauses, but by the still more unequivocal testimony of tears'.[67]

One of the most obvious ways in which Wakley endeavoured to stir emotions in his readers was his extensive use of epithet and insult. Most of those individuals, groups, or institutions who were a frequent target of his ire earned what Sprigge calls 'galling and offensive' nicknames.[68] Hence, the hospital 'pures' were often referred to as 'Bats' or 'Hole and Corner' surgeons for their tendency to avoid the 'light' of public scrutiny, while the Society of Apothecaries, whose authority over general practice was greatly resented by

[65] *Lancet* 1:1 (5 October 1823), p. 33. The position of poet laureate had traditionally been rewarded with a 'butt of sack', or some 105 gallons of sherry, yearly. This attack was contained in Robert Southey, *A Vision of Judgement* (London: Longman, Hurst, Rees, Orme, and Brown, 1821), pp. xix–xxi. Byron's parodic *Vision of Judgement* (1822) mocked Southey's High Tory politics. See Geoffrey Carnall, 'Southey, Robert (1774–1843)', *ODNB*.
[66] *Medico-Chirurgical Review and Journal of Medical Science* 4:16 (1 March 1824), p. 976.
[67] *Lancet* 1:2 (12 October 1823), p. 57. See also *Lancet* 1:3 (19 October 1823), p. 86.
[68] Sprigge, *Wakley*, p. 68. See also 'Pladek, '"Variety"', p. 580; Brown, '"Bats, Rats"', p. 191.

men who considered themselves more than mere tradesmen, were derided as 'the Old Hags of Rhubarb Hall'.[69] This latter phrase testifies to the importance of literary allusion. The apothecaries were initially cast either as the 'Old Ladies' or 'gentle Dames of Rhubarb Hall', a moniker that simultaneously effeminised them while emphasising the traditional associations between the apothecary's trade and that of the grocer (the two companies having split in 1617).[70] Soon, however, they became the 'Old Hags', a name that perhaps evoked *Macbeth*'s three witches and their 'charmed pot' of 'poysond Entrailes'.[71] The same intertextuality shaped Wakley's use of personal nicknames. For example, his use of 'The Three Ninnyhammers' to describe the St Thomas' surgeons Benjamin Travers, Joseph Henry Green, and Frederick Tyrrell was, according to Sprigge, 'hallowed by Sterne, Swift, Arbuthnot and, indirectly, Shakespeare', evoking 'the forcible-feeble behaviour to be expected from persons so designated'.[72] The influence of literary culture is likewise evident in the nicknames that he gave to his rivals in the world of print. For example, Roderick Macleod (1795–1852), Wakley's arch-nemesis and editor of the reactionary *London Medical Gazette*, was designated 'the Goth', an allusion to the hated Southey's epic poem *Roderick the Last of the Goths* (1814), while James Johnson's (1777–1845) *Medico-Chirurgical Review* was known as the 'Quarterly Journal', not simply because of its periodicity, but also in reference to the conservative and anti-reformist *Quarterly Review*.

The use of such names allowed Wakley to cast his political opponents as villains and fools. As argued elsewhere, it 'reinforced the moral indignation of radical opposition, promoting and sustaining a culture of collective outrage'. This use of nicknames likewise depersonalised 'the principal beneficiaries of medical corruption [...] rendering them "at one" with the system they perpetuated'.[73] However, when viewed through the prism of melodrama, it also performed another function, for 'disguised identities', 'hidden relationships', and malign stratagems plotted by 'masked personages' and 'secret societies' were some of the key features of the melodramatic imagination.[74]

As Peter Brooks points out in his classic study, nineteenth-century melodrama was characterised by a number of things, including 'hyperbolic figures' and 'lurid and grandiose events'. Above all, perhaps, it was defined by

---

[69] For example, see *Lancet* 17:422 (10 October 1829), p. 2 and *Lancet* 3:56 (23 October 1824), pp. 82–5. For an extended meditation on the term 'Bat', see *Lancet* 17:422 (1 October 1831), pp. 1–6.

[70] For example, see *Lancet* 6:152 (29 July 1826), p. 564 and *Lancet* 6:153 (5 August 1826), p. 594.

[71] *Lancet*, 6:153 (5 August 1826), p. 596. A digital facsimile of the First Folio of Shakespeare's plays, Bodleian Arch. G c.7, 'The Tragedy of Macbeth', Act 4, Scene 1, p. 143. https://firstfolio .bodleian.ox.ac.uk/text/753 (accessed 15/09/21).

[72] Sprigge, *Wakley*, p. 111. See also Pladek, '"Variety"', p. 580.

[73] Brown, '"Bats, Rats"', p. 191.

[74] Peter Brooks, *The Melodramatic Imagination: Balzac, Henry James, Melodrama and the Mode of Excess*, 2nd ed. (New Haven: Yale University Press, 1995), pp. 3, 5.

a Manichean 'polarization into moral absolutes', a world 'charged with the conflict between lightness and darkness', of 'overt villainy, persecution of the good, and final reward of virtue'.[75] Anyone familiar with *The Lancet*'s prose will recognise these qualities, particularly when it comes to the weekly editorials penned by Wakley himself. There are, indeed, too many instances to recount, but the following example, published in January 1831, is illustrative. Expounding upon the baleful effects of nepotism and corruption, Wakley wrote:

The medical Colleges and Companies are the pest-houses of the profession [...] yet in no instance has the profession come forward as a body [...] determined to rid themselves of the cankers which had been preying upon their vitals, to effect their annihilation, or even their partial overthrow [...] If the members of the profession had not breathed the foul air generated by collegiate impurities; If they had not been most foolishly taught to yield to slavish obedience, and to view with submissive respect, the self-appointed dispensers of medical law, and patronage, they would long since have been freed from the galling shackles of their thraldom [...] Strong, powerful, masculine minds, at once shrink back, flushed with rage and indignation on beholding the tyranny of our Colleges, and the hideous effects of corporate misrule. Hence it is, that the well-informed portion of the public, men of liberality and learning, are shocked and indignant beyond expression, at the exposure of those abuses which have been communicated to the public in the last few years [...] But thus it ever has been, and ever will be, where "the few" have the power to domineer over "the many".[76]

Wakley often claimed that his principal targets were systems, rather than individuals.[77] However, his moral outrage was perhaps never more forcibly expressed than when attacking those whom he deemed to have profited by that system. As he continued:

Of all the monsters, of all the abandoned and stony-hearted creatures, that wear the human form, or infest society, there are none to equal in black ingratitude and treacherous debasement, those who [...] live upon the fruits of corruption [...] At once the betrayers of their friends [...] they are the bitterest enemies of human kind. They are spies, traitors, villains [...] Public indignation, like the lightning's flash, should scare the heartless wretches, should mark them out as guilty offenders against GOD and man, and blight their every hope of enjoyment, even amidst the fascinating and sumptuous allurements of collegiate banquets.[78]

Wakley's rhetorical world was one of monsters, spies, and villains, of fetid dungeons and the chains of bondage. It was also a world of perpetual conflict with an enemy forever teetering on the brink of defeat. In an 1828 editorial about the Royal College of Surgeons, for example, he claimed:

---

[75] Brooks, *Melodramatic*, pp. 4, 5, 11–12.
[76] *Lancet* 15:386 (22 January 1831), pp. 564–5. Note the reference to Percy Bysshe Shelley's (1792–1822) *Masque of Anarchy* (1819) and its now famous line, 'Ye are many – they are few'.
[77] Brown, '"Bats, Rats"', p. 191.   [78] *Lancet* 15:386 (22 January 1831), p. 565.

The oligarchy is expiring. The Hydra of medical corruption is at its last gasp, and one well-directed blow may rid us of a monster, whose noxious influence has retarded the progress of science, disgraced the character of British surgery, and rendered the profession an object of public scorn, or of public apprehension.

The College has once more set in motion the base tool of its infamous power; and its members are to be again traduced and vilified, in order that an imbecile and worthless faction may triumph over the rights of their professional brethren; but we have possession of the field, and THE LANCET IS UNBROKEN.[79]

Even in *The Lancet*'s more ironic moments, such language and imagery were ever-present. Joseph Henry Green, one of the 'Three Ninnyhammers' of St Thomas', was a friend and disciple of Samuel Taylor Coleridge and sought to apply Coleridge's conservative, paternalistic, and fundamentally anti-democratic philosophy to the governance of surgery.[80] In 1831, he published a pamphlet entitled *Distinction without Separation* in which he proposed a top-down and essentially hierarchical reform of the Royal College of Surgeons. Wakley, who despised Green's politics and ridiculed his sophistry, nonetheless thought that he possessed a 'natural goodness of heart' and thus, perhaps, greeted his entry into the sphere of reform with that 'mock-heroic bombast' noted by his opponents.[81] Wakley struggled to understand how a man 'who could exhibit so much acuteness and accuracy of perception, vigour of thought, and power of reasoning, should at the same time betray so much confusion and obscurity in all matters connected with hospital government':

But the riddle is now solved. The mind of MR GREEN has not been permitted to enjoy a free scope. It has been encumbered by prejudices, and darkened by theories, which he could neither object to, nor expose, nor control. The poison stole upon him imperceptibly; and at a moment when he expected to find himself in the high road to preferment, and in the full sunshine of professional popularity, he discovered alas! when almost too late, that he was plunged into the very dungeon of nepotism, bound hand and foot by the demon monopoly [...]

Impatient under the tortures of this unnatural bondage, and viewing with disgust the mazes of iniquity in which he had so long been imprisoned, by one heroic effort he has cast aside his fetters, escaped his abhorred tyrants and companions and now stands before the profession, at once a humble supplicant, and an instructive monitor.[82]

Clearly, it was not always a straightforward matter to tell when Wakley was being serious: when the monsters and dungeons of his imagination were

---

[79] *Lancet* 9:228 (12 January 1828), p. 561. For more on the martial metaphor in reforming medical discourse, see Michael Brown, '"Like a Devoted Army": Medicine, Heroic Masculinity, and the Military Paradigm in Victorian Britain', *Journal of British Studies* 49:3 (2010), 592–622.

[80] Desmond, *Politics*, pp. 260–75; Desmond, 'Lamarckianism and Democracy: Corporations, Corruption and Comparative Anatomy in the 1830s', in James R. Moore (ed.), *History, Humanity and Evolution: Essays for John C. Greene* (Cambridge, UK: Cambridge University Press, 1989), 99–130.

[81] Desmond, *Politics*, pp. 261–2.   [82] *Lancet* 16:413 (30 July 1831), pp. 568–9.

intended to generate anger, mirth, or indeed both. But this was not the only ambivalence attendant upon his use of the melodramatic mode. *The Lancet*'s entry into the field of medical journalism in 1823 prompted a conservative reaction in the form of Macleod's *London Medical Gazette* (founded in 1827). At the same time, existing journals, such as the *Medico-Chirurgical Review* (founded in 1820), adopted a more powerful editorial voice in order to challenge, or at least mitigate, the force of Wakley's 'democratic celebrity'.[83] These rival journals, particularly the *Gazette*, deployed melodramatic devices of their own in presenting *The Lancet* as 'the Antichrist of the Apocalypse' and Wakley as 'Satan himself'.[84] In June 1828, for example, Macleod penned an editorial in which he denounced 'that system of literary plunder and personal abuse which had degraded medical literature', claiming that 'we have not hesitated to tear the mask from the face of the imposter, and [show] him in his native hideousness'.[85] In response, *The Lancet*'s Irish correspondent, 'Erinensis', charged Macleod with addressing himself 'more to the imagination and the passions than to the understanding'.[86] And yet, in critiquing Macleod's appeal to feeling, 'Erinensis' could seemingly find no other literary mode himself, as he compared Macleod to that most melodramatic of villains, the poisoner, who in adapting 'the virulence of his comments to the conjectured capacity of his constituents for slander […] gradually increases the strength of the dose as he proceeds'. In this 'foul reservoir of envious scurrility', he claimed, somewhat extravagantly, of Macleod's rather tepid editorial, 'we have collected […] the pure, unadulterated essence of hatred and revenge'.[87]

We shall say more, in due course, about the ambivalences surrounding *The Lancet*'s use of melodramatic forms. For the moment, it is important to note that melodrama was not simply used to caricature Wakley's enemies; it was not simply a device for provoking ridicule or exciting rage. Rather, it shaped Wakley's own political identity, for if the Manichean dualism of the *mélodrame* presented his opponents as villains, then it also framed his supporters, and more especially himself, as heroes. What is more, these heroic forms of representation were not confined to the printed page, but extended out into the world of public political performance.[88] Despite the prominence of his editorial

---

[83] Desmond, *Politics*, p. 15–16; Berkowitz, *Charles Bell*, pp. 79–81. The term 'democratic celebrity' comes from the editor of the *Black Dwarf*, Thomas Jonathan Wooler (1786?–1853): Kevin Gilmartin, *Politics*, pp. 38–40.

[84] *Lancet* 13:321 (24 October 1829), p. 159.

[85] *London Medical Gazette* 7 June 1828, pp. 25–6.

[86] At the time, the identity of Erinensis was not revealed. It is now known to have been Peter Hennis Green (1803–70): Charles Alexander Cameron, *History of the Royal College of Surgeons in Ireland* (Dublin: Fannin, 1886) p. 339; Clarke, *Recollections*, pp. 150–1.

[87] *Lancet* 11:289 (14 March 1829), p. 742.

[88] Of course, for most at the time (as for historians in the present), these performances were mediated by print in the form of textual reports.

voice, *The Lancet* rarely promoted Wakley as an individual, even if it alluded to its own role as a torchbearer for truth and liberty. However, in its reporting of meetings involving its editor, the tope of heroic individualism was inescapable. In late September 1830, for example, a dinner was held at that most radical of 'Romantic taverns', the Crown and Anchor on the Strand, to celebrate Wakley's 'able and manly advocacy of the cause of justice' during his unsuccessful attempt to be elected as Coroner for East Middlesex.[89] In introducing the guest of honour, the chair of the meeting, the French-trained radical anatomist Thomas King (1802–39), stated:

> You are all acquainted with his entry upon public life, the obstacles he has had to encounter, the difficulties with which he has been surrounded. Alone and unsupported, Mr Wakley has withstood the efforts of the most powerful public body in the state. You have seen how nearly he has been overthrown – you must have feared he would have been entirely overpowered; but Gentlemen, by pursuing one honest, straight-forward, manly course he has surmounted every one of the surrounding dangers, and risen superior to his enemies.[90]

This was pure political theatre, and King spoke as if he were addressing a theatrical audience. Given that this audience included none other than Henry 'Orator' Hunt (1773–1835), they were most likely well versed in the conventions of radical melodrama and would have recognised the tropes of trial, tribulation, and ultimate triumph that King deployed. The line 'you must have feared he would have been entirely overpowered', in particular, speaks to the emotional machinations of the melodramatic mode, the audience anxiously rooting for its hero in the midst of peril, knowing, ultimately, that he must prevail. Moreover, Wakley seems to have been reading from the same script, for in his speech he claimed that 'I have often been assailed, I am still assailed, on the right hand and the left; I am abused from behind, but few there are who ever venture to meet me in front. My dirty foes are ever at their work in secret'.[91] Wakley was thus cast, and cast himself, as the quintessential melodramatic hero, his honest, upright manliness set in stark contrast to the conspiratorial tactics of his opponents.

No doubt, Wakley's status as a heroic figure was enhanced by his physical appearance. As Joanne Begiato's work on emotionalised bodies in the nineteenth century has shown, men, especially public men like Wakley, were often judged on their physical appearance and their approximation to a manly ideal.[92] For certain political figures, like the Irish nationalist Daniel O'Connell

---

[89] *Lancet* 15:370 (2 October 1830), p. 45. On the Crown and Anchor, see Newman, *Romantic Tavern*, ch. 2.
[90] *Lancet* 15:370 (2 October 1830), p. 43. On Thomas King, see Desmond, *Politics*, pp. 96, 424.
[91] *Lancet* 15:370 (2 October 1830), p. 45.
[92] Joanne Begiato, *Manliness in Britain, 1760–1900: Bodies, Emotion and Material Culture* (Manchester: Manchester University Press, 2020), ch. 1.

(1775–1847), or the Chartist leaders Feargus O'Connor (1796?–1855) and Henry Vincent (1813–78), their authority was underwritten by their handsome features, open countenance, and/or muscular physiques.[93] The same was true of Wakley. According to Sprigge, he excelled at that most manly of early nineteenth-century pursuits, boxing, and at over six feet tall cut an imposing figure in public:

All who saw Thomas Wakley striding along in the streets [...] asked who he was, and once seen his was a figure and face not easily to be forgotten. Tall, erect, square-shouldered, and perfectly proportioned – a man of bulk, but yet of lightness – his frame bore the proofs of his great muscular strength and incessantly active life. His clean-shaven, florid face was replete with expression [...] His golden hair, worn in natural and lengthy clusters nearly down to his coat collar, was fine and waved in the little breeze that his energetic and sprightly gait stirred up around him.[94]

Such attention as we have thus far paid to the specifics of language, both in print and in performance, might seem excessive. But in actual fact, the language used by Wakley and *The Lancet* is of critical importance because, in many ways, *The Lancet*'s politics *was* a politics of language. As Robert Poole has suggested of Romantic radicalism in general, 'bold language *was* [...] rebellion'.[95] Not only did it provide 'a script for popular protest', but, given the imbalance of power between the forces of reform and those of reaction, illicit or inflammatory language was often the sole means of active defiance to the authorities, something that is evident from the place of blasphemy and seditious libel within the cultures of popular radicalism.[96] Moreover, within the radical imagination, with its Manichean moral polarities, the mere act of bringing corruption and tyranny to light and exposing them to the full force of popular outrage was thought sufficient to bring about their defeat. The same was true of *The Lancet*. Indeed, given that few of Wakley's political schemes, such the London College of Medicine, ever got off the ground, *The Lancet*'s political power can be said to have been almost entirely rhetorical and ideational. Moreover, like the radical political press more broadly, it imagined that the power of print could, by itself, produce significant structural change. As an editorial of January 1831 put it, 'The foundation of these institutions

---

[93] For O'Connell, see Katie Barclay, 'Performing Emotion and Reading the Male Body in the Irish Court, c.1800–1845', *Journal of Social History* 51:2 (2017), 293–312, at p. 299; Barclay, *Men on Trial*. For O'Connor, see Sanders, 'Platform', p. 51. For Vincent, see Tom Scriven, *Popular Virtue: Continuity and Change in Radical Moral Politics, 1820–1870* (Manchester: Manchester University Press, 2017), p. 59.

[94] Sprigge, *Wakley*, pp. 21–2, 327–8.   [95] Poole, '"Last Drop"', p. 38.

[96] Poole, '"Last Drop"', p. 39. On blasphemy and seditious libel, see Smith, *Politics of Language*; McCalman, *Radical Underworld*; Epstein, *Radical Expression*; Gilmartin, *Politics*; Joss Marsh, *Word Crimes: Blasphemy, Culture and Literature in Nineteenth-Century England* (Chicago: Chicago University Press, 1998).

172   'Scenes of Cruelty and Blood'

(the Colleges, etc.) is so rotten and [...] so corrupt, that they would fall, never to rise again, before a single well-directed impulse of public opinion'.[97]

Wakley's invocation of the 'public' here is interesting. As we have heard, *The Lancet* sought to draw together the interests and agency of students and general practitioners. But it also sought to appeal to a broader political audience. At one level, Wakley's comments bring to mind the insights of Jürgen Habermas concerning the emergence of a public sphere of discourse in the eighteenth and nineteenth centuries.[98] But we must be cautious for, as has been argued elsewhere, Wakley's relationship to the 'people', as a body with political agency, as opposed to the 'public', as an object of professional guardianship, was complex and ambivalent.[99] Even so, and as we shall now see, the campaign to reform metropolitan hospital surgery maintained that students and general practitioners were not the only victims of corruption and tyranny. Indeed, by extending its rhetorical concerns to the fate of patients undergoing operations at the hands of supposedly incompetent surgeons, *The Lancet* deployed perhaps its most melodramatic and emotive forms of critique. As Wakley wrote:

If this system of nepotism in the abstract be so detestable that every liberal mind must shrink from it in disgust, with what horror must the humane and intelligent practitioner reflect upon its consequences! The poor patients! Alas for the unfortunate patients. A, B, or C, is not made a hospital surgeon because he has signalized himself in the practice of his profession; because he is remarkable for the knowledge and principles of surgery; because he is noted for kindness of disposition, punctuality, or industry, – but because he happens to have been the apprentice of D, E, or F, a surgeon of the hospital [...] [The patients] may be neglected, mutilated, and slaughtered, but their agonising groans and cries can never reach the hard-hearted supporters of nepotism.[100]

The Emotional Politics of Radical Scrutiny

If Wakley was determined to make audible the 'agonising groans and cries' of the suffering surgical patient, or even, as he claimed in another editorial, to 'Alarm and instruct the nation with [their] tales of blood', he did not necessarily start out with that intention.[101] There was no explicit mention of a plan to publish regular accounts of metropolitan hospital surgery in the opening preface to the first issue of *The Lancet* on 5 October 1823. Indeed, it was not until the sixth issue, on 9 November, that such case reports first appeared, heralded by neither fanfare nor justification. For the first three weeks of their existence,

[97] *Lancet* 15:386 (22 January 1831), p. 565.
[98] Jürgen Habermas, *The Structural Transformation of the Public Sphere: An Inquiry into a Category of Bourgeois Society*, trans Thomas Burger (Cambridge, UK: Polity Press, 1989).
[99] Brown, '"Bats, Rats"', pp. 204–7.   [100] *Lancet* 15:386 (22 January 1831), p. 567.
[101] *Lancet* 27:690 (19 November 1836), p. 302.

they ran as largely factual accounts, devoid of editorial commentary. Later, in 1830, Wakley suggested that 'accurate descriptions of diseases [...] as they really occur in our hospitals [...] furnish materials for supplying a knowledge of the principles and practice of medicine inferior only to those which can be derived from personal observation and experience'. It was, he claimed, 'under this impression that we commenced the publication of hospital reports in the autumn of 1823'. However, while Wakley sought to justify the publishing of case histories largely on epistemological grounds, he also suggested an emotional imperative for the practice, writing that 'By the sufferings of the patient, the observer becomes sympathetically interested in his welfare, and impressions painfully produced are long fixed upon the memory'.[102]

Such words recall the sentiments of John Bell, quoted at length in Chapter 2. But, in addition to being personally and professionally edifying, this practice of publishing case reports soon came to serve another function, initiating what Wakley called a 'kind of medical police'.[103] The first indication of this strategy came on 30 November in the course of a case report from St Thomas' Hospital. The patient in question, known simply as 'Tho[ma]s. H.', was a 44-year-old drayman who had suffered a compound fracture of the left leg after being run over by a cart. He was taken under the care of Benjamin Travers, who performed an amputation. The operation itself passed off reasonably well, although the patient was later to suffer 'jumping and starting of the limb'. It was in terms of aftercare, however, that *The Lancet* found especial cause for concern. As it noted at the end of its report, the patient suffered a haemorrhage some three days after the operation 'in consequence of [...] being obliged to move his body for the purpose of allowing a bed-pan to be passed under him'. In this way, it claimed, 'the life of a patient has been endangered for want of a simple contrivance that might have enabled him to pass his stools without disturbing [...] the limb'. As it concluded:

We have seen so many instances of this kind in the Borough Hospitals, that we shall take every opportunity of giving publicity to them when they occur, in the expectation that a cause of so much mischief will soon be removed. It is, however, melancholy to state that this is but one of many evils in the Metropolitan Hospitals, which are a disgrace to those who allow them to exist – in due time we shall expose them all.[104]

It should perhaps come as little surprise that Wakley's *alma mater*, St Thomas', came in for particular scrutiny in these early numbers of *The*

[102] *Lancet* 15:369 (25 September 1830), p. 3.
[103] *Lancet* 15:369 (25 September 1830), p. 3. Clearly, Wakley did not intend to use the term 'medical police' in its conventional contemporary sense, i.e. as pertaining to the relations between medicine and the state, in terms of either the law or public health. Rather, he intended it to suggest a function of surveillance and regulation.
[104] *Lancet* 1:9 (30 November 1823), pp. 310–11.

Lancet. While Astley Cooper's practice at Guy's elicited mostly praise, his acolyte Travers' practice at its sister hospital was held up in stark contrast, as was that of his fellow 'Ninnyhammers', Green and Tyrrell. Indeed, *The Lancet*'s frequently critical reports of operations conducted at St Thomas' were part of a broader campaign waged against the 'Hole and Corner' surgeons of the Borough. This included its scathing coverage of a January 1824 anniversary dinner in which Travers praised the system of English medical education for being 'both elaborate and expensive', thereby restricting it to 'persons, who have a certain stake in the country, with respect to property and respectability'.[105] *The Lancet* likewise ridiculed Green's meditations on friendship and the 'gladsome feelings of boyhood', delivered at the same dinner, calling them 'tawdry puerilities, which he has culled from second-rate novels and romances'.[106]

For their part, the surgeons of St Thomas' actively resisted any attempts to publicise their cases and sought to 'suppress' *The Lancet*, banning Wakley from attending the hospital (which he ignored) and threatening to expel any student suspected of reporting operations (which it was not in their power to do).[107] In fact, the response from Travers and his colleagues, together with the active opposition of the *Medico-Chirurgical Review*, only encouraged Wakley in his endeavours and heartened his supporters. In a letter published in February 1825, for example, a correspondent remarked upon the apparent alarm and suspicion that *The Lancet* had aroused among the surgeons of St Thomas', asking Wakley if he possessed 'the wonderful faculty of splitting yourself into quarters, and sprouting up entire "*Dramatis Personae*", in as many distant places at the same time? Or is your presence, the "terror of evil doers", imaginary only, the mere false creation of perturbed minds and misgiving consciences?' Continuing in this theatrical vein, he claimed to have come across a surgeon 'soliloquizing by a window' on the wards of St Thomas', asking: 'Is this a *Lancet* which I see before me; – / Or art thou but a dagger of the mind [...]?' The correspondent concluded by thanking Wakley for his services and requesting 'for the benefit of the younger members of the profession, that you will shortly explore other *dark places of the earth*, and rid them of their malpractices as effectually as you have done the "hole and corners" of St Thomas' Hospital'.[108]

As it happened, Wakley was already doing just this, for while St Thomas' provided the initial focus for his strategy of radical scrutiny and exposure, it soon broadened out to encompass other institutions. Most notably, during the late spring and summer of 1825, two cases of alleged neglect were reported at

[105] *Lancet* 1:15 (11 January 1824), p. 56; *Lancet* 1:16 (18 January 1824), pp. 90–4.
[106] *Lancet* 1:15 (11 January 1824), p. 61; *Lancet* 2:38 (19 June 1824), p. 371.
[107] *Lancet* 2:38 (19 June 1824), pp. 371–2.
[108] *Lancet* 3:74 (26 February 1825), p. 250. Emphasis in original.

St George's Hospital. In the first instance, the Coroner for the City of London found that James Wheeler, a 32-year-old patient, had died 'from the want of proper attention' given to him at the hospital. He had initially come into St George's for a cough and was bled by an unnamed student dresser who accidentally punctured his artery. His arm was subsequently bandaged too tightly, stopping the circulation. After three days, it was found to be 'in the most horrid state of inflammation and mortification'. According to his servant, Wheeler was convinced he would die from the injury, stating that he was 'A MURDERED MAN'. His wife likewise testified that he had said 'HE KNEW IT WAS ALL OVER WITH HIM' and that 'HIS ARM WOULD KILL HIM'. *The Lancet* welcomed the coroner's findings, lamenting that it was far from being 'a solitary instance of a human being having lost his life through ignorance and inattention in one of our Public Hospitals'.[109]

As if to prove its point, in July a second coroner's inquest was held into a remarkably similar case. The deceased was John Hammond, a 21-year-old servant who had fallen upon broken glass and cut his knee. He had been attended by the senior surgeon, Henry Jeffreys, and the house surgeon, a 'Mr Pitman'. Pitman had, like the dresser in the previous case, bound the wound too tightly, to the great pain and discomfort of the patient. It remained in this state for several days, despite Hammond's protestations, and when it was finally removed, it was clear that 'though the external wound had closed and healed, matter had formed and burrowed underneath' so as to 'reduce his system, and to make his case hopeless'. In a remarkable hearing, reported by the *Morning Chronicle* and reprinted in *The Lancet*, one of the jurors gave his opinion that 'this young man died by gross neglect and improper surgical treatment', arguing that such 'mismanagement and improper treatment ought to be made public'. The coroner warned him that such an accusation 'may be a libel', but the rest of the jury concurred, finding that Hammond died 'from the effects of IMPROPER SURGICAL TREATMENT AND NEGLECT'.[110]

In addition to St Thomas' and St George's, the surgical practice at the Middlesex Hospital also came under early scrutiny. In May 1825, *The Lancet* drew attention to the case of John Moore, who had died from an inflammation of the stomach while under the care of the senior surgeon John Joberns (d.1832). Joberns (known to *The Lancet* by his nickname 'Joe Burns') was said to have delayed performing a vital operation, costing the patient his life.[111] Meanwhile, in November of the same year, John Shaw (1792–1827), the brother-in-law of his fellow Middlesex Hospital surgeon Charles Bell, performed a lithotomy on a 57-year-old 'robust healthy looking countryman' by

[109] *Lancet* 4:87 (28 May 1825), pp. 228–9.
[110] *Morning Chronicle* 26 July 1825, p. 2; *Lancet* 4:96 (30 July 1825), pp. 113–15.
[111] *Lancet* 4:87 (28 May 1825), 230–7.

the name of John Fletcher. The patient suffered a severe haemorrhage during the operation and died some ten hours afterwards, the result, or so Shaw
claimed, of his having 'an irregular distribution of the arteries' around the
bladder. *The Lancet* was not convinced, questioning Shaw's experience and
suggesting that he had 'never performed the operation on the living subject,
until he operated on the poor man whose case we have just given'. 'Mr. Shaw
may be a good anatomist', it acknowledged, 'but his knowledge of practical
surgery is about equivalent to that of Joe Burns'.[112] Reflecting on the first case,
The Lancet asked whether 'all the supporters of this Institution [are] deaf to the
voice of humanity – to the cries of the afflicted? and will they still permit this
incompetent creature to practise upon the objects of their charity?' 'Our language may appear harsh', it conceded, 'but we cannot repress the ardour of our
indignation when we contemplate the "sad work" of the Senior Surgeon'.[113]

The phrase 'ardour of [...] indignation' well describes the emotional register
of *The Lancet*'s campaign of scrutiny, which continued in earnest for the next
decade. So far in this book we have heard about a range of emotions and affective states, from anxiety and compassion to despondency and sympathy. But
the emotion that characterised *The Lancet*'s coverage of metropolitan surgery
for much of the later 1820s and early 1830s was anger, often mixed with pity.
The forms of its expression varied: sometimes it came in curt, offhand remarks,
such as in relation to the St Bartholomew's surgeon Henry Earle (1789–1838),
whose amputation was said to have been performed with 'such bungling' as was
'generally believed to be confined to the surgical tyro in the dissecting room'. At
other times, the descriptions were considerably more emotionally involved.[114] In
Chapter 1, we heard an account of the operation undertaken at St Bartholomew's
in May 1829 to remove a tumour from the knee of a 25-year-old woman named
Mary Hayward. Things started badly when she was called into the theatre and
'walked to the operating table, wet with the stream of blood on the floor that had
issued from the patient who had just been removed'. She was poised to lay herself on the table, 'which was still covered by a sheet upon which the operation of
lithotomy had been performed, and of which a considerable proportion was actually drenched in blood'. At this point, however, she began to lose her composure:

The poor thing having stepped first upon the chair at the lower end of the table, also
besmeared with blood, stood wringing her hands, and throwing her eyes first upon the
floor, next upon the operating table, then across the theatre, and next towards the ceil-
ing, trembling and weeping in the most pitiable manner, until, at length, a dresser on
each side *humanely* took her by the arms and assisted in lying her down on the table
thus conditioned.[115]

[112] *Lancet* 5:115 (12 November 1825), pp. 217–22.
[113] *Lancet* 4:96 (30 July 1825), p. 125.   [114] *Lancet* 7:176 (13 January 1827), p. 495.
[115] *Lancet* 12:298 (15 May 1829), p. 220.

Chapter 2 showed how Romantic surgeons were expected to make operations as palatable to the patient as possible, in part through the exercise of their own moral authority, and in part through the arrangement of the operating space itself. In Chapter 3, meanwhile, we heard that the reciprocal obligation of the patient in such idealised circumstances was fortitude and emotional self-control. In this instance, however, such expectations and obligations had broken down in the most egregious manner imaginable. Instead of comforting their charge, the two surgeons, John Painter Vincent (1776–1852) and William Lawrence, stood at 'some distance from the patient', conversing between themselves, while two of the hospital's nurses 'were joking and laughing at the fireplace with some of the pupils'. Meanwhile, 'in the midst of it, was this young female elevated on the chair and crying most bitterly'. To make matters worse, the operation itself was badly performed. The tumour was 'picked out piece-meal' and the procedure needlessly drawn out, to the extent that the already distressed patient began to cry out in pain and fear to 'let it alone!'[116]

If the nature and form of *The Lancet*'s exposure of metropolitan surgical incompetence varied, its tone largely did not. In reporting such incidents, and, more especially, in its editorial commentary on them, it consistently sought to arouse anger and indignation in its readers, using language that was melodramatic and censorious in the extreme. In commenting on the deaths at St George's in 1825, for example, Wakley claimed that 'Charity is degraded into a loathsome, execrable and sordid passion, that rankles amidst the havoc of its victims. Some of these places are human slaughterhouses [...] conducted by crafty, designing, mercenary medical men, whose knowledge of the sciences is not more contemptible than the motives by which their general conduct is governed'.[117] Elsewhere, *The Lancet* referred to metropolitan hospitals as 'mutilating man-traps' that the public 'never enter without feelings of horror and dread'. This was because of the 'scenes of cruelty and blood, so constantly presented by the inexperienced and misguided hands of the neveys and noodles' who, 'under the flimsy shield of sham elections, [are] forced into the offices of surgeon'.[118] In many cases it also sought to arouse pity and sympathy, not only for the direct 'victims' of such incompetence, but also for their dependants, often invoking sentimental ideals about the family as well as practical economic realities. Thus, in commenting on the death of James Wheeler, it reminded its readers that 'The wife of the unfortunate man is now, with two helpless children, deprived of the succour and protection of an industrious husband and the latter of an affectionate father'.[119]

---

[116] *Lancet* 12:298 (15 May 1829), p. 220.   [117] *Lancet* 5:115 (12 November 1825), p. 259.
[118] *Lancet* 14:363 (14 August 1830), p. 788; *Lancet* 14:350 (15 May 1830), p. 243.
[119] *Lancet* 4:87 (28 May 1825), p. 230. For the trope of the tender and providing father in the Romantic era, see Joanne Bailey, *Parenting in England, 1760–1830: Emotion, Identity*

Such language clearly had the desired effect on its audience. As has been argued elsewhere, *The Lancet* functioned as an intertextual space within which its readers might establish a dialogic relationship with the journal's contents and agendas.[120] Thus it was that they occasionally wrote letters to *The Lancet*, reflecting or commenting on its reporting of instances of surgical incompetence. In July 1825, for example, one correspondent opened his missive by stating that 'With great indignation I read, in your last Number, an account of the shocking occurrence which lately took place at St. George's Hospital, and by which an unfortunate man has lost his life'.[121] Meanwhile, in December 1830, *The Lancet* itself observed that 'There stands before us a pile of letters, all couched in terms of indignation and abhorrence, on the subject of the operation performed the other day at St Bartholomew's by Mr. HENRY EARLE'.[122] Even more significantly, perhaps, as was common in the early years of *The Lancet*, several readers took Wakley's metropolitan campaign as a cue to demand investigations into their own local hospitals. Thus, in October 1828, a correspondent from Birmingham, a 'constant reader of your valuable journal', expressed himself 'astonished' that his native city 'should have escaped your investigations'. Being of the opinion that 'the evil doings of our "Hole and Corner" Gentlemen should be circulated far and wide', he claimed that he would 'rejoice, when [...] the doors [of the Birmingham General Hospital] shall be opened to show the "hell that's there"'.[123] Moreover, in 1833 a correspondent from Scotland reported on an operation at the Glasgow Royal Infirmary that was performed in so 'bungled a manner' that 'no man of feeling and humanity [...] could allow it to pass without the severest censure'. 'What better is the man', he asked, 'who unskilfully lifts the operating knife than an inhuman butcher, under whom the living subject is but a carcase, and the operating table less desirable than the shambles?'[124]

While the campaign to expose the alleged incompetence and cruelty of metropolitan hospital surgeons lasted well into the 1830s, it can be said to have reached its apogee in 1828 with Bransby Cooper's notoriously bungled operation for lithotomy, performed at Guy's Hospital on a 53-year-old labourer by the name of Stephen Pollard. This case has been explored in detail elsewhere, but it bears further consideration in this context, not only for what it reveals about melodramatic forms of radical critique, but also for

---

and Generation (Oxford: Oxford University Press, 2012); Bailey, 'A Very Sensible Man: Imagining Fatherhood in England c.1750–1830', *History* 95:319 (2010), 267–92; Bailey, 'Masculinity and Fatherhood in England c.1760–1830', in John H. Arnold and Sean Brody (eds), *What Is Masculinity? Historical Dynamics from Antiquity to the Contemporary World* (Basingstoke: Palgrave, 2011), 167–86.
[120] Brown, 'Medicine', pp. 1377–80.   [121] *Lancet* 4:92 (2 July 1825), p. 405.
[122] *Lancet* 15:381 (18 December 1830), p. 403.   [123] *Lancet* 11:268 (18 October 1828), pp. 84–5.
[124] *Lancet* 20:516 (20 July 1833), pp. 537–8.

the questions it raises about the emotional politics of this strategy.[125] Indeed, if previous instances of exposure made extensive use of melodramatic language, then *The Lancet*'s reporting of the Pollard case took the melodramatic mode to its logical extreme. The original report, which was penned by Guy's student James Lambert and published on 29 March 1828, was simply titled 'Guy's Hospital' in the manner of a conventional case report. In actual fact, it presented the account of the procedure as a literal 'tragedy' in two acts.[126] The first act saw Cooper and his staff blundering in their attempts to insert the sound into Pollard's bladder and locate the stone. The second recorded Cooper's increasingly desperate attempts to cut into the bladder and remove it, 'the stillness of death, broken only by the horrible squash, squash of the forceps in the perineum'.[127]

In many ways, the Pollard case was the *ne plus ultra* of *The Lancet*'s entire campaign. Its target, Bransby Cooper, was the quintessence of surgical nepotism, a man who owed his position almost entirely to the influence of his uncle, Astley Cooper, over the Guy's Hospital treasurer, Benjamin Harrison (1771–1856).[128] Likewise, the case positively dripped with pathos and, at least as far as *The Lancet* was concerned, presented a cast composed of clear-cut victims and villains. Pollard, the vulnerable protagonist, was referred to as a 'poor fellow' and a 'poor man' who had 'left behind a wife and six children'. His optimism at having '[come] to town to be operated on by the "Nevey" of the great Sir Astley' was contrasted with his subsequent agony and constant cry of 'Oh! let it go – pray let it keep in'. Cooper's team were likewise cast in the role of villains. 'Never shall we forget', the author stated, 'the triumphant manner in which the Assistant Surgeon raised his arms and flourished the forceps over his head with the stone in their grasp' even as Pollard lay exhausted and dying, still bound to the table.[129]

If the Pollard case distilled the stylistic extravagance of *The Lancet*'s assault on alleged incompetence and corruption within metropolitan surgery, it also intensified the anxieties and ambivalences that attended the use of such emotive forms of professional critique. Lambert's report generated a great deal of debate and, ultimately, led to Wakley being found guilty of libel, albeit in circumstances in which he could claim a moral victory.[130] However, what many objected to was not so much the factual content of the report as its framing in intensely melodramatic and theatricalised terms. Writing to *The Times*,

---

[125] Brown, '"Bats, Rats"', pp. 192–204.   [126] *Lancet* 9:239 (29 March 1828), pp. 959–60.
[127] *Lancet* 9:239 (29 March 1828), p. 959. In reality, Pollard did not expire on the operating table, though he would indeed die just over a day after his hour-long ordeal.
[128] Brown, '"Bats, Rats"', p. 194. The etymology of the word 'nepotism' derives from the Latin for nephew.
[129] *Lancet* 9:239 (29 March 1828), pp. 959–60.   [130] Brown, '"Bats, Rats"'.

one correspondent decried the 'extraneous matter in which the report itself is embodied', arguing that it mocked 'the agonies of afflicted humanity by burlesque associations'. The operation for lithotomy, he claimed, was 'necessarily harrowing to the feelings' and thus 'unfitted for indiscriminate and promiscuous public discussion'.[131] Two days later, *The Times* published another letter, this one signed by 178 students of the Borough hospitals, who likewise alleged that 'the spirit in which the report is written plainly disproves the sincerity of the publication'.[132] Meanwhile, at the trial itself, Wakley asked a witness to the operation whether the report in *The Lancet* was correct or incorrect. 'Generally speaking it is [correct]', the witness responded, before adding, 'The form of the report is objectionable; if you want an opinion, the form of the report is objectionable'.[133]

Doubtless, Wakley's greatest critics with regard to style were his rivals in the world of print. Shortly before *The Lancet* published its account of Cooper's lithotomy, *The London Medical Gazette* had observed, in reference to another case report, that the author had 'a heart and imagination, filled with the foulest images and the darkest passions'.[134] In the immediate aftermath of the Pollard case, meanwhile, the attacks on *The Lancet* that regularly graced its pages turned into a veritable torrent, as correspondents charged Wakley with all manner of outrages, up to and including blasphemy.[135] Writing in an editorial of April 1828, Roderick Macleod stated that 'we are of the opinion that, in its long course of falsehood and abuse, the Lancet has never outraged the feelings of the profession more grossly than in the account of Mr. Bransby Cooper's recent case of Lithotomy'. Once again, it was the style of the report that elicited the greatest condemnation. If a medical journal were to 'make exposures', Macleod claimed, 'it ought to be done at least with a spirit of reluctance'. *The Lancet*, by contrast, had dressed its critique with '*theatrical* accompaniments' and demonstrated an 'unfeeling brutality' and 'malignant pleasure' in describing 'the embarrassment of the surgeon'.[136]

This last charge alerts us to an essential point of contention concerning *The Lancet*'s use of emotion. As we have seen, the deployment of sympathy and pity on behalf of the patient-victim was one of the hallmarks of Wakley's melodramatic style. His rivals, however, rejected this tactic. Writing in *The London Medical Gazette*, Macleod questioned Wakley's 'judgement in presenting such scenes to the public gaze', criticising his 'endeavours to excite the

[131] *Times* 31 March 1828, p. 2.   [132] *Times* 2 April 1828, p. 4.
[133] Thomas Wakley, *A Report of the Trial of Cooper v. Wakley for an Alleged Libel* (London: 1829), p. 56.
[134] *London Medical Gazette* 15 March 1828, p. 445.
[135] *London Medical Gazette* 12 April 1828, pp. 567–70.
[136] *London Medical Gazette* 5 April 1828, pp. 539–40. Emphasis in original.

sympathy of the unprofessional public by tales of horror'.[137] For Macleod and others, such 'sympathy' was misplaced and should, instead, have been directed to the feelings of the operator. As we have heard, the performance of surgery in this era was attended with great anxiety. Thus, as Macleod claimed:

Mr. Cooper will be regarded as having met with one of those difficult and perplexing cases where the efforts of the most expert and skilful surgeons are not always crowned with success till after much anxiety and delay – an anxiety so great to sensitive minds, that Cheselden [...] tells us that he used to feel it "even to sickness" [... and which has] been known to unnerve some of the most experienced and skilful men in the profession [...] To all reflecting men it must be a matter of serious apprehension to think what the consequences may be, if the difficulties and fearful responsibility attending capital operations are to be yet further increased by the consciousness on the part of the surgeon, that there are present those who, instead of participating in his anxious efforts, gloat with fiendish delight on his embarrassment, ready to caricature, to exaggerate, and to pervert.[138]

It is interesting to contrast this passage with the letter to *The Lancet* with which we began this chapter. In the one, the observer effects an intersubjective engagement with the feelings of the patient. In the other, that engagement is with the feelings of the surgeon. It is important not to be drawn too readily to essentialist explanations here, to assume that *The Lancet* and its readers cared *only* for patients while *The London Medical Gazette* and its readers cared *only* for surgeons. Indeed, one might go even further and suggest that it would be problematic to assume that *The Lancet actually* cared for patients or that *The London Medical Gazette actually* cared for surgeons. As we have suggested, following Reddy, emotions are not only a lived experience but also a system of symbolic meaning.[139] For the sake of interpretative clarity, it might therefore be best to regard these positions as fundamentally rhetorical and discursive in nature. By seeking to defend the surgical establishment from the emotive and populist forms of radical critique advanced by *The Lancet*, conservative forces such as *The London Medical Gazette* deployed their own language of emotion to refocus sympathy on the figure of the surgeon.

Roderick Macleod's apparent concern for the feelings of the operative surgeon is in keeping with the broader ideological contours of medical reform, whereby *The Lancet*'s modernist 'vision of the medical profession as an abstract body of public servants dedicated to the social good [...] founded upon the inchoate middle-class values of meritocracy, duty and reward' contrasted with the medical conservatives' individualism and its 'aristocratic

---

[137] *London Medical Gazette* 28 June 1828, p. 120.
[138] *London Medical Gazette* 29 December 1828, p. 99.
[139] William Reddy, *The Navigation of Feeling: A Framework for the History of the Emotions* (Cambridge, UK: Cambridge University Press, 2001), chs. 3 and 4, particularly pp. 128–9.

values of character, breeding and reputation'.[140] Indeed, while they may have been brought to the fore by the Pollard case, such ambivalences of character, compassion, and sympathy had attended *The Lancet*'s campaign of scrutiny and exposure from the very beginning. Among the reasons given against the publication of hospital case reports was the idea that they might injure the reputations of surgeons, especially young and inexperienced ones. Hence the *Medico-Chirurgical Review* castigated those who would 'lacerate the feelings of an individual', claiming that 'No man can command success in surgical operations – and if a surgeon fail from want of dexterity, he suffers mortification enough, Heaven knows, in the operation-room, without being put to the cruel and demoniacal torture of seeing the failure blazoned forth in the public prints'.[141] Wakley, for his part, dismissed such arguments, suggesting that they were based not on principles of 'public utility' but rather on the 'private interests of the operating surgeon'. For his conservative opponents, he maintained, the 'suffering and destruction of the patient go for nothing, and it is only the mortification endured by the Surgeon, from the consciousness of his own ignorance, which excites their sympathy and commiseration'. Meanwhile, referring to the potential damage to the reputation and character of young surgeons, he responded:

All we have to say in answer to this objection is, that if a young man is elected to fill the office of surgeon to a public hospital, the public have a right to know in what manner he performs his duty. If the objection be urged as an *argument* against publicity, this, we apprehend is a sufficient answer; if it be taken as an appeal to our compassion, then we reply, that there is a compassion due to patients as well as to surgeons, and that if the reputation, or finances, of the latter plead for suppression, the safety of the former calls imperiously for publicity.[142]

We might ascribe these contrasting evocations of pity and sympathy to ideological differences between the forces of reform and those of reaction, and we would be right to do so. But at the same time, it is important to acknowledge the inconsistencies and ambivalences within *The Lancet*'s own use of emotive and melodramatic tropes. We have already seen how the language employed by Wakley and his colleagues was deliberately inflammatory, regularly skirting close to, and oftentimes overstepping, the threshold of libel. We have also seen how this language was calculated to stir emotions in its readers and encourage emulative forms of expression and action. Yet there was always a risk that *The Lancet* could lose control over the very feelings it sought to promote and, on occasion, it even had to manage the emotional fallout of its own invective. For

[140] Brown, '"Bats, Rats"', p. 200. See also Brown, 'Surgery, Identity and Embodied Emotion: John Bell, James Gregory and the Edinburgh "Medical War"', *History* 104:359 (2019), 19–41.
[141] *Medico-Chirurgical Review and Journal of Medical Science* 4:16 (1 March 1824), p. 975.
[142] *Lancet* 2:39 (26 June 1824), pp. 395, 397.

example, in August 1826 it ran an editorial on the mismanagement of hospitals in which it referred to the 'horrid secrets of the charnel house', claiming that it could tell 'a tale whose lightest word would harrow up the soul and freeze the blood'. Most notably, it referred to incompetent surgeons as 'murderers', stating 'these men deserve no better title'.[143] And yet, three years later it had cause to question the tone of one of its own correspondents who had seemingly submitted an account of an operation conducted at Bury St Edmunds, stating that the account 'must be authenticated' and that if it 'be correct, the operation was certainly performed in a very unscientific, violent, and bungling manner; but the patient was *not murdered*'.[144]

Moreover, while *The Lancet*'s own appeals to feeling served to underscore the righteousness of its cause and the authenticity of its sentiment, when it came to its opponents the 'testimony of tears' was markedly less 'unequivocal'. For instance, in August 1825, the surgeon Henry Jeffreys wept during his speech to the St George's Hospital Committee meeting convened to inquire into the death of John Hammond; he expressed pity for those patients whose 'unfortunate circumstances' brought them to the hospital and declared his heartfelt desire, 'lest any patient should feel aggrieved at being attended by me', that he should 'have every thing like an imputation against my surgical character wiped away'. Far from being moved by such expressions of feeling, however, *The Lancet* mocked him in a predictably ostentatious and theatrical manner. Quoting from the scene in Shakespeare's *As You Like It* in which 'the melancholy Jacques' weeps over the death of a deer, it described Jeffreys 'heav[ing] forth such groans', the 'big round tears' coursing down 'his innocent nose / In piteous chase'. As it observed, 'The *old ladies* [meaning the Committee members] were very much affected by this touch of the pathetic'.[145]

Conclusion

As both William Reddy and Thomas Dixon have shown, tears occupied an ambivalent place as markers of emotional sincerity and authenticity within Romantic culture. For *The Lancet*, as for others in this period, they might function as an 'unequivocal testimony' of true feeling; yet they might also raise suspicions of artifice, effeminacy, even unreason.[146] Moreover, the evidence of

[143] *Lancet* 6:156 (26 August 1826), p. 693.
[144] *Lancet* 13:322 (31 October 1829), p. 200. Emphasis added.
[145] *Lancet* 4:97 (6 August 1825), pp. 141, 149–50.
[146] Reddy, *Navigation*, chs. 5 and 6; Thomas Dixon, *Weeping Britannia: Portrait of a Nation in Tears* (Oxford: Oxford University Press, 2015), chs. 7 and 8; Dixon, 'The Tears of Mr Justice Willes', *Journal of Victorian Culture* 17:1 (2012), 1–23. See also Markman Ellis, *The Politics of Sensibility: Race, Gender and Commerce in the Sentimental Novel* (Cambridge, UK: Cambridge University Press, 1996), ch. 6.

The Lancet suggests a broader anxiety about the place of emotion within radical medical discourse in the 1820s and early 1830s. At one level, the melodramatic mode served as a powerful means to express outrage against institutional corruption, to excite anger at the supposed incompetence of surgical office holders and encourage pity at the fates of those innocent patients on whom they operated. At the same time, however, such rhetorical appeals to feeling could also potentially undermine the credibility of one's political position, exposing the tensions identified by Reddy between 'liberal reason' and 'Romantic passions'.[147] This is not a simple story of *The Lancet* being outflanked by cultural ambiguity or cultural change. As we have seen, the appeal of emotive, and even explicitly melodramatic, forms of discourse was such that they could be utilised and admonished in equal measure by those on either side of the political divide. Thus, following the report of John Shaw's botched lithotomy in 1825, a number of correspondents wrote to *The Lancet* to comment on the case. In one instance, a correspondent signing himself 'Impartiality' sought, while defending Shaw's professional reputation, to reconcile the emotional politics of surgical failure, suggesting that 'no medical man, of humane feelings' could have read the account in *The Lancet* 'without his pity being roused at the fate of the unfortunate patient, and his sympathy excited for the unfortunate operator'.[148] For his respondent, however, such claims to emotional equitability would not do. Gently mocking 'Impartiality's' appeal to feeling, he questioned whether such sentiments had made the report any less *true*, for 'facts', he claimed 'are stubborn things'.[149] Such comments are suggestive of the ways in which these tensions between emotion and reason would come increasingly to prominence in this period, for as we shall see in the next chapter, the 1820s and 1830s would give rise to another form of medical discourse, one whose arch-rationality would seek, albeit with mixed success, to purge surgery of feeling and subject it to the operations of an instrumentalist logic.

---

[147] Reddy, *Navigation*, ch. 7.   [148] *Lancet* 5:118 (3 December 1825), p. 363.
[149] *Lancet* 5:120 (17 December 1825), p. 426.

5   Quiescent Bodies
Utilitarianism and the Reconfiguration of Surgical Emotion

Introduction

Within Astley Cooper's archive at the Royal College of Surgeons of England is a file collated by his nephew, Bransby Cooper.[1] After Astley's death in 1841, Bransby assumed responsibility for preparing his uncle's biography and, in the course of his research, wrote to a number of Astley's friends and associates, particularly those who had known him in his youth, in order to solicit anecdotes and reminiscences illustrative of the great man's character. One of the responses he received was from Samuel Sherrington (1776–1845), who had attended school in Brooke, the small village just to the south of Norwich where Astley's father, the Rev. Samuel Cooper (bap. 1739, d. 1800), then occupied the manor house. In Bransby's two-volume biography of his uncle, published in 1843, he quotes at length from Sherrington's letter, including his account of first meeting Astley. According to Sherrington, one of his schoolmates had seized the hat of another pupil and thrown it into a nearby pond: 'The boy, lamenting the loss of his hat, and fearing he should be punished for his absence from school, was crying very bitterly' when along came the young Astley, dressed in a 'scarlet coat, a three-cocked hat [...] and white silk stockings – his hair hanging in ringlets down his back'. Seeing the boy's tears, Astley strode into the pond and fetched his hat, emerging with his fashionable attire soaking wet and caked in mud 'much above his knees'. As Sherrington writes, he and Astley fell into conversation and 'from that period he seemed to have taken a fancy to me, and selected me as his companion. We were both of us frolicsome, mischievous boys and played many pranks together in the village'.[2]

If Bransby was happy to relate this story of the dashing young Astley, suggesting as it did his inherent sympathy with the distresses and misfortunes of others, he was somewhat more circumspect with another of Sherrington's

---

[1] RCSE, MS0008/2/2/1, File of letters giving descriptions of cases, 1813–41.
[2] RCSE, MS0008/2/2/1, Letter from Samuel Sherrington to Bransby Cooper, 29 March 1841; Bransby Blake Cooper, *The Life of Sir Astley Cooper, Bart.*, vol. 1 (London: John W. Parker, 1843), pp. 51–2.

anecdotes. In fact, he passed over this story, which saw the two friends 'engaged against a tailor in the village, to whom Astley owed a slight grudge', in some haste, claiming that 'in the detail [...] of the principal event, – an attack upon the poor man's windows, – there is nothing worthy of publication, nor characteristic of my uncle, excepting proof of the natural kindness of his disposition, from his having subsequently [...] remunerated him for the fright and injury to which he had been subjected'.[3]

Clearly, Bransby Cooper was keen to manage his uncle's posthumous reputation: to ensure that his narrative of Astley's transformation from, in his father's words, a 'sad rogue' into a 'shining character' accorded with the morally edifying ideal of Romantic *Bildung*, and that any account of Astley's youthful misbehaviour was balanced by a clear demonstration of his heartfelt sensibility.[4] To that end, it might seem peculiar that Bransby chose to quote quite as extensively as he did from another letter in the archive, this one sent by Peter Holland (1766–1855), an 'intimate associate' of Astley during his time as a surgical apprentice, when both boys lived in the house of Henry Cline. According to Holland:

During this time Astley, who was always eager to add to his physiological and anatomical knowledge, made a variety of Experiments on living animals. I recollect one day walking out with him when a dog followed us [...] home, little perceiving the fate that awaited him. He was confined for a few days till [Astley] had ascertained that no owner would come to claim him – He was then brought up to be the subject of various operations. The first of these was the tying one of the femoral arteries. When poor Chance – for so we named the dog, was sufficiently recovered from this, one of the humeral arteries was subject to a similar process. After the lapse of a few weeks the ill-fated animal was shot, the vessels injected and preparations were made from each of the limbs.[5]

Aside from substituting the word 'killed' for the specific (and perhaps more brutal) 'shot' in his description of the poor dog's fate, Bransby reproduced this anecdote almost verbatim in his published biography.[6] And yet this brief reference to the young Astley's practice of vivisection necessitated a two-page apologia, lest its inclusion 'lead those, who are unconscious of its necessity, to attribute a disposition devoid of feeling to my uncle and his friend'. 'In order to remove such an impression', Bransby continued, 'it becomes incumbent on me to say a few words on the advantages which this source of knowledge alone offers, and the consequently necessary sacrifice of our feelings in embracing them'.[7]

---

[3] Cooper, *Life*, vol. 1, pp. 52–3; RCSE, MS0008/2/2/1, Letter from Samuel Sherrington to Bransby Cooper, f. 1.
[4] Cooper, *Life*, vol. 1, p. 81.
[5] RCSE, MS0008/2/2/1, Letter from Peter Holland to Bransby Cooper, undated, unpaginated.
[6] Cooper, *Life*, vol. 1, p. 142.   [7] Cooper, *Life*, vol. 1, p. 144.

Vivisection was not the only unsavoury activity that Bransby chose to address in his biography. Another anecdote, also taken from Holland, involved the dissection of cadavers in Cline's house, away from the 'common dissecting room' of St Thomas' Hospital. One day, Holland claims, he and Astley were 'busily engaged with a subject on the table' when they noticed several men, who had been replacing some tiles on the building opposite, 'eagerly watching our operations' through the window. 'At that time', he notes, 'a mob was readily collected in the streets' and so they 'thought it prudent to convey our subject into a more private part of the house'.[8] Holland makes no specific mention of the fact that these bodies were illicitly acquired, but the implication is clear enough. Indeed, the last three chapters of the first volume of Bransby's biography are entirely dedicated to those 'Resurrection Men' who supplied Astley, and others like him, with the disinterred corpses of the poor.[9]

Both vivisection and anatomical dissection were highly contentious issues at the height of Astley Cooper's career in the 1820s. In June 1825, for example, the recently founded Society for the Prevention of Cruelty to Animals held a meeting at the Crown and Anchor on the Strand to consider the issue of animal experimentation. Several testimonies from leading London surgeons were read out and, while all acknowledged what John Abernethy called 'the unwarrantableness of such experiments, unless to determine some important question', opinion varied from Everard Home's conviction that 'the Lord has blessed his creatures for our use' to Charles Bell's incredulity that 'Providence should intend that the secrets of nature are [to] be discovered by means of cruelty'. Others were even less equivocal. Bell's fellow Paleyite, the Oxford professor John Kidd (1776–1851), questioned 'whether anyone can habitually inflict pain on even a brute, without impairing that sensibility, for the possession of which we ought to be most thankful'. Philip Crampton (1777–1858) likewise argued that 'The natural feelings of commiseration which we entertain for the sufferings of a helpless and inoffensive animal, are entwined with the best and tenderest sympathies of our nature' and 'we cannot part with the one without tearing up the others by the very roots'.[10] As Rob Boddice has demonstrated, the moral and emotional politics of vivisection were vociferously contested throughout the century, and for Bransby Cooper, writing in the early 1840s, the use of animals in physiological experiment clearly remained a highly sensitive topic, requiring extensive justification.[11] By contrast, the issue of anatomical

---

[8] Cooper, *Life*, vol. 1, pp. 141–2.   [9] Cooper, *Life*, vol. 1, chs. 18–20.
[10] *Morning Chronicle* 30 June 1825, pp. 3–4.
[11] Rob Boddice, *The Science of Sympathy: Morality, Evolution and Victorian Civilization* (Urbana: University of Illinois Press, 2016), ch. 4; Boddice, *The Humane Professions: The Defence of Experimental Medicine, 1876–1914* (Cambridge, UK: Cambridge University Press,

dissection was, by this time, seemingly settled. 'When the dead can be rendered subservient to the most important interests of the living, however much humanity may shudder at the idea of a beloved relative being disturbed from the stillness of the tomb', Bransby asked, 'who is there that would not sacrifice those feelings of repugnance, which, though so common, in truth can [...] be traced only to selfish motives?'[12]

That Bransby Cooper was willing to address issues such as vivisection and grave-robbing in a biography ostensibly concerned to present his uncle as a gentleman of exquisite feeling suggests something about the contours and boundaries of sentiment and sensibility in relation to surgery, the shifting delineations of which are the subject of this chapter. The first half of this book has been concerned to demonstrate the extent to which the emotional regime of early nineteenth-century surgery was shaped by the cultures of Romantic sensibility and defined by an idealised emotional intersubjectivity between surgeons and their patients. In Chapter 4, we considered how those cultures of sensibility and sentiment were 'weaponised' by radical reformers in an effort to undermine the political hegemony of the metropolitan surgical elites. In this chapter, we shall continue our exploration of the ambiguities of surgical emotion by charting the beginnings of a shift, whereby the appropriateness of feelings such as sympathy and pity, as well as their imagined objects, came to be questioned and, ultimately, reconfigured. We shall do this by focusing on two key moments in surgical history, separated by some twenty years. They are, firstly, the debates surrounding the practice of anatomical dissection that came to the fore in the 1820s and culminated in the passage of the Anatomy Act in 1832, and, secondly, the introduction and early use of inhalation anaesthesia in the later 1840s. Both have extensive historiographies of their own, but they have rarely been examined together, let alone treated as cognate phenomena. Indeed, they could hardly be viewed more differently. One is regarded, generally speaking, as a political assault upon the dignity and rights of the poorest in society, while the other, despite waves of more nuanced scholarship, retains its status as a triumphant moment of scientific discovery: a deliverance from pain and suffering that marks the birth of modern surgery.[13]

2020). See also Alan W. Bates, *Anti-vivisection and the Profession of Medicine in Britain: A Social History* (London; Palgrave Macmillan, 2017); Paul White, 'Sympathy under the Knife: Experimentation and Emotion in Late Victorian Britain', in Fay Bound Alberti (ed.), *Medicine, Emotion and Disease, 1700–1950* (Basingstoke: Palgrave Macmillan, 2006), 100–24.

[12] Cooper, *Life*, vol. 1, pp. 446–7.

[13] In terms of the Anatomy Act, this is particularly true of Ruth Richardson, *Death, Dissection and the Destitute* (London: Routledge and Kegan Paul, 1987). For subsequent scholarship, see Tim Marshall, *Murdering to Dissect: Grave-Robbing, Frankenstein and the Anatomy Literature* (Manchester: Manchester University Press, 1995); Michael Sappol, *A Traffic of Dead Bodies: Anatomy and Embodied Social Identity in Nineteenth-Century America* (Princeton: Princeton University Press, 2002); Helen MacDonald, *Human Remains: Dissection and Its Histories* (New

However, what connects these two episodes is the process by which the 'emo-tional object' at the heart of the Romantic surgical encounter, namely the body, either as the writhing, anguished agent of an agonised consciousness or as the object of professional pity, sympathy, and emotional self-reflection, came to be silenced: rendered quiescent and subservient to a more abstract emotional logic.[14] More specifically, what also unites them (and, indeed, the period as a whole) is the powerful political, cultural, and ideological influence of utilitari-anism, the consequentialist moral philosophy propounded by Jeremy Bentham (1747–1832) and his acolytes, whose ideas about the social good allowed early nineteenth-century medical practitioners to reimagine the relations between 'knowledge, expertise and civil and state governance'.[15]

At one level, the influence of utilitarianism could hardly be more widely acknowledged than in the literature on the Anatomy Act. Ruth Richardson's pioneering account, *Death, Dissection and the Destitute* (1987), presents the utilitarians and their Parliamentary advocates, particularly Henry Warburton (1784–1858), as the prime movers behind the Act. And yet, while Richardson acknowledges the vital role played by surgical interests in pushing for legis-lation, she does not explore the ideological dimensions of early nineteenth-century surgery in especially close detail, nor does she consider the influence of utilitarianism on surgical culture more generally. Indeed, within her analysis, surgery is, to borrow the Latourian concept, 'black-boxed', its internal dynam-ics reduced to broad characterisation (even caricature).[16] This is a corollary of Richardson's underlying belief that, for all surgeons stood to gain from the Act, it was not fundamentally a piece of surgical legislation but rather 'a class repri-sal against the poor', which only 'incidentally [...] endorse[d] the respectability

Haven: Yale University Press, 2005); Elizabeth Hurren, *Dying for Victorian Medicine: English Anatomy and Its Trade in the Dead Poor, c.1834–1929* (Basingstoke: Palgrave Macmillan, 2011); Fiona Hutton, *The Study of Anatomy in Britain, 1700–1900* (London: Pickering and Chatto, 2013). On anaesthesia, see Martin S. Pernick, *A Calculus of Suffering: Pain, Professionalism and Anaesthesia in Nineteenth-Century America* (New York: Columbia University Press, 1985); Stephanie Snow, *Operations without Pain: The Practice and Science of Anaesthesia in Victorian Britain* (Basingstoke: Palgrave Macmillan, 2006); Snow, *Blessed Days of Anaesthesia: How Anaesthetics Changed the World* (Oxford: Oxford University Press, 2008).
[14] For an introduction to the concept of 'emotional objects', and the ways in which objects might be imbued with, and divested of, emotional meaning, see the essays in Stephanie Downes, Sally Holloway, and Sarah Randles (eds), *Feeling Things: Objects and Emotions through History* (Oxford: Oxford University Press, 2018). The embodied quality of emotions has recently been explored in Dolores Martín-Moruno and Beatriz Pichel (eds), *Emotional Bodies* (Urbana: University of Illinois Press, 2019), while 'emotionalised bodies' and their relation to other material objects is the subject of Joanne Begiato, *Manliness in Britain, 1760–1900: Bodies, Emotion and Material Culture* (Manchester: Manchester University Press, 2020).
[15] Michael Brown, 'Medicine, Reform and the "End" of Charity in Early Nineteenth-Century England', *English Historical Review* 1214: 511 (2009), 1353–88, at p. 1356.
[16] Bruno Latour, *Science in Action: How to Follow Scientists and Engineers through Society* (Cambridge, MA: Harvard University Press, 1987), pp. 1–17.

of scientific medicine'.[17] Without seeking to contest the general point about the social, political, and humanitarian implications of utilitarian thought, it is clear that Richardson's approach mirrors that of E. P. Thompson, especially his 'rationalist' conception of social relations, wherein the 'emotional' appeal of charismatic preachers like Joanna Southcott is rendered 'delusional' in the very same sentence as his celebrated rejection of historical 'condescension'.[18] Such tendencies are similarly evident in Richardson's treatment of emotion, which features prominently, yet obliquely, in her book. She acknowledges that 'The Anatomy Act was an emotive issue' and she regularly situates the cold rationalism of utilitarianism in opposition to 'popular sentiment' surrounding the corpse.[19] However, she regards all discussion of 'feeling', especially when deployed by Parliamentary proponents of the Act, as a mere cover for 'real' economic and political motives.[20] Pitting callous liberals against the perse-cuted poor in a morally unambiguous class war, she views emotions as 'valid' or 'authentic' only when deployed by (or, more commonly, on behalf of) the potential 'victims' of the Act. Hence surgeons, who are as much the villains of the piece as their political allies, are, in emotional terms, entirely defined by the idea of clinical detachment, and their appeals to feeling either ignored or dismissed as inherently cynical and disingenuous.[21]

As we have seen, the monolithic and transhistorical concept of clinical detachment does little to explain the emotional cultures of Romantic surgery. And, as we shall see in this chapter, it likewise does nothing to capture those shifts in the emotional regime of surgery that were underway in the 1820s and that were exacerbated by the debates around anatomical dissection. In Chapter 4, we saw that the 1820s and early 1830s witnessed what we might call the crescendo of surgical sentiment when, in pursuit of specific politi-cal ends, surgical reformers invested the bodies of surgical patients with heightened emotional significance, publicising their sufferings and deaths in order to provoke pity, outrage, and anger. And yet, at precisely the same moment, many of those self-same reformers were seeking to divest other bodies, namely dead bodies and, more especially, the dead bodies of the poor, of much of their emotional significance, presenting them as a corporeal *terra nullius* that might be appropriated for the education and edification of surgeons and their pupils. There was no inherent contradiction in this posi-tion. Indeed, sympathy for the patient's sufferings, and a desire to alleviate their plight, was not infrequently invoked as the very reason why that same

[17] Richardson, *Death*, p. 266.
[18] Richardson, *Death*, p. 192; E. P. Thompson, *The Making of the English Working Class* (New York: Pantheon Books, 1964), pp. 12, 385.
[19] Richardson, *Death*, p. 230.   [20] Richardson, *Death*, p. 186.
[21] Richardson, *Death*, pp. 30–1, 50–1, 95, 132.

patient's body might cease to have any emotional meaning at the moment of their death. However, what *was* of profound and lasting significance for the emotional cultures of surgery was the way in which the feelings of the individual, once the principal nexus of the surgical ideal, were subordinated to an abstract conception of the social good. This act of sublimation is clearly evident in Bransby Cooper's appeal to emotional *sacrifice*, as are its utilitarian roots. But what is instructive about this example is that Cooper was no utilitarian and neither were many of those surgeons who advocated for the appropriation of 'unclaimed' bodies from hospitals and workhouses. Indeed, one of the great ironies of the Anatomy Act is how pervasive such rhetoric was even among the most conservative of surgical commentators, while those who were more closely aligned with the utilitarian political agenda often found it hardest to reconcile themselves. Hence, while the Anatomy Act was hugely important in shifting the emotional focus of surgery away from the individual and towards the social, it was by no means a straightforward process, not only, as we shall see, because utilitarians often made appeals to emotion themselves, but also because those contortions of logic that sought to render the dead bodies of the poor uniquely free of emotional association only served to enhance their pathos.

By contrast with the practice of surgical anatomy, the role of utilitarianism is somewhat less well acknowledged in the scholarship on anaesthesia. To be sure, in his ground-breaking revisionist history of anaesthesia in the United States, Martin S. Pernick frequently uses the term 'utilitarianism' and invokes a form of reasoning reminiscent of Bentham's famous 'felicific calculus'. However, Pernick's conception of utilitarianism is more akin to a pragmatic process of clinical decision-making than to an historically contingent and contextually specific moral philosophy or cultural ideology.[22] Stephanie Snow, meanwhile, has notably less time for utilitarianism in her account of the development of anaesthesia in the United Kingdom, and the same is true for Bourke and Moscoso in their respective histories of pain.[23] This is perhaps surprising, given Bentham's explicit identification of pain as 'in itself an evil; and, indeed, without exception, the only evil'.[24] One of the few historians to make a firm connection between utilitarianism and the advent of anaesthesia is Christopher Lawrence, in a relatively obscure

---

[22] Pernick, *Calculus*.
[23] Snow makes one brief reference to Bentham's idea of pain as an 'inherent evil', but does not expand on it: Snow, *Operations*, p. 33. Moscoso has only two references to Bentham in his book and Bourke not one: Javier Moscoso, *Pain: A Cultural History* (Basingstoke: Palgrave Macmillan, 2014), pp. 72, 76; Joanna Bourke, *The Story of Pain: From Prayers to Painkillers* (Oxford: Oxford University Press, 2014).
[24] Jeremy Bentham, *An Introduction to the Principles of Morals and Legislation* (London: T. Payne and Son, 1789), p. 98.

article from 1997.[25] This chapter takes up Lawrence's suggestive reasoning, arguing that utilitarianism was as implicit in the making of anaesthesia as it was explicit in the making of the Anatomy Act. I say *implicit*, because few commentators of the period necessarily identified Bentham or his philosophy by name in decrying the pain of operative surgery or imagining its abolition. But that, I contend, is because, from around the time of the debates surrounding anatomical dissection, utilitarian values had become so deeply embedded in medical and surgical thinking, as well as in much social and political thought more generally, that they hardly required identification. Having said this, the place of pain in surgical culture was not necessarily a straightforward or clear-cut one, as historians of anaesthesia have recognised.[26] The same, as we shall see, was true of the emotional and intersubjective qualities of surgery in the years immediately before and after the advent of anaesthesia. Indeed, while this chapter seeks to demonstrate the ways in which the operative subject was culturally and emotionally silenced by the practice of anaesthesia, rendered a quiescent pseudo-presence in the operating theatre, it is important to recognise that this process was, in common with the debates surrounding anatomical dissection, replete with complexity and ambivalence. Indeed, one of the principal purposes of my argument is to demonstrate how, as with anatomical dissection, the figure of the anaesthetised patient as a de-emotionalised object, akin to a corpse or, more palatably perhaps, a person asleep, had to be *made*, forged from a set of messy, complex, and culturally problematic associations with other 'altered states'. Moreover, as well as considering how the patient was emotionally and culturally reconfigured by the advent of anaesthesia, the chapter also explores its implications for surgical identity and self-presentation, ultimately demonstrating how anaesthesia paved the way for a techno-scientific conception of surgery in which the thoughts, feelings, and experiences of the individual patient were subordinated to a more abstract ideological rationale as the emotional regime of Romantic sensibility gave way to one of scientific modernity.

This argument about the switch of emotional focus from the individual to the broader social good has clear parallels with Boddice's arguments about later nineteenth-century vivisection, vaccination, and eugenics. Indeed, at one point in *The Science of Sympathy* (2016), Boddice digresses into a brief discussion of anaesthetics and surgery, although he posits an opposition between the surgeon caring for the individual patient and the vivisecting physiologist 'whose

---

[25] Christopher Lawrence, 'Anaesthesia in the Age of Reform', *History of Anaesthesia Proceedings* 20 (1997), 11–16. See also Donald Caton, 'The Secularization of Pain', *Anesthesiology* 62 (1985), 493–501.

[26] This is particularly true of Pernick, *Calculus*, but is also a feature of much of the best literature on the topic.

operations were for the good of everybody'.[27] As we shall see in this chapter and, more especially, Chapter 6, such observations could increasingly be made of surgeons too. This chapter therefore bears out Boddice's argument about the shifting terrain of scientific sympathy. However, whereas Boddice is concerned to locate this shift within a post-Darwinian discourse, and presents a somewhat two-dimensional characterisation of the emotional cultures of the Romantic era, this chapter demonstrates the importance of the period from the 1820s to the 1850s, at least as concerns the practice of surgery, and argues for the ideological significance of utilitarianism, of which Boddice is generally dismissive.[28]

There are also parallels, albeit somewhat slighter, between my argument and that of William Reddy, who suggests that the displacement of sentimentalism by 'liberal reason' and 'Romantic passions' in Restoration France provided for a more 'stable' emotional regime.[29] I make no such claims for the stability or otherwise of the two emotional regimes at work here, namely those of Romantic sensibility and scientific modernity. For one thing, there was evidently a greater continuity between sentimentalism and Romanticism in Britain than in France, where the former became so closely intertwined with the fervid political cultures of the Revolution. Nor do I completely share Reddy's opinion that Romanticism relegated sentiment to 'a private realm of personal reflection, artistic endeavour, and interior, noncivic spaces'.[30] After all, we have already seen the extent to which sentiment shaped interpersonal relations and political discourse within Romantic surgical culture. Most importantly of all, however, while Reddy is inclined to downplay the persistence of sentiment within his own schema, I think it is important to acknowledge the inconsistencies and incompleteness of the transition from one emotional regime to another.[31] As we shall see, neither utilitarian rationalism nor anaesthetic oblivion entirely eliminated emotional intersubjectivity between surgeon and patient. Nor did they end the discourse of sentiment in surgery. What they *did* do was lay the groundwork for a surgical identity whose social and moral authority derived less from emotional authenticity than from techno-scientific rationality.

The 'Struggles of Natural Feeling':
Emotions and the Dead

Of all John Bell's pupils, John Lizars (1791/2–1860) was perhaps the most closely formed in his master's image. Born shortly after Bell opened his Edinburgh anatomical school, and three years before he published his *Discourses on the Nature and Cure of Wounds* (1795), he was only 5 or so

[27] Boddice, *Sympathy*, p. 87.   [28] Boddice, *Sympathy*, p. 71.
[29] William Reddy, *The Navigation of Feeling: A Framework for the History of Emotions* (Cambridge, UK: Cambridge University Press, 2001), ch. 7.
[30] Reddy, *Navigation*, p. 236.   [31] Reddy, *Navigation*, p. 217.

when Bell treated the wounded from the Battle of Camperdown (1797).[32] And yet, such was the duration of the French wars, combined with the youth of contemporary surgical initiates, that he completed his apprenticeship in time to gain his own experience of wartime surgery, serving aboard a frigate off the Iberian Peninsula from 1810 to 1814. Like Bell, Lizars was renowned as a 'bold and accomplished operator', the first Scottish surgeon to excise the upper jaw and the first British surgeon to perform an ovariotomy.[33] Like Bell, he was also a master anatomist and the author of a beautifully illustrated and highly regarded anatomical work in five volumes, published between 1822 and 1826. The second volume of this work opens with Lizars quoting from his former master, who had died only three years before. 'When I began the First Part of this Work', he writes, 'I little thought that I should live to witness the sentiments of my late worthy preceptor Mr John Bell so completely verified'. These sentiments, originally published in 1794, were that Edinburgh had become a place 'where it is not praise-worthy, but even dangerous to propose dissections'.[34] 'When I read this in my early years of study', Lizars continues, 'I conceived it to be the sentiment of a disappointed man, and never dreamt that this literary city, and this enlightened age, would endeavour to suppress a study which has been universally allowed to form the basis for all surgical and medical science'.[35]

As Lawrence has shown, anxieties about the declining importance of Edinburgh as a centre for medical and surgical education stretched back to the time when Bell was writing in the 1790s, but they were becoming increasingly pronounced in the 1820s when Lizars could imagine that 'the City of Edinburgh, which has extended its fame for literature, philosophy, and medicine, to the most distant regions of the earth, is doomed to dwindle into comparative insignificance'.[36] The reason for this decline, according to Lizars, was the rise of a 'miserable prejudice', a tide of 'ignorance, bigotry and superstition' by which the authorities, in their 'zeal, that bodies should remain undisturbed

---

[32] Malcolm Nicholson, 'Lizars, John (1791/2–1860)', *ODNB*. For John Bell's treatment of the wounded, see Michael Brown, 'Wounds and Wonder: Emotion, Imagination, and War in the Cultures of Romantic Surgery', *Journal for Eighteenth-Century Studies* 43:2 (2020), 239–59, at pp. 242–5.

[33] Nicholson, 'Lizars', *ODND*. One of the first ovariotomies had been performed by another of Bell's former pupils, the American surgeon Ephraim McDowell (1771–1830): Sally Frampton, *Belly-Rippers, Surgical Innovation and the Ovariotomy Controversy* (London: Palgrave Macmillan, 2018), pp. 49–50.

[34] John Lizars, *A System of Anatomical Plates ... Part II. Blood Vessels and Nerves of the Head and Trunk* (Edinburgh: Daniel Lizars, 1823), p. vii, quoting John Bell, *Engravings Explaining the Anatomy of the Bones, Muscles and Joints* (Edinburgh: John Patterson, 1794), p. xi.

[35] Lizars, *System ... Part II*, p. vii.

[36] Lizars, *System ... Part II*, p. viii; Christopher Lawrence, 'The Edinburgh Medical School and the End of the "Old Thing" 1790–1830', *History of Universities*, 1 (1988), 259–86.

in their progress to decomposition', had 'laboured to destroy [...] that art, whose province it is to free living bodies from the consequences [of] accident and disease'.[37] Lizars was one of the earliest surgeons to publicly express his concerns about the increasing practical and legal difficulties of acquiring subjects for anatomical dissection, but he was not quite the first. That distinction is often accorded to John Abernethy who, in his Hunterian Oration of 1819, drew inspiration from continental European practices, most notably those of post-Revolutionary France, to suggest that either 'the body of any person dying in [public] institutions, unclaimable by immediate relatives', or, at a push, 'the body of any person of whatsoever rank or fortune, unclaimable by immediate relatives', should be subject to dissection.[38]

The history of grave-robbing and anatomical dissection is too well known to warrant extensive repetition here. Suffice it to say that, while the practice of exhuming bodies for the purposes of dissection was of long standing, the marked expansion in anatomical education discussed in Chapter 4, and the move away from anatomical *demonstration* towards hands-on *dissection* initiated by the Hunters, Bells, and others, saw an increased demand for cadavers in the later decades of the eighteenth and early decades of the nineteenth century. This was a demand that could not be met by the legal provisions of the Murder Act of 1752, which allowed for the public dissection of hanged felons.[39] As Lizars' lament suggests, the shortage of bodies in Edinburgh was particularly acute and encouraged attempts to import cadavers from Ireland, where they were more readily obtainable. But even in London, the situation by the early 1820s had become untenable. As we heard in the previous chapter, in his testimony to the 1828 Select Committee on Anatomy, Astley Cooper estimated that around 700 pupils attended one or more of the anatomy schools in the metropolis and, by Warburton's calculations, these students required access to at least 2,000 bodies each year.[40] Various estimates were given by contemporaries as to the number of cadavers available via statutory means, but as records suggest that only 25 people were executed for murder in London between 1800 and 1820 (some 29 per cent of the 87

---

[37] Lizars, *System ... Part II*, pp. viii–ix.

[38] John Abernethy, *The Hunterian Oration for the Year 1819* (London: Longman, Hurst, Rees, Orme, and Brown, 1819), p. 36; Richardson, *Death*, p. 108.

[39] For an account of attempts to increase the availability of corpses for dissection through penal provision, see Richard M. Ward, 'The Criminal Corpse, Anatomists and the Criminal Law: Parliamentary Attempts to Extend the Dissection of Offenders in Late Eighteenth-Century England', *Journal of British Studies* 54:1 (2015), 63–87.

[40] *Report from the Select Committee on Anatomy* (1828), p. 16; *Hansard*, HC Deb vol. 19, col. 16 (22 April 1828). See also *Morning Chronicle* 23 April 1828, p. 1. These figures were contested. Joshua Brookes thought the number of students in 1823 to be closer to 1,000, while Cooper thought that only about 450 bodies were dissected in any one season: *Report*, pp. 4, 17.

sentenced to death at the Old Bailey), this provided, on average, just over one body a year.[41]

As a result of this demand, the early nineteenth century saw the rise of a commercial trade in grave-robbing to supply bodies to the anatomy schools. In turn, this encouraged greater vigilance on the part of families and parish authorities, particularly in places like Edinburgh, making bodies harder to obtain and raising their price. According to Cooper, the price per body in London had risen from two guineas at the time of his first entry into practice in the 1790s to eight guineas by 1828 and, in times of especial privation, had reached as much as fourteen.[42]

The legal status of this trade was not entirely clear. As corpses had no monetary value in English law, disinterring them was not technically theft. The case of *Rex* v. *Lynn* in 1788 had established that it was a misdemeanour, *contra bones mores*, to carry away a body from a churchyard for the purposes of dissection, and surgeons could be charged as accessories to that offence. Meanwhile, the case of *Rex* v. *Young* had seen the master of a workhouse, a surgeon, and another party convicted of conspiracy for preventing the burial of a former inmate.[43] However, such prosecutions were rare and most surgeons were unaware that their actions contravened the law in any way, at least until 1828, when a jury at the Lancaster Assizes found two students guilty of a misdemeanour for possessing the body of one Jane Fairclough.[44]

Such were the economic, pedagogical, and legal circumstances of the early 1820s that encouraged practitioners to imagine a new system whereby a regular supply of cadavers might be provided by the state. As has been argued elsewhere, such imaginings were an early expression of the reformist impulse in medicine and surgery, whereby the interests of the profession and those of the state were figured as increasingly congruent, and by which a rhetoric of decline was harnessed to an ideology of progress.[45] The varied configuration of these imaginings serves to illuminate the emotional regime of surgery and its shifting norms. Hence, what is notable about Lizars' and Abernethy's early contributions to the debate is how tentative they seem in comparison to other, later projections. Lizars was perhaps too coy to propose anything concrete in

---

[41] Calculated using the *Digital Panopticon* website, www.digitalpanopticon.org (accessed 12/08/20).
[42] *Report*, p. 17. According to the National Archives currency converter, 14 guineas in 1820 was equivalent to 98 days' wages for a skilled labourer or £844.23 in 2017: www.nationalarchives .gov.uk/currency-converter/#currency-result (accessed 12/08/20).
[43] *Report*, pp. 6, 147–50.   [44] *Report*, pp. 18–19; Richardson, *Death*, p. 107.
[45] Michael Brown, *Performing Medicine: Medical Culture and Identity in Provincial England, c.1760–1850* (Manchester: Manchester University Press, 2011), pp. 129–37; John Harley Warner, 'The Idea of Science in English Medicine: The "Decline of Science" and the Rhetoric of Reform, 1814–1845', in Roger French and Andrew Wear (eds), *British Medicine in the Age of Reform* (London: Routledge, 1991), 136–64.

the preface to his second volume of *A System of Anatomical Plates* (1823).[46] He even suggested that his work might 'form some substitute' for access to real bodies, something that was, in principle, roundly refuted by later commentators.[47] Meanwhile, Abernethy's early advocacy for a French-style system of institutional supply was hedged by a desire to give 'no offence to common decency and humanity'. '[B]etter would it seem to me', he claimed, 'that medical science should cease, and our bodily sufferings continue, than that the natural rights and best feelings of humanity should not be equally respected in all classes of society'.[48]

And yet, at the same time, these early interventions set the template for much subsequent debate, not least by the way in which they appealed to a higher emotional register, pitting heartfelt professional and patriotic *sentiment* against vulgar and indulgent popular *sentimentality*. As a former naval surgeon, Lizars was in a particularly strong position to do this, drawing on his wartime experiences to evoke the frisson produced by imagining the practical consequences of anatomically deficient physicians and surgeons:

Who does not shudder when he thinks of the number of young medical gentlemen who, after a year or two of grinding, obtain a degree or a diploma, and who thus, ignorant of the very elements of their profession, annually go to the East and West Indies, and to the army and navy, where they have the charge of hundreds of their suffering fellow-creatures[?] Little are these individuals aware of the fearful responsibility which awaits them in the hour of sickness, or on the field of battle; and little do the public think that they are the instruments of such cruelty and murder.[49]

If neither Lizars nor Abernethy offered a substantive proposal for a system of cadaver supply, it was not long before someone did. That man was William Mackenzie (1781–1868), a Scottish surgeon who had attended Abernethy's lectures at St Bartholomew's Hospital in the later 1810s and who, by the mid-1820s, was Professor of Anatomy and Surgery at Anderson College in Glasgow. In 1824, the year after Lizars' lament, he published *An Appeal to the Public and the Legislature on the Necessity of Affording Dead Bodies to the Schools of Anatomy, by Legislative Enactment*. This thirty-six-page pamphlet was the first sustained intervention into the emerging debate on the acquisition of anatomical subjects and the first comprehensive proposal for legislative reform. It is notable for many things, not the least of which was the emphasis it placed on *surgical* anatomy. That surgeons were the professional constituency most directly interested in these matters was implicit in much

---

[46] He did, however, hint at possible solutions in subsequent volumes, e.g. *A System of Anatomical Plates ... Part IV. The Muscles of the Trunk* (Edinburgh: Daniel Lizars, 1824), p. ix.
[47] Lizars, *System ... Part II*, p. xii.   [48] Abernethy, *Hunterian Oration*, pp. 35–6.
[49] Lizars, *System ... Part II*, pp. x–xi. The parallels here with John Bell's writing are very strong. See Brown, 'Wounds', p. 244.

of the discussion surrounding the practice of anatomical dissection. Even so, anatomy encompassed a range of meanings, including the kinds of demonstrative instruction sufficient for would-be physicians, and it was these forms that allowed opponents to claim that access to bodies might be supplemented, or even supplanted, by illustrated plates, wax models, and other simulacra.[50] For Mackenzie, however, anatomy was of a different order of importance for surgeons, because in order to operate successfully, and with confidence, on a living patient, it was necessary, as John Bell had argued, to have an intimate, *'practical acquaintance'* with the human body. 'No doubt', Mackenzie wrote, 'there is a manual address in the performance of surgical operations, which actual practice only can give; but it is evident that practice on the living ought, from the very first, to be under the guidance of a clear and well-understood system of rules, which the surgeon has already put to the test [...] on the dead body'.[51]

Needless to say, providing multiple bodies to each and every student would require a far more extensive system of procurement than was necessary for demonstrative purposes only. In order to convince his readers of the necessity for such provision, therefore, Mackenzie drew upon the cultures of Romantic surgical intersubjectivity to evoke sympathy for the prospective plight of both patient and surgeon. Thus, he conjured the spectre of 'a man tormented with the stone' whose 'excruciating sufferings' and 'anguish' could not be 'adequately' described, and only alleviated by skilful surgical intervention. Likewise, he imagined the embodied experience of the ill-prepared surgeon as he confronts his operative subject: 'his hand trembles, and his heart fails, he hears the frightful cries of his victim, and sometimes sees him expire under his hand'.[52]

As we have already seen, such imaginings were typical of Romantic surgical discourse, and owed much to the influence of John Bell. However, rather than simply functioning as a demonstration of the profound sensibility, and hence cultural credibility, of the surgeon, Mackenzie's appeal to emotion was explicitly intended to counter, and ultimately displace, another set of emotional associations, namely those attached to the bodies of the dead. From the very beginning of his pamphlet, Mackenzie asserted surgery's status as a social good.[53] Hence, while he acknowledged the 'struggles of natural feeling' that might result from supplying surgeons with 'unclaimed' bodies,

---

[50] For example, see Henry Hunt's comments in *Hansard*, HC Deb vol. 9, cols 1279–7 (8 February 1832). For a good account of these different styles of anatomy, see Carin Berkowitz, *Charles Bell and the Anatomy of Reform* (Chicago: Chicago University Press, 2015), ch. 2.
[51] William Mackenzie, *An Appeal to the Public and the Legislature on the Necessity of Affording Dead Bodies to the Schools of Anatomy, by Legislative Enactment* (Glasgow: Robertson and Atkinson, 1824), pp. 11–14. Emphasis in original.
[52] Mackenzie, *Appeal*, pp. 6–8.   [53] Mackenzie, *Appeal*, p. 4.

he maintained that 'the subject is of the deepest interest to humanity [...] almost *too deep* indeed to admit of *personal feelings*'.[54] By figuring the emotional regime of surgery as commensurate with the interests of 'humanity', Mackenzie was able to dismiss opponents of anatomical dissection as 'worshippers of ignorance' indulging in 'idolatry of the dead' who should 'listen to reason, not to passion'.[55]

Despite Mackenzie's contrast between 'reason' and 'passion', he did not seek to exclude emotion from the debate. Rather, he intended to sublimate 'personal feelings' into a higher emotional logic. In so doing, however, he figured certain feelings as valid and others as invalid, discriminating between authentic sentiment and what he called the 'mask of tender-heartedness'.[56] This concern with inauthentic sentiment, or *sentimentality*, had its roots in later eighteenth-century debates about the limits of sensibility, but what distinguished Mackenzie's conception of emotional authenticity was that it was determined not simply, as had been the case before, by the profusion or otherwise of its expression, or, indeed, by the object of its focus, but by the extent to which it accorded with the interests not just of 'humanity', but, more specifically, of the state.[57]

By the nineteenth century, the interests of the state were perhaps most obviously manifest in the prosecution of war and imperial conquest and it was these twin endeavours with which medical practitioners increasingly sought to imaginatively align themselves.[58] For Mackenzie and his contemporaries, the battles of the French wars, most especially Waterloo, were a recent memory. Hence, like Lizars before him, he capitalised on the imaginative and emotional appeal of the military, albeit in a somewhat more ambiguous manner. Addressing those who 'would reject the present appeal, on the ground that [...] this humane and religious nation forbids such cruel butchery of the human body', he begged leave to 'in imagination [...] convey these persons to the dissecting room, where a single dead body lies under the minute knife of the anatomist, who in his hidden and silent retreat [...] is preparing to instruct perhaps a hundred young and ardent minds, in a knowledge of those facts which are to prove, in their hands, the salvation of innumerable lives'. He then proposed

---

[54] Mackenzie, *Appeal*, p. 36. Emphasis added.   [55] Mackenzie, *Appeal*, pp. 16–17.
[56] Mackenzie, *Appeal*, p. 34.
[57] Markman Ellis, *The Politics of Sensibility: Race, Gender and Commerce in the Sentimental Novel* (Cambridge, UK: Cambridge University Press, 1996), ch. 6; Michael Brown, 'Surgery, Identity and Embodied Emotion: John Bell, James Gregory and the Edinburgh "Medical War"', *History* 104:359 (2019), 19–41, at pp. 35–6.
[58] Brown, 'Wounds'; Brown, '"Like a Devoted Army": Medicine, Heroic Masculinity, and the Military Paradigm in Victorian Britain', *Journal of British Studies* 49:3 (2010), 592–622; Christopher Lawrence and Michael Brown, 'Quintessentially Modern Heroes: Surgeons, Explorers, and Empire, c.1840–1914', *Journal of Social History* 50:1 (2016), 148–78.

to convey them from a scene which they loathe so much and know so ill, to one which they have heard more of, and have loved better – to the battle-field [...] the red and living blood is pouring in torrents, the air is rent with agonizing cries, and [...] the ground is covered with weltering corpses. We have seen the day, when Britain, reckoning up the slain, coolly subtracted the number of her own sons whose blood had drenched a foreign soil [...] The *humane* and *feeling* public received the estimate of slaughter with rapture. It was the estimate of what they had won. The youth, the vigour, and the beauty of the fallen were forgotten. The loud lamentations of the widow, the mother, and the sister, refusing to be comforted, were lost to a deafening cry of victory. The hour was given to madness, and midnight's darkness could not hide the wantonness of mirth and triumph.[59]

Mackenzie's intensely melodramatic prose paints a deeply ambivalent picture of 'victory' at Waterloo, an ambivalence that, as Philip Shaw and others have shown, was by no means uncommon within Romantic culture.[60] But in Mackenzie's hands, this ambivalence served a distinct purpose, highlighting what he perceived to be the emotional hypocrisy of the public (or elements thereof) in celebrating wartime sacrifice while 'raising their hands in well-affected horror' at the proposition of anatomical dissection.[61] Both, he argued, were of equivalent importance to the state, for if 'the end of war, which is the defence of our country, is sufficient to justify the adoption of a mean[s] so terrible as the destruction of hosts of living men, surely the end of anatomical study, which is the assuagement of human suffering, is ten times sufficient to justify the dissection of the dead!'[62]

There is nothing in Mackenzie's biography to suggest that he was an avowed utilitarian. However, his claim that in order to 'discover whether any action [...] be right or wrong, we have to inquire into its tendency to promote or diminish the general happiness', bears the unmistakable stamp of utilitarian thought.[63] So too does the unflinching rationality of his legislative proposals (he was, as far as I know, the only major commentator who suggested sourcing bodies from *foundling* hospitals alongside infirmaries, workhouses, and prisons).[64] Jeremy Bentham had a long-standing interest in the legal status, and potential utility, of the dead and, during the mid-1820s, corresponded with the Home Secretary Robert Peel (1788–1850) about legislative reform on the

[59] Mackenzie, *Appeal*, pp. 33–4. Emphasis added.
[60] Philip Shaw, *Suffering and Sentiment in Romantic Military Art* (Aldershot: Ashgate, 2013), pp. 158–69. See also Barbara Leonardi, 'Hunger and Cannibalism: James Hogg's Deconstruction of Scottish Military Masculinities in *The Three Perils of Man, or War, Women and Witchcraft!*', in Michael Brown, Anna Maria Barry, and Joanne Begiato (eds), *Martial Masculinities: Experiencing and Imagining the Military in the Long Nineteenth Century* (Manchester: Manchester University Press, 2019), 139–60.
[61] Mackenzie, *Appeal*, p. 34.
[62] Mackenzie, *Appeal*, p. 35. Mackenzie's statement is an early example of the ambivalent alignment of medicine and war, discussed in Brown, '"Devoted Army"', pp. 614–17.
[63] Mackenzie, *Appeal*, p. 19.   [64] Mackenzie, *Appeal*, pp. 24–5, 29.

matter of obtaining subjects for anatomical dissection.[65] However, rather than Bentham, it was his close associate, the physician and sometime Unitarian minister Thomas Southwood Smith (1788–1861), who would make the single biggest contribution to shaping public and professional discourse on this subject. In 1824, Smith published an anonymous review of Mackenzie's pamphlet in the *Westminster Review* under the title 'Use of the Dead to the Living'. Like Mackenzie, Smith was keen to establish from the outset that medicine and surgery were an inherent social good, claiming that 'An enlightened physician and a skilful surgeon, are in the daily habit of administering to their fellow men more real and unquestionable good, than is communicated, or communicable by any other class of human beings to another'.[66] Again, like Mackenzie albeit even more so, Smith was also concerned to reconcile this social good with popular sentiment, elaborating an emotional logic by which the interests of the living were prioritised over their feelings *towards* the dead. In the published version of his 1832 lecture over Bentham's corpse, Smith reminded his readers of Bentham's distinction between the twin fallacies of 'asceticism' and 'sentimentalism'. Whereas asceticism approved of an action 'in as far as it tends to diminish happiness', sentimentalism judged actions not by their tendency to enhance or diminish happiness, but according to the subject's feelings about the act itself. It was as a *via media* between these two extremes that Bentham proposed his famous principle of 'felicity', whereby actions were judged solely by their 'CONDUCIVENESS TO THE MAXIMUM OF THE AGGREGATE OF HAPPINESS'.[67]

For Smith, Bentham's principle was to 'moral science' what Isaac Newton's law of universal gravitation was to natural philosophy, and necessitated a thoroughgoing reconfiguration of understandings of emotion and sentiment.[68] John Stuart Mill (1806–73) maintained that Bentham was both philosophically and personally immune to emotion, stating that 'In many of the most natural and strongest feelings of human nature he had no sympathy'. Likewise, describing his father, and Bentham's close friend, James Mill, he claimed: 'For passionate emotions of all sorts, and for everything which has been said or written in exaltation of them, he professed the greatest contempt'.[69] Smith, by contrast, was seemingly less averse. Indeed, in the 'Use of the Dead to the Living' he acknowledged that one of the most 'formidable obstacles' to 'the prosecution of anatomical investigations' was a 'feeling which is natural to the heart of

[65] David McAlister, *Imagining the Dead in British Literature and Culture, 1790–1848* (London: Palgrave Macmillan, 2018), pp. 81–88; Richardson, *Death*, pp. 109–10.
[66] [Thomas Southwood Smith], 'Use of the Dead to the Living', *Westminster Review* 2:3 (July 1824), 59–97, at p. 59.
[67] Thomas Southwood Smith, *A Lecture Delivered over the Remains of Jeremy Bentham Esq.* (London: Effingham Wilson, 1832), pp. 8, 25–6.
[68] Smith, *Lecture*, pp. 8–9.   [69] Quoted in McAlister, *Imagining*, p. 8.

man', namely an emotional attachment to the bodies, and even material possessions, of our loved ones. We cannot, he alleged, 'separate the idea of the peculiarities and actions of a friend from the idea of his person':

everything that has been associated with him acquires a value from that consideration; his ring, his watch, his books, and his habitation. The value of these as having been his is not merely fictitious; they have an empire over my mind; they can make me happy or unhappy; they can torture and they can tranquilize; they can purify my sentiments and make me similar to the man I love; they possess the virtue which the Indian is said to attribute to the spoils of him he kills, and inspire me with the powers, the feelings, and the heart of their preceding master.[70]

These were not Smith's own words. He was quoting (albeit without attribution) from William Godwin's (1756–1836) *Essay on Sepulchres* (1809), a meditation on the dead and a call for a system of national memorialisation that was, in part, shaped by Godwin's own grief at the loss of his wife Mary Wollstonecraft (1759–97).[71] As David McAlister has shown, while they shared many of the same utilitarian principles, Godwin and Bentham entertained very different conceptions of the emotions attached to the dead. By quoting as extensively as he did from Godwin, both in his *Westminster Review* article and in his later lecture, McAlister suggests that Smith was acknowledging 'what Godwin had got right and Bentham wrong; the importance of emotion and its capacity to stimulate progressive reform'.[72] There is much truth to this observation, for Smith did indeed appeal to the emotions in making his argument. For example, like Lizars and Mackenzie before him, he sought to conjure feeling through imagination:

We put it to the reader to imagine what the feelings of an ingenious young [surgeon] must be who is aware of what he ought to do, but whose knowledge is not sufficient to authorise him to attempt to perform it, and who sees his patient die before him, when he knows that he might be saved and that it would have been within his own power to save him, had he been properly educated. We put it to the reader to conceive what his own sensations would be, were an ignorant surgeon [...] to undertake an important operation [...] suppose it were his mother, his wife, his sister, his child, whom he thus saw perish before his eyes, what would the reader then think of the prejudice which withholds from the surgeon that information without which the practice of his profession is murder?[73]

Smith did not valorise emotions for their own sake, however. Rather, like Mackenzie, he valued them only insofar as they were conducive to social utility, to the realisation of a greater good. Thus, he followed up his quotation from Godwin by claiming that 'It is not the eradication of these feelings that

---

[70] [Smith], 'Use of the Dead', p. 80.
[71] McAlister, *Imagining*, p. 90. See also Thomas W. Laqueur, *The Work of the Dead: A Cultural History of Mortal Remains* (Princeton: Princeton University Press, 2015), pp. 49–54.
[72] McAlister, *Imagining*, p. 109.   [73] [Smith], 'Use of the Dead', pp. 91–2.

can be desired, but their control: it is not the extinction of these natural and useful emotions that is pleaded for, but that they should give way to higher considerations when these exist'.[74] And yet, Smith does not follow through on his philosophical premise. He does not invoke the character of the bereaved friend so that he might ask them to sacrifice their tender feelings for the greater good and hand the body of their loved one over to the surgeons. Rather, he proposes to use *other people's bodies*, notably, as suggested by Mackenzie and Abernethy, those dying, unclaimed by relatives, in hospitals, workhouses, and other institutions. Richardson has charted the complex and contested meanings of the term 'unclaimed' within the debates surrounding the Anatomy Act: whether, for example, it meant those with no living relatives, those whose relatives did not immediately present themselves, or simply those who could not, or would not, pay for a funeral.[75] What is notable about Smith's contribution to the debate is that he cast this category in fundamentally emotional terms. To be sure, he made the claim that the bodies of the poor (or rather *paupers*, though Smith did not admit a distinction) were, *in principle*, 'public property', stating that 'no maxim can be more indisputable than that those who are supported by the public die in its debt, and that their remains might, without injustice, be converted to the public use'. He also argued that it would be the poor themselves who would benefit from the resulting improvements in surgical standards, as the wealthy could always afford the most experienced and skilled attendants, whereas the poor had little choice about who treated them. However, he maintained that 'it is not proposed to dispose in this manner of the bodies of *all the poor*; but only of that portion of the poor who die unclaimed and *without friends*, and whose appropriation to the *public service* could, therefore, *afford pain to no one*'.[76]

The concept of *friendlessness* has received little consideration within the scholarship on the Anatomy Act, but it is vital to understanding how the Act was justified in emotional terms. More will be said about its ambiguities and contradictions in due course, but for the moment it is important to reiterate that Smith highlighted the ties of friendship not in order to demonstrate the emotional sacrifice demanded of the rational citizen, but, rather, to present a contrast to the emotion*less* quality of those bodies that would be taken in 'the public service'. As Smith saw it, the body only possessed emotional meaning within a nexus of interpersonal relationships; it had no *intrinsic* emotional value and any body that could be said to have fallen outside of this nexus could therefore be appropriated without compunction. Such a measure, he concluded, would 'tranquilize the public mind. Their dead would rest undisturbed:

---

[74] [Smith], 'Use of the Dead', p. 81.   [75] Richardson, *Death*, pp. 121–9, 186–9.
[76] [Smith], 'Use of the Dead', p. 94. Emphasis added.

the sepulchre would be sacred: and all the horrors which the imagination connects with its violation would cease for ever'.[77]

Smith's essay exerted a huge influence over subsequent debates concerning the procurement of subjects for anatomical dissection. Indeed, while disagreements persisted over issues such as the stigma of juridical dissection, the exact institutions from which bodies might be taken, or the disposal of remains, the maxims established by Smith in 1824 remained remarkably unchallenged throughout the later 1820s and early 1830s, at least among proponents of reform. Thus, the *Report from the Select Committee on Anatomy* (1828) claimed that 'If it be an object deeply interesting to the feelings of the community that the remains of friends and relations should rest undisturbed, – that object can only be effected by giving up for dissection a certain portion of the whole, in order to preserve the remainder from disturbance'.[78] This should perhaps come as little surprise. As Richardson points out, the Select Committee was composed either of 'first degree Benthamites' such as Warburton and Joseph Hume (1777–1855), or of 'keenly sympathetic' radicals like John Cam Hobhouse (1786–1869).[79] And, indeed, Smith was one of the witnesses who testified before the Committee. What is notable, however, is the number of other witnesses who would not have been considered utilitarians, but who nonetheless followed Smith's maxims to the letter. Astley Cooper, for example, who provided some of the most extensive testimony, repeated, among other things, Smith's claims about the benefits of dissection falling upon the poor and his belief that, when it came to the appropriation of unclaimed bodies, 'As no person's feelings would be outraged, there would be no reasonable objection to it'.[80] Similar sentiments were expressed by Benjamin Brodie, who claimed that 'the fittest persons in society for dissection, are those who have no friends to care about them', adding 'the dead body [...] does not feel either injury or disgrace, and where there are no friends to feel it, the mischief to society can be none at all'.[81]

Even more remarkable was the extent to which Smith's utilitarian ideas permeated sections of the medical press that were otherwise actively hostile to the politics of Bentham and his circle of 'Philosophical Radicals'. The conservative *London Medical Gazette*, for example, fell well and truly in behind the reformist party line, railing against 'popular prejudice' and advocating a resolutely instrumentalist approach to the dead body. In January 1829, for example, it asked 'What is the boasted march of intellect good for, if [...] the most useful of arts is to be sacrificed to imaginary fears?', while in May 1828 it struck a resonantly utilitarian tone when it proclaimed that 'venerate the dead as we

---

[77] [Smith], 'Use of the Dead', p. 95.   [78] *Report*, p. 10.   [79] Richardson, *Death*, p. 109.
[80] *Report*, pp. 16, 19.   [81] *Report*, p. 24.

may, we should never forget that veneration for the living is a duty of superior obligation: the promotion of human happiness is a duty from which we cannot be exonerated'.[82] In many ways, the issue of anatomical dissection can be said to have functioned as a kind of conceptual looking glass, through which the usual politics of the *Gazette* were inverted. Thus, it might find itself advocating a materialist understanding of the body, in which the corpse was merely a 'residue of molecules' with 'no intrinsic value', or praising the post-Revolutionary French surgical system when it normally deprecated the Francophilia of radical reformers.[83] The *Gazette* even attacked the conservative stalwart and Waterloo veteran George Guthrie (1785–1856), for daring to break ranks with surgical orthodoxy and declare his objection to the Anatomy Bill. Referring to one of Guthrie's lectures in which he expressed 'his abhorrence of having [dissection] performed on his body after death', the *Gazette* queried the emotional sincerity of his remarks, stating:

As an individual confession of undefinable and superstitious horror (for we cannot call it by any other name), it is curious [...] But it is only curious. Upon its announcement, in the lecturer's energetic and fluent tones, it excited in his auditory no feeling but that of surprise – no sympathy; and as it appeared to us, the fact seemed to be communicated rather for the sake of producing *effect*, than for any other perceptible reason. If this was really Mr G.'s design, he was very successful; but if he intended more – to excite or to encourage a kindred horror and antipathy in the bosom of any of his hearers – he must have been sadly disappointed.[84]

However, while practitioners and the medical press sought to regulate professional opinion, public sentiment could not be so easily disciplined. In the face of attempts to render the 'friendless' dead body an emotionless object, Guthrie's comments were a reminder of the capacity of the imagination to generate intense feelings of dread. Even if some commentators suggested that 'No man of even ordinary intellect shrinks from the thought of being anatomised himself [for] the senseless man can suffer nothing', Guthrie's example suggested otherwise, and affirmed that the living subject (rich or poor, friendless or otherwise) might yet imagine their body being eviscerated after death and feel abhorrence, revulsion, and fear.[85]

Writing shortly before the Anatomy Bill became law in August 1832, a contributor to *The Times* reflected on Bentham's decision to have his body dissected and preserved for posterity, stating that 'it becomes the duty of all

---

[82] *London Medical Gazette* 24 January 1829, p. 269; 3 May 1828, p. 669. Indeed, this was a paraphrase of [Smith], 'Use of the Dead', p. 81.
[83] *London Medical Gazette* 3 January 1829, p. 162; 27 February 1830, p. 695.
[84] *London Medical Gazette* 5 March 1831, p. 724. Emphasis in original.
[85] 'Supply of "Subjects" for Dissection to the Students of Anatomy', *Monthly Magazine* 5:29 (May 1828), p. 473.

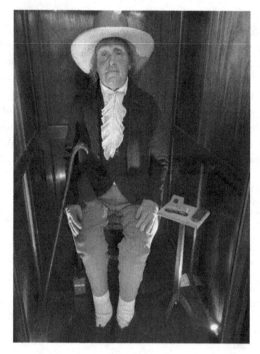

Figure 5.1 Jeremy Bentham's 'Auto-Icon', housed in Thomas Southwood
Smith's consulting room before being moved to University College
London in 1850. Wikimedia Commons: CC-BY-SA 2.0. https://commons
.wikimedia.org/wiki/File:2016-01-15_Jeremy_Bentham_Auto-icon.jpg

those who are interested in the happiness of mankind, to oppose the progress
of such injurious opinions' as expressed by Guthrie and other opponents of
the proposed legislation. 'Mr Bentham', they continued, 'impressed with this
idea […] determined to devote his own body to the public good'.[86] Bentham's
'Auto-Icon' was by far the most extravagant expression of mortuary rationalism in this period (Figure 5.1). Even so, many other like-minded individuals
sought to do their 'duty' in challenging what they believed to be popular superstition and sentimentality. For some, such as the radical Liverpudlian surgeon
George Rogerson, public lectures provided an ideal opportunity to preach the
rationalist creed. At one of a series of lectures at the Mechanics' School of Arts
in 1830, for example, he castigated the 'foolish objections against dissections',
exclaiming 'Begone with such prejudices, with such *childish feelings*; they are

---

[86] *Times* 12 June 1832, p. 6.

a disgrace to the age we live in'. On receiving a hearty applause from his arti-sanal audience, he was evidently gratified: 'Gentlemen', he proclaimed, 'I hear this applause with feelings of real pleasure, for it is a proof that the members of this institution have minds enlightened and superior to vulgar prejudices. This is creditable to you'.[87]

Others promoted what, to use Richardson's phrase, we might call an 'alter-native necrology'.[88] These utopian visions were occasionally so far removed from reality that they might easily have passed for satire. Thus, one com-mentator imagined a state in which the donation of one's body for dissec-tion was heralded as a form of civic sacrifice for which the rational citizen would be celebrated in both life and death, their urn 'distinguished by some mark' and heralded to the grave by 'a train of children [...] with garlands and songs of thanks'.[89] The radical proto-socialist Pierre (Peter) Baume (1797–1875), meanwhile, was probably only half joking when, in denouncing the 'ROMANTICISM OF THE GRAVE', he decreed that not only should his body be dissected, but 'even the least particle of my extinguished frame should be rendered subservient to some useful purpose', his skin tanned and used for furniture and his bones transformed into 'knife-handles, pin-cases, small boxes [and] buttons'.[90]

Nonetheless, such efforts to 'tranquilize the public mind' faced significant challenges, especially after the discovery of William Burke (1792–1829) and William Hare's (b. 1792/1804) heinous crimes in Edinburgh in late 1828.[91] The Burke and Hare case transformed the terrain of debate, invoking the spectre of a whole new form of bodily appropriation in which cadavers were not merely disinterred but manufactured through murder. At one level, this merely gave added impetus to legislative efforts to establish a legal supply of anatomical subjects. For large sections of the public, however, it intensified the emotive qualities of the issue and made the rationalist argument harder to sell. For one thing, it raised the possibility that, under any system of bequest or appropriation, the relatives of the dead might sell their bodies for profit, just as Burke and Hare had done their victims. This violation of precisely those emotional ties that the proposed legislation was supposed to protect excited a great consternation that was never fully resolved, not even after the passage of the Act in August 1832.[92]

---

87 *Kaleidoscope, or Literary and Scientific Mirror* 10:504 (23 February 1830), p. 270. Emphasis added.
88 Richardson, *Death*, ch. 7.
89 'Subjects for Dissection', *The Companion* 17 (30 April 1828), p. 229.
90 [Pierre Baume], 'Speech of Our French Scholar', *Lion* 3:13 (27 March 1829), p. 397. For more on Baume, see Roger Cooter, 'Baume, Pierre Henri Joseph (1797–1875)', *ODNB*; Richardson, *Death*, pp. 168–9.
91 For the best account of the Burke and Hare case, see Lisa Rosner, *The Anatomy Murders* (Philadelphia: University of Pennsylvania Press, 2010).
92 For the persistence of the body trade after 1832, see Hurren, *Dying*.

Thus, the Bill's most implacable Parliamentary opponent, the radical MP for Preston, Henry Hunt, asked 'What could be said in favour of a Bill which gave to a father the power of selling the dead body of a child – which gave to a husband the power of selling the dead body of a wife'.[93] In a similar vein, the conservative MP for Worcester, George Richard Robinson (c.1781–1850), claimed that the Bill held out an 'inducement to the most poor and miserable class of the community to dispose, by public sale, of the dead bodies of their nearest relatives. A husband, for instance, might sell the body of his wife, the mother of his children'.[94] Even more significantly, the Burke and Hare murders further amplified the ambivalences surrounding the concept of friendlessness that was so central to the rationalisation of bodily appropriation, for, as many commentators noted, it was precisely these people, itinerant, unknown, unlooked for, who were chief among Burke and Hare's victims. As Thomas Babington Macaulay (1800–59), an ardent champion of the Bill, put it, 'What man, in our rank of life runs the smallest risk of being Burked? That a man has property, that he has connections, that he is likely to be missed and sought for, are circumstances which secure him against the Burker [...] The more wretched, the more lonely, any human being may be, the more desirable prey is he to these wretches'.[95]

Macaulay's comments highlight the pitfalls of using friendlessness as the essential category for determining which bodies should be appropriated for surgical use. Friendlessness was not a semantically empty vessel into which the utilitarians might pour their own meaning. It was, on the contrary, a well-established cultural motif. The association of poverty with friendlessness can be traced back to the Bible, specifically Proverbs 14:20, which claimed that 'The poor is hated even of his own neighbour: but the rich hath many friends'.[96] Such language found its way, via biblical paraphrase, into hymns such as 'Rulers of Sodom! Hear the Voice', which enjoined 'Do justice to the friendless poor, / and plead the widow's cause'.[97] A quick survey suggests that use of the term 'friendless' increased markedly over the later eighteenth century, before reaching its peak between 1820 and 1850.[98] Friendlessness

---

[93] *Hansard*, HC Deb vol. 10 col. 378 (15 February 1832).

[94] *Hansard*, HC Deb vol. 12 col. 665 (18 April 1832).

[95] *Hansard*, HC Deb vol. 10 col. 842 (15 February 1832).

[96] www.kingjamesbibleonline.org/Proverbs-14-20 (accessed 20/08/20).

[97] *Translations and Paraphrases in Verse, of Several Passages of Sacred Scripture Collected and Prepared by a Committee of the General Assembly of the Church of Scotland, in Order to be Sung in Churches* (Edinburgh: Hunter, Blair, and Bruce, 1809), p. 7. This was actually a paraphrase of Isaiah 1:17, the King James rendering of which is 'relieve the oppressed, judge the fatherless, plead for the widow'.

[98] https://books.google.com/ngrams/graph?content=friendless&year_start=1750&year_end=2019&corpus=26&smoothing=3&direct_url=t1%3B%2Cfriendless%3B%2Cc0#t1%3B%2Cfriendless%3B%2Cc0 (accessed 20/08/20).

was a concept widely deployed both by the poor themselves, notably in pauper letters, and also by charities, such as the Friendless Poor Society, founded in Newcastle-upon-Tyne in 1797.[99] The concept of friendlessness therefore served to sharpen political discourse around a Bill that many opponents saw as a calculated attack on the dignity of the poor. As another implacable opponent of the Bill, William Cobbett, noted, 'It is curious that the WHIG REFORMERS *are for this bill*, and that TORIES are *against it!*'; and, indeed, it was true that Parliamentary opposition forged an unlikely alliance between popular radicals like Hunt and ultra Tories like Charles Sibthorp (1783–1855).[100] The language of friendlessness could thus be deployed in both a defiant and a paternalistic manner. The Earl of Harewood (1767–1841), for example, claimed that he 'did not see why the bodies of the poor and friendless should be particularly selected for the dissecting-knife'.[101] Meanwhile, in a neat example of the double meaning that the term had by then acquired, *Cobbett's Weekly Register* ran a piece from the *Leeds Mercury* ahead of the highly contested election of 1832, protesting the 'DEAD BODY BILL' and addressed to 'THE RATE PAYERS OF LEEDS, BUT ESPECIALLY TO THE FRIENDLESS POOR'.[102]

However, the ultimate irony of the utilitarian use of friendlessness was that, in seeking to divest the anatomical body of affective meaning, they only succeeded in investing it with greater emotional significance than might have been the case for the legally more problematic, but culturally less resonant, term 'unclaimed'. Indeed, far from being the emotive vacuum that men like Smith had imagined, the friendless poor were in actual fact the most pitiable and pathetic of all possible people. By definition, of course, such individuals were largely unknown, if not unknowable, precisely because they lacked social capital, but this only encouraged opponents of what one commentator called the 'philosophy of the shambles' to imagine the people they *might* have been or the lives they *might* have led.[103] Due to their powerful association with personal nobility, bodily proficiency, and state service, soldiers and sailors were a favoured subject of such fantasies. Thus, *The London Medical Gazette* dismissed as a 'pseudo-pathetic story' the *Morning Herald*'s imagined account of a soldier who had 'fought battles for his country' only to be 'brought to the "human shambles" and exposed to the knife of the anatomist,

---

[99] K. D. M. Snell, 'Belonging and Community: Understanding of "Home" and "Friends" among the English Poor', *Economic History Review* 65:1 (2012), 1–25; Eneas Mackenzie, *A Descriptive and Historical Account of the Town and County of Newcastle upon Tyne ... Vol. 1* (Newcastle-upon-Tyne: Mackenzie and Dent, 1827), p. 546.

[100] *Cobbett's Weekly Register* 28 January 1832, p. 267.

[101] *Hansard*, HL Deb vol. 13 col. 827 (19 June 1832).

[102] *Cobbett's Weekly Register* 10 November 1832, p. 342.

[103] 'On the Necessity of Anatomical Subjects', *Imperial Magazine* 12:34 (February 1830), p. 170.

and the "rude gaze of rabble boys"'.[104] Even more elaborately, in the immediate aftermath of the passage of the Act, *Fraser's Magazine* published a story entitled 'Dialogues of the Dead', which imagined a reckoning in the afterlife for utilitarians, surgeons, and their Parliamentary allies. Representing the 'victims' of the Act was a sailor who had 'done nothing but served [his] country in three quarters of the globe'. As Charon, the ferryman of Hades, announced:

> Well! here's a fellow come down, who swears that they denied him the common right to his own body, when he died, merely because he was unfortunate! that he led a hard life in their service; by serving them, he was cut off from all connexions of father, husband, friend; and because he was thus cut off, they refused him burial, used his poor remains of a body as they have used their criminals in time out of mind – dissected it! in a word, that because he had no friend on earth, he should neither have mercy nor justice.[105]

It was because of these political and cultural complexities that *The Lancet* ultimately found itself unable to support the Anatomy Bill. As has been argued elsewhere, Thomas Wakley trod a careful path through the political cultures of the 1820s, balancing the philosophical radicalism of Bentham and his circle against the popular radicalism of Hunt, Cobbett, and their ilk.[106] In the early days of the debate, *The Lancet* took a decidedly utilitarian stance on the issue of anatomical dissection. In February 1824, for instance, it decried the existence of a 'prejudice' against dissection among the higher orders, by which means it 'becomes more deeply rooted in the minds of the ignorant and uninformed who are not able to think for themselves'. In order to advance the practice of anatomy and thereby 'increase the happiness and lessen the misery of mankind', it called upon the profession to 'come forward and devise some means by which the present impediments may be removed'. It even recommended Abernethy's suggestion that bodies should be sourced from 'those persons who die in London without friends' as 'deserving of consideration'.[107] *The Lancet* maintained this line throughout the succeeding five or so years. In 1826, for example, it urged surgeons to undertake public demonstrations of anatomy, arguing that it was 'useless to *reason* on a circumstance which is purely a matter of *feeling*. SHOW the people the utility of dissections – SHOW them the benefits which are conferred upon their fellow creatures [...] and they will [...] consider them the laudable means by which the greatest public good can be accomplished'.[108] Like other proponents of reform, it also adhered to

---

[104] *London Medical Gazette* 21 March 1829, p. 513.
[105] 'Dialogues of the Dead. On Sepulchral Rites and Rights', *Fraser's Magazine* 6:36 (December 1832), p. 730.
[106] Michael Brown, '"Bats, Rats and Barristers": The Lancet, Libel and the Radical Stylistics of Early Nineteenth-Century English Medicine', *Social History* 39:2 (2014), 182–209, at pp. 204–7.
[107] *Lancet* 1:19 (18 February 1824), pp. 194–5.
[108] *Lancet* 7:171 (9 December 1826), pp. 323–4. Emphasis in original.

the idea that the bodies of the 'friendless' were emotionally neutral, maintaining that 'it is the feelings of survivors only, which the legislature is called upon to respect' and arguing that 'however averse an individual may be in his life time to the dissection of his body after death, if he has no surviving relatives to respect this prejudice, [...] no reason can be urged against the dissection of such a person's body, nor could public feeling possibly be outraged by it'.[109]

During the later 1820s, however, Wakley's position began to shift, at first slightly, then completely. When the report of the Select Committee was released in 1828, Wakley declared it to be 'upon the whole, a satisfactory document', but objected to Abernethy's claim that the bodies of the institutionalised poor were, by rights, public property, arguing, somewhat expediently, that 'though it is obvious that none but the bodies of the poor are likely to be unclaimed', the law should avoid making dissection 'inseparable from poverty'.[110] But with the discovery of Burke and Hare's crimes, all such nuance was abandoned. In an editorial of January 1829, Wakley stated that 'It is fearful and humiliating to reflect on the enormities of which wretches wearing the human form are capable' and called for the immediate closure of all dissecting rooms in Britain. 'The injury to medical science, [and] the inconvenience to medical teachers' were, he claimed, 'all insignificant considerations compared with the overwhelming necessity of protecting the public against assassins, who traffic in the dead bodies of their victims'.[111] Perhaps unsurprisingly, neither the authorities nor the profession followed Wakley's lead, and, in a subsequent editorial, he expressed his 'indignation and disgust' at 'the chilling apathy with which the greater number of our teachers of anatomy, have regarded the late unparalleled disclosures'.[112] As such comments suggest, the crimes of Burke and Hare, together with those of John Bishop and Thomas Williams in the summer of 1831, pushed *The Lancet* firmly into the camp of popular radicalism and fuelled the kinds of melodramatic outrage explored in Chapter 4. This is not to say that Wakley rejected dissection in principle; indeed, he continued to dismiss opposition to pathological anatomy as an irrational and 'sentimental' prejudice.[113] However, he increasingly came to see the Bill itself as the work of corporate monopoly and political tyranny and professed 'common feeling' with the friendless poor.[114] Hence *The Lancet* celebrated the failure of the first Anatomy Bill in 1829 and, as the second neared the end of its passage through Parliament, predicted 'popular fury and violence'.[115] Moreover, when it finally passed into law, Wakley declared, in characteristic style, that 'This foul, this disgusting, this

---

[109] *Lancet* 10:245 (10 May 1828), pp. 179–80.
[110] *Lancet* 10:262 (6 September 1828), pp. 722–3.
[111] *Lancet* 11:279 (3 January 1829), p. 433.   [112] *Lancet* 11:283 (31 January 1829), p. 562.
[113] *Lancet* 11:291 (28 March 1829), p. 820.   [114] *Lancet* 12:297(9 May 1829) p. 182.
[115] *Lancet* 12:302 (13 June 1829), p. 338; 17:438 (21 January 1832), p. 594.

anti-humanising, this blood-stained ANATOMY ACT, must be remodelled, or it will bring the profession into everlasting disgrace with the public'.[116]

The Lancet's response to the Anatomy Act is instructive, and suggests the limits of generalisation. Even so, Wakley was well aware that he was an outlier.[117] Popular opposition to the Act, which was soon to become intimately bound up with the iniquities of the New Poor Law, continued for some time, but the issues that were debated throughout the 1820s were, by 1832, effectively settled. The vast majority of the profession, from conservatives to radicals, were united in their belief that surgeons should be supplied with the bodies of friendless paupers whose appropriation for the purpose of anatomisation was both socially beneficial and emotionally inoffensive. Of course, it should be noted that surgeons and anatomists had long held a dualistic view of the human body as something to be both healed and used; it was nothing new to view the cadaver as an object. But what *was* new was that, during the 1820s, surgeons articulated a public discourse that actively positioned itself against popular sentiment, stripping the bodies of the dead of emotional association and rendering them subservient to a surgical project that was figured as congruent with the interests of the state. As their greatest political ally, Henry Warburton, put it to his fellow MPs:

They must recollect [...] that there were cases, in which the feelings and wishes of mankind were made to succumb to the service of the state. What could be more savage than war? And yet when the service of the State, the preservation of the nation, and the welfare of the people were at stake, we set aside private feelings, and scenes of bloodshed and suffering were the consequence [...] in such instances, the wishes and feelings of individuals were held as nothing, when compared with the interests of the nation at large. Why, then, should they hesitate to make some sacrifice when a question was at issue which so materially affected the welfare of every human being?[118]

This is not to say that the dead body was entirely denuded of all emotional meaning, not even within surgical culture. Two documents in Bransby Cooper's file, with which we began, indicate the continued emotional complexities of the cadaver. One is a short note sent to Astley Cooper by an unnamed individual who wrote that, having heard 'you are in the habit of purchasing bodys [*sic*]' and 'knowing a poor woman that is desirous' of selling hers, 'I have taken the liberty of calling to know the truth'. Cooper's curt, incredulous response, written on the back, reads: 'The truth is that you deserve to be hanged for such an unfeeling offer'.[119] The second is a far more elaborate bequest sent to Cooper by one William Williams in the aftermath of the Anatomy Act. In lengthy and tortuous legalese, Williams promised his body to Cooper for the

---

[116] *Lancet* 19:482 (24 November 1832), p. 275.   [117] *Lancet* 18:465 (28 July 1832), p. 537.
[118] *Hansard*, HC Deb vol. 9, col. 301 (15 December 1831).
[119] RCSE, MS0008/2/2/1, unsigned and undated letter. Emphasis in original.

sake of the 'public benefit derived from anatomy'. He states that, should he die a 'bachelor and unmarried', his 'mortal remains may be at your disposal for the aforementioned purposes of dissection'. However, he makes an exception in the event of his marriage, in which case 'I beg it to be understood [...] that [...] my said wife's approbation or disapprobation may be obtained and ascertained and according as she shall or may approve or disapprove of the said dissection the approval or disapproval of and by her [...] is to [...] be considered as [...] my will and earnest desire and pleasure'.[120] Clearly then, despite all attempts to render the subject one of pure reason, transcending sentiment, the emotional ties of love and marriage could not easily be 'put asunder'. Even an individual's stated desire as to the fate of their mortal remains could be countermanded by precisely those emotional attachments that Smith had sought to mitigate through the dictates of a higher duty. In death, as in life, the biblical and legal injunction that the married couple were of 'one flesh' was, it seemed, as much literal as figurative. As we shall see in the next section, however, it was not only the dead body that would undergo an uncertain emotional reconfiguration at the hands of surgeons in this period; some fifteen years after the passage of the Anatomy Act, another transformation in practice and perception would render the living body of the operative subject similarly quiescent and, in the eyes of some, uncannily reminiscent of the cadaver on the dissection table.

Constructing the 'Chamber of Sleep': Emotions and the Unconscious

In 1900, Frederick Treves (1853–1932), the recently appointed Surgeon Extraordinary to the elderly Queen Victoria, gave a lecture to the annual meeting of the BMA in which he looked back over the preceding century to a time when the surgeon 'was but a sorry element in social life'. 'The operator of olden times', he claimed, 'stepped into the arena of the operating theatre as a matador strides into the ring':

Around him was a gaping audience and before him a conscious victim, quivering, terror-stricken, and palsied with expectation. His knife was thrust through living flesh and acutely-feeling tissue, and the sole kindness of his mission was to be quick. In spite of moans for mercy from gagged lips the knife had to move its way steadily and, undeterred by struggles and bursts of haemorrhage, the blade must needs pass without faltering or sign of hesitancy.

'There is less need for such qualities now', Treves continued; 'The operating theatre of the present day has lost its horrors and has changed from a shambles to a chamber of sleep'. For Treves, the advent of anaesthesia in 1846 had not

[120] RCSE, MS0008/2/2/1, William Williams to Astley Cooper, 20 June 1833.

only changed the nature of operative practice, allowing the surgeon to proceed 'leisurely without fear of being regarded as timorous', it had transformed the very 'personality' and 'bearing' of the surgeon, losing, perhaps, some of the 'dash' of earlier days, but 'gain[ing] much in the direction of the sympathetic handling of his patient and in the culture of gentleness'.[121]

By the time of Treves' talk in 1900, the narrative of surgery's transformation from an age of filth, disorder, and suffering to one of cleanliness, painlessness, and techno-scientific rationality was firmly established, as was anaesthesia's pivotal place within it. What is more, and as Treves' words suggest, this transformation was often couched in terms of emotional deliverance. Pernick observes that 'anaesthesia made possible a greater range of medical sentiment toward patients – both more routine callousness and more benevolent sensitivity', but he also suggests that the associated rise of modern bureaucratic medicine 'limited the expression of sympathy and full concern for the individual'.[122] In Chapter 6, we shall examine in more detail the emotional ambivalences and complexities of later nineteenth-century techno-scientific surgery. In this chapter, we are concerned with that very specific historical moment in the mid-nineteenth century when the patient, as a conscious, agentive individual, effectively disappeared from the emotional space of the operating theatre, rendered quiescent by anaesthetic oblivion. As we shall see, this process was far from being as simple as Treves' metaphor of the 'chamber of sleep' suggests. Indeed, the phenomena of ether and chloroform were many, potentially far more troubling, things before they were rendered as innocuous as sleep. As Pernick, Snow, and others have demonstrated, though remarkable in its effects, anaesthesia was no magic bullet. Rather, it was a dramatic chemical and technological intervention into well-established practice whose professional, social, and cultural acceptance was conditional and contested. Pernick's account provides an invaluable insight into the implications of anaesthesia for measuring pain, for rationalising care, and for shaping clinical judgement in the context of the United States.[123] Snow, meanwhile, tells the story from the British perspective, demonstrating the vital role played by John Snow (1813–58) in making anaesthesia a distinct branch of surgical practice, as well as exploring the varied aspects of its professional and social contestation.[124] However, although much of this work alludes to the complex emotional dimensions of anaesthesia, few historians have focused specifically on its role in reshaping the cultures of surgical subjectivity and intersubjectivity.[125] This is precisely what this section

[121] *Lancet* 156:4014 (4 August 1900), pp. 313–15.   [122] Pernick, *Calculus*, p. 235.
[123] Pernick, *Calculus*.   [124] Snow, *Operations*.
[125] The exceptions to this include Mary Poovey, '"Scenes of an Indelicate Character": The Medical "Treatment" of Victorian Women', in *Representations* 14 (1986), 137–68, and Moscoso, *Pain*, ch. 5.

seeks to do; but, in order to do so, it is first necessary to address one of the most puzzling and long-standing questions in the history of anaesthesia.

It is virtually impossible to talk about the 'discovery' (or invention) of anaesthesia without acknowledging the fact that the chemist Humphry Davy recognised the potential utility of nitrous oxide for pain relief nearly half a century before inhalation anaesthesia became standard practice. In his *Researches Chemical and Philosophical* (1800), Davy observed that as 'nitrous oxide in its extensive operation seems capable of destroying physical pain, it may probably be used with advantage during surgical operations in which no great effusion of blood takes place'.[126] Many early advocates for the use of ether and, later, chloroform felt compelled to note Davy's abortive discovery, even if they were at a loss to explain why it was not taken up. John Gardner (1804–80), for example, could only opine that 'Numberless instances might be cited where men have held in their hands, looked at with their bodily eyes, but without perceiving, the elements of great discoveries'.[127]

By contrast with contemporaries, historians have actively sought to understand why the palliative possibilities of nitrous oxide (and other gases) were not fully realised until the later 1840s. Margaret C. Jacob and Michael J. Sauter suggest that Davy and his associates lacked the technical capability to develop nitrous oxide as an effective anaesthetic agent. More importantly, they also contend that these people lacked the conceptual and ideological capacity to perceive nitrous oxide as anything other than a powerful *enhancer* of sensation, intimately associated with either 'pleasure or danger'.[128] Jacob and Sauter situate themselves, in part, against the argument, advanced by E. M. Papper, that anaesthesia was a direct product of Romantic sensibility, which, by giving birth to subjectivity and interiority, made physical suffering inherently insufferable.[129] In many ways, Papper's argument runs directly counter to my own. As we have seen in this book, Romantic surgeons were powerfully alive to the sufferings of their patients and were concerned to do what they could to ease them where possible. And yet, as we have also seen, pain was part of a wider cultural sensorium that sustained emotional intersubjectivity and encouraged forms of personal reflection that, though often productive of 'emotional suffering', also stimulated 'good' emotions such as pity, sympathy, and reverence. For instance, in 1807, Charles Bell wrote to his brother George to share with

[126] Humphry Davy, *Researches Chemical and Philosophical, Chiefly Concerning Nitrous Oxide or Dephlogisticated Nitrous Air and Its Respiration* (London: J. Johnson, 1800), p. 556.
[127] *Lancet* 49:1231(3 April 1847), pp. 352–3.
[128] Margaret C. Jacob and Michael J. Sauter, 'Why Did Humphry Davy and Associates Not Pursue the Pain-Alleviating Effects of Nitrous Oxide', *Journal of the History of Medicine and Allied Sciences* 57:2 (2002), 161–76, at p. 176.
[129] E. M. Papper, *Romance, Poetry and Surgical Sleep: Literature Influences Medicine* (Westport, CT: Greenwood Press, 1995).

him a revelation he had experienced during a stay in the rural residence of a patient on whom he was to operate. One day, Charles claimed, he rose at five in the morning and 'leaped the garden wall, and ran in full chase through the country, making acquaintance with every living thing I met. I found three young horses, an ass, a tame fox, and an owl, particularly conversable'. Driven inside by rain, he 'enjoyed a waking dream' in which 'all was right in the system of the universe – that consistent with our desires and passions was the shortness of our life and our being liable to suffering and disease' and that, without this, 'we should have been inanimate, cold, and heartless creatures'. 'I thought I perceived two great objects of admiration and love', he continued, the first being 'the intimate creation' of life itself, the other being the 'still higher enjoyment in the contemplation of mind [...] strengthened by communication and sympathy'.[130] For Romantics like Charles Bell, then, sensation was everything, and pleasure and pain so inextricably intertwined in the complexities of sympathy and intersubjectivity that the notion that one specific form of pain might be extinguished from the world was barely conceivable.[131] This is not to say that Bell or his contemporaries lauded pain and suffering, or would necessarily have rejected anaesthesia had it been offered them. Rather, it is to suggest that, for them, pain was an ineluctable and largely irreducible feature of the human condition that, by necessity perhaps, had its moral and emotional compensations.

Clearly, it would require a far more reductionist understanding of pain in order to imagine the possibility of its abolition and, indeed, this is exactly what would come to pass in the second quarter of the nineteenth century. Stephanie Snow argues that 'by the 1830s, the radical view that pain was purposeless began to emerge', and she makes brief reference to Bentham's conception of pain as an 'inherent evil'.[132] However, she does not locate the origins of anaesthesia in these broader social and cultural shifts so much as in the specific conceptual transformations of medicine itself. In particular, she points to the clinical revolution of Parisian medicine at the turn of the nineteenth century and the ascendancy of what, following Owsei Temkin, Erwin Ackerknecht called the 'surgical point of view'.[133] There is much to recommend this argument, and there is much truth in Snow's assertion that the physiological researches of men like Marshall Hall promoted the idea that the vital functions of the body

---

[130] Charles Bell to George Bell, 11 May 1807, *Letters of Sir Charles Bell* (London: John Murray, 1870), pp. 94-5. See also Brown, 'Wounds', p. 251.
[131] Jacob and Sauter make a similar observation that, for Thomas Beddoes, 'the pain presented by surgical procedures did not move him any more than the pain caused by consumption or depression': 'Humphry Davy', p. 170.
[132] Snow, *Operations*, pp. 21, 33.
[133] Snow, *Operations*, pp. 22-3; Erwin Ackerknecht, *Medicine at the Paris Hospital, 1794–1848* (Baltimore: Johns Hopkins University Press, 1967), p. 25.

might be uncoupled from conscious volition.[134] But the clinical revolution does not, in itself, account for changing surgical understandings of pain, for it was perfectly possible for surgeons invested in clinical medicine to believe in the moral or physiological benefits of pain. The only way to fully account for this shift is to acknowledge the ascendancy of a moral and political philosophy that regarded pain as an 'evil' to be eradicated. Here we encounter difficulties, for, as I have suggested, it is rare to find surgeons directly invoking utilitarianism in their efforts to eradicate the pain of operative surgery, even if later commentators acknowledged the connection.[135] Nevertheless, there is enough material to constitute a reasonably robust version of what Dror Wahrman has called the 'weak collage' of cultural change.[136] For example, by 1840, one finds comments such as these from Charles Aston Key who, during a lecture on the 'Principles and Practice of Surgery' at Guy's Hospital, questioned the long-held view that pain was a reliable indicator of the presence of disease:

Do we find that pain is the first impression made in every instance by a morbid cause acting on the whole frame or a part of the human frame? Certainly not. You may have a morbid cause with pain or without it [...] Pain is, therefore, merely an *accidental concomitant*; and diseased action may cause an impression on the nervous system unaccompanied by pain.[137]

Meanwhile, in the same month, at the same hospital, Samuel Ashwell (1798?–1852) told his students:

Pain and disease, whatever may have been said to the contrary by philosophers, are great evils, apart only from their power to discipline the mind and soften the heart: they cover with darkness the activities and enjoyments of existence. We fly from them instinctively, as we fly from death; of which we all know they are too often the servants and harbingers.[138]

These quotations suggest something about shifting conceptions of pain in this period but, evidently, they do not refer explicitly to utilitarianism. Indeed, Ashwell specifically positioned himself against those 'philosophers' who advocated the moral virtues of pain without mentioning the very philosopher whose ideas underwrote his own argument. And yet, I would contend that such comments testify to the *implicit* influence of utilitarian thought within contemporary British medicine and surgery. We have already seen evidence of its role in shaping ideas about anatomical dissection, even among non-avowed

---

[134] Snow, *Operations*, pp. 28–9.
[135] For example, see Frances Power Cobbe, 'Vivisection and Its Two-Faced Advocates', *Contemporary Review* 41 (April 1882), 610–626, at p. 617.
[136] Dror Wahrman, *The Making of the Modern Self: Identity and Culture in Eighteenth-Century England* (New Haven: Yale University Press, 2004), p. 45.
[137] *Lancet* 35:896 (31 October 1840), p. 170. Emphasis added.
[138] *Lancet* 35:895 (24 October 1840), pp. 137–8.

Benthamites, and elsewhere I have demonstrated its influence in reconfiguring notions of medical charity in the 1830s.[139] We might also appeal to the pervasive presence of utilitarian ideas in British social thought more generally from the 1830s onwards. In 1839, for instance, one critic decried what he called 'the vile spirit of Utilitarianism which is creeping like a plague over the land and over the age', while more than thirty years later, another commentator claimed that 'Utilitarianism [...] may be described as practically the dominant creed of our time'.[140]

Having said this, it would be misleading to suggest that the influence on surgery of the utilitarian conception of pain as 'in itself an evil' was sudden, complete, or unambiguous.[141] After all, even in his denunciation of pain, Ashwell held to the idea that it had some residual moral qualities, namely its 'power to discipline the mind and soften the heart'. In the latter we detect the continued resonance of Romantic sensibility. In the former, meanwhile, we find evidence for the existence of an alternative model of pain that flourished in the decade or so immediately before the advent of anaesthesia and existed alongside utilitarian conceptions of pain as a morally vacuous evil.

In Chapter 3, we saw how the rhetoric of operative fortitude was routinely used to shape an ideal of the surgical patient as 'bodily acquiescent and emotionally self-controlled'. This concept was of long standing, but by the 1840s it was increasingly figured as a signifier of physical hardiness and moral superiority, and those displaying such qualities were often contrasted with others who, in giving expression to their pain, fear, or suffering, failed to show the requisite degree of resolve.[142] There was, moreover, an increasingly gendered aspect to this culture of surgical self-possession. As we have seen, women had long been thought capable of equal, if not greater, displays of surgical fortitude compared to men, but by the 1840s surgical stoicism was increasingly figured as a masculine (often military) virtue, while displays of emotion were both feminised and pathologised. Of particular importance here is the spectre of hysteria; this began to re-enter medical and surgical discourse in a very pronounced way in the 1840s, spurred by works like Thomas Laycock's *Treatise on the Nervous Diseases of Women* (1840), which located hysteria in women's physiology and sexuality.[143] Such associations of femininity with pathological

---

[139] Brown, 'Medicine'.
[140] 'On the Present State of Utilitarianism', *Penny Satirist* 2:104 (13 April 1839), p. 3; [John Morley], 'Mr Lecky's First Chapter', *Fortnightly Review* 5:29 (May 1869), p. 538.
[141] Bentham, *Principles*, p. 98.
[142] For popular expressions of this sentiment, see 'Triumphs over Bodily Suffering, Including an Account of the Mandarins of North America', *Saturday Magazine* 17:523 (29 August 1840), pp. 78–80; 'Female Fortitude', *Mirror* 1:25 (18 June 1842), p. 400.
[143] Thomas Laycock, *A Treatise on the Nervous Diseases of Women* (London: Longman, Orme, Brown, Green, and Longmans, 1840). For a classic account of nineteenth-century hysteria as

displays of emotion and inherent physiological weakness also found popular expression in such contemporary works as *The Daughters of England* (1842) by Sarah Stickney Ellis (1799–1872), which claimed that 'woman, from her very feebleness is fearful; while from her sensitiveness she is particularly sensitive to pain'.[144]

The influence of hysteria on surgical attitudes towards patients in general, and their expressions of pain in particular, is evident in the archives of Benjamin Travers junior (1808–68), who succeeded his father as surgeon to St Thomas' Hospital in 1841. His four volumes of casebooks, which cover the period from 1843 to 1859, offer a valuable insight into the quotidian realities of surgical practice at mid-century and are remarkable for his repeated identification of moral failings in his male patients, particularly in terms of physical appearance, alcohol consumption, and propensity to masturbate.[145] As Joanne Begiato has argued, Victorian notions of manliness were rooted in forms of bodily and emotional self-mastery and a failure to conform to these ideals could, for surgeons like Travers, produce serious illness.[146] Travers made an explicit link between male expressions of emotion and the disease of hysteria, whose manifestation in women was a notable feature of his casebooks.[147] For example, in September 1843 he recorded the case of a 'butcher's lad' who was 'struck with a saw which inflicted a severe wound upon his right cheek':

> He was so restless with frequent hysteric sobbing that I bled him to a full pint from the arm although he had lost a great deal of blood from the face. Soon afterwards he became tranquil and slept for some time. He answered questions initially when he awoke, but the hysteric condition continued for some time. This is a sign of <u>severe shock</u> in young people and if it continues highly dangerous. It is allied to and is illustrative of the passio hysterica in Women.[148]

Clearly then, from around the 1830s but especially in the 1840s, we see the articulation of two models of surgical pain that were, in essence, contradictory: one that viewed pain as a purposeless blight on human happiness, the other that considered it to be a test of character and virtue, particularly

---

a gendered phenomenon, see Elaine Showalter, *The Female Malady: Women, Madness and English Culture, 1830–1980* (New York: Pantheon Books, 1985). For a more recent general account, see Andrew Scull, *Hysteria: The Biography* (Oxford: Oxford University Press, 2009).

[144] Sarah Stickney Ellis, *The Daughters of England: Their Position in Society, Character and Responsibilities* (London: Fisher and Son, 1842), p. 383.

[145] RCSE, MS0276/1, Benjamin Travers [junior], Manuscript case books (4 volumes), 1843–1859.

[146] Joanne Begiato, 'Punishing the Unregulated Manly Body and Emotions in Early Victorian England', in Joanne Ella Parsons and Ruth Heholt (eds), *The Victorian Male Body* (Edinburgh: Edinburgh University Press, 2018), 46–64; Begiato, *Manliness*, ch. 2.

[147] For more on the history of male hysteria, see Mark S. Micale, *Hysterical Men: The Hidden History of Male Nervous Illness* (Cambridge, MA: Harvard University Press, 2008).

[148] RCSE, MS0276/1, Casebook 1 (February 1843–July 1844), 21 September 1843, unpaginated. Emphasis in original.

for men. The first of these regarded pain as something to be eliminated, the other as something to be endured. Neither model held complete sway and indeed, as we have seen in the case of Samuel Ashwell, it was possible for practitioners to subscribe to both simultaneously. And yet, despite their evident ambiguities, both were, in their own way, equally far removed from the Romantic conception of pain as an intersubjective social experience, productive of edifying emotions in the beholder as much as the sufferer. Moreover, in the dialectic tension between them, there emerged, if not a resolute determination that surgical pain *should* be eliminated, then perhaps a growing consensus that it *could* be.

As many historians have recognised, despite the narrative of abortive discovery associated with anaesthesia, the period between Davy's observations on nitrous oxide and the American dentist William T. G. Morton's (1819–68) first public demonstration of ether in October 1846 was not entirely devoid of attempts to induce a state of insensibility in those required to submit to what *The Lancet* called the 'hard doom' of operative surgery.[149] In 1819, for example, James Wardrop bled a female patient to a state of syncope in order to remove a tumour from her head.[150] Revealingly, Wardrop's experiment attracted relatively little interest until 1833, when he referred to it in one of his lectures, stating that it was 'a great desideratum in surgery to discover a mode by which the pain of surgical operations could be either alleviated or diminished'.[151]

However, by far the most promising, if also the most contested, form of anaesthesia that emerged in the period before ether was mesmerism. There is no space here to do full justice to the conceptual richness and cultural complexities of mesmerism. For our purposes, it is important to note that histories of mesmerism and inhalation anaesthesia have often set the two firmly in opposition. As we have already heard, Robert Liston probably did not say of ether that 'this Yankee dodge beats mesmerism hollow', though he did, in a letter to James Miller composed in the immediate aftermath of his famous December 1846 operation, write: 'Hurrah! Rejoice! Mesmerism, and its professors, have met with a "heavy blow and great discouragement"'.[152] As Alison Winter has shown in her peerless history of the subject, Liston's antipathy to mesmerism owed much to a personal dislike of John Elliotson, his rival at University College London and its most high-profile medical advocate. The same might be said of Thomas Wakley, whose friendship with Elliotson was

[149] *Lancet* 49:1232 (10 April 1847), p. 393.
[150] *Medical and Chirurgical Transactions* 10:1 (1819), pp. 273–7.
[151] *Lancet*, 20:518 (3 August 1833), pp. 596–8, at p. 596. See also Snow, *Operations*, p. 24.
[152] This letter is transcribed in 'Painless Operations in Surgery', *North British Review* (May 1847), pp. 176–7.

destroyed by his radical exposure of the alleged fraudulence of Elliotson's favourite mesmeric subjects, Elizabeth and Jane Okey.[153]

Despite vociferous opposition, however, there were many practitioners who regarded mesmerism as worthy of serious study. Thus, in 1840 Thomas Laycock claimed that it had 'engaged the attention, not merely of the unthinking multitude, but of learned professors of medicine' and necessitated 'a thorough revision' in 'the relations of mind to body'.[154] Moreover, by 1842 it was being used with increasing frequency as a means of alleviating the pain of operative surgery. In his Harveian Oration to the Royal College of Physicians, given just six months before Liston's first operation using ether, Elliotson claimed that 'anaesthesia, is but a form of palsy [...] If this condition can be induced temporarily by art, we of necessity enable persons to undergo surgical operations without suffering'. Elliotson 'fearlessly declare[d] that the phenomena' of mesmerism, including 'the prevention of pain under surgical operations [were] true' and he 'implore[d]' his audience to 'carefully investigate this important subject'.[155] In many ways, Elliotson was beseeching the wrong audience. Generally speaking, physicians were more inclined to embrace the operative use of mesmerism than were surgeons, not least because it did not have the same potential to undermine their established practice and professional authority. Commenting on the lack of surgical attendees at a demonstration of mesmeric dentistry in June 1846, for example, the Bath physician and mesmerist Henry Storer questioned whether 'painless operations in surgery' might 'prove too great a shock to their nervous systems, having been so long accustomed to witnessing the contrary'.[156]

Winter has documented what she calls the 'ambivalent' support for surgical mesmerism in the years immediately preceding the introduction of ether, suggesting that, by late 1846, it was 'on the brink of gaining acceptance among constituencies that had long resisted' it.[157] There were even some who thought that the 'discovery' of ether, far from disproving the reality of mesmerism, only confirmed its veracity. For one contributor to *Blackwood's Edinburgh Magazine*, this extended to all mesmeric phenomena, including clairvoyance, while others, such as Charles Radclyffe-Hall (1820–79), were more conditional

---

[153] Alison Winter, *Mesmerized: Powers of Mind in Victorian Britain* (Chicago: Chicago University Press, 1998), pp. 95–100, 180–1. See also Wendy Moore, *The Mesmerist: The Society Doctor Who Held Victorian Society Spellbound* (London: Weidenfeld and Nicholson, 2017), pp. 93–4, 188–9.

[154] Laycock, *Nervous Diseases*, p. 3.

[155] John Elliotson, *The Harveian Oration, Delivered before the Royal College of Physicians, London, June 27 1846* (London: H. Baillière, 1846), p. 68.

[156] Henry Storer, 'Mesmerism in Surgical Operations', *Critic* 3:78 (27 June 1846), 754.

[157] Winter, *Mesmerized*, p. 173.

in their acceptance.[158] The 'so-called higher phenomenon of mesmerism', such as 'the sublime absurdities of clairvoyance and prevision', were 'impossible and quite incredible', he claimed. Nonetheless, ether confirmed the essential truth that 'sensibility may be entirely suspended for a time by artificial means'.[159]

The fundamental problem with mesmerism, as Winter has shown, was that it was beset by intractable issues of subjectivity and authority. The reality of the mesmeric trance was virtually impossible to verify, being entirely dependent on observable (but easily faked) phenomena or the testimony of experimental subjects. Even Radclyffe-Hall remained unsure as to whether the mesmeric trance was 'feigned', 'real', or 'an hysterical vagary'. Thomas Wakley, on the other hand, was far less equivocal. For him, it was the fundamentally subjective and intersubjective qualities of mesmerism that made it at once ludicrous and dangerous. Citing the example of the Okey sisters, together with the more recent clairvoyant 'Arsenic Prophetess' Mrs Bird, he grounded mesmerism in a supposedly feminine capacity for deceit and a 'morbid desire' for attention. At the same time, he also regarded mesmerism as, in itself, a pathology of the emotions, stating that 'The production of [...] morbid conditions of the nervous system, through the influence of the emotions of the mind, is – we repeat it emphatically – one great trunk, if not the root, of the mesmeric infamy'.[160]

Winter astutely observes that, compared to the intersubjectivity of mesmerism, ether and chloroform offered a more objective foundation upon which surgeons might stake their claim to professional authority. As she puts it, 'mesmeric effects explicitly involved the relationship between two people; one might even say they *consisted of* that relationship. The power of ether to produce an anaesthetic state lay in a chemical, not a social relationship. Ether avoided the disturbing and sometimes subversive associations that attended the mesmeric relationship'.[161] In a profoundly important way, Winter is right. Many received the news of ether in the same way as a correspondent to *The London Medical Gazette*, who saw it as the death knell for mesmerism and proof that 'their boasted power is a deception, or, at most, has no influence but over the minds of a few hysterical females'.[162] But at the same time, Winter overstates the extent to which chemical anaesthesia constituted an objective phenomenon, free from potentially 'subversive associations'. Ether was no 'clean break' from the intersubjectivity of Romantic surgery, nor from the ontological 'messiness' and personal idiosyncrasy that characterised the pre-anaesthetic

[158] 'Mac Davus', 'Letters on the Truths Contained in Popular Superstitions', *Blackwood's Edinburgh Magazine* 62:382 (August 1847), 166–77.
[159] *Lancet* 49:1234 (24 April 1847), p. 437.
[160] *Lancet* 49: 1224 (13 February 1847) pp. 178–83, at p. 178.
[161] Winter, *Mesmerized*, p. 180. Emphasis in original.
[162] *London Medical Gazette* 16 April 1847, p. 669.

operative subject. Rather, the figure of the quiescent surgical patient, rendered emotionally absent by induced insensibility, was one that had to be forged from the chaotic and complex free-for-all of early anaesthetic practice.

In the aftermath of Liston's first operation using ether, surgeons up and down the country sought to explore the remarkable effects of the new vapour for themselves. As a consequence, the medical and popular press published hundreds of articles, letters, and case reports on the topic in the first six months of 1847. Though this ether 'mania' had subsided by the summer of 1847, there was a revived interest in anaesthetic experiment, though not perhaps at quite the same level of fervid excitement, following James Young Simpson's first use of chloroform in November of the same year. What is notable about many of these early accounts of the use of ether is not the *absence* of the operative subject but rather their powerful vocal, physical, and emotional *presence*. In some cases, of course, the patient was put into 'a perfectly quiescent state, without motion or sound', but in others, the uncertain effects of the vapour made for a far less placid scene.[163] At St George's Hospital in January 1847, for example, surgeons attempted several operations under ether in front of a large audience including Liston, Benjamin Brodie, and even Jérôme Bonaparte (1784–1860). The first patient, a 'weakly lad of 19 or 20', could not be made to inhale an adequate quantity of the vapour due to a combination of 'fright' and 'coughing', and the procedure was terminated. The second patient, by contrast, inhaled the ether '*con amore*' but 'appeared to suffer a great deal from it, turning very red, or rather purple in the face and resisting at times somewhat violently'. 'The effect on the bystanders', *The Times* noted, 'was anything but favourable, several declaring that ether was as bad as the operation, or worse'. Things did not improve for, the patient having become seemingly insensible, the surgeon proceeded to remove his diseased finger, at which point he was 'at once restored to his senses, and shouted so loudly, and snatched his hand from the operator so vigorously as to leave no doubt that he suffered pain as acutely as if no steps had been taken to deaden it'. Unsurprisingly, the operation was declared 'a total failure'.[164]

Even in less dramatic cases, patients under ether would often flinch, lash out, or exhibit other convulsive movements. For instance, in January 1847 an 'Irishman' having his leg removed at the London Hospital gave 'sly winks and facetious nods to those surrounding him [...] forcing from the bystanders involuntary laughter, and converting that which was to the poor fellow a most tragic event into a scene little short of a farce'. Even so, when the effects of the ether passed off, the patient 'could scarcely believe that his leg had been

---

[163] 'The Use of Ether in Surgery', *Examiner* (9 January 1847), p. 129.
[164] *Times* 15 January 1847, p. 3. See also *London Medical Gazette* 22 January 1847, p. 168.

so painlessly removed'.[165] Such cases raised profound doubts, which remain to this day, as to what exactly it was that patients experienced while under the influence of anaesthetic. Though some practitioners firmly believed that ether brought about 'a complete obliteration of existence', others were not so sure.[166] One commentator claimed that there were numerous instances where patients could not move but 'had been conscious all the time, and have witnessed every step of the operation performed on them'.[167] Even after the introduction of chloroform, the chemist William Thomas Brande (1788–1866) remained uncertain:

A question had been raised whether sensibility was really annihilated under the influence of these vapours, or whether the patient did not suffer at the time, but had no recollection of the pain on his recovery. This was rather a metaphysical than a physiological part of the inquiry; and there were no facts by which the question could be solved. Some patients had undoubtedly a consciousness of the operation during its performance.[168]

As with mesmerism, then, the early use of ether was marked by disruptive behaviour and uncertain facts. It was, moreover, characterised by equally unreliable testimony. According to *The Lancet*, 'As a measure of insensibility to pain, we must be entirely guided by the credibility of the patient, and his own subsequent account of the matter'.[169] However, when patients were asked to give account of their experiences, which was virtually routine in the early months of 1847, they hardly offered much clarity. For one thing, the ubiquitous expressions of surprise and incredulity elicited from patients who had no recollection of having a leg amputated could easily make ether seem like a cheap parlour trick.[170] For another, what patients described was, in many cases, unnervingly reminiscent of the more extreme manifestations of mesmeric phenomena. Patients' experiences under ether ranged from 'optical illusions' to full-on hallucinations.[171] One fourteen-year-old boy, upon regaining consciousness after an eye operation, 'exclaimed, in a high tone of voice, and with great energy "I have been going to heaven; I have been seeing the angels, and I don't know what all! I have been going to heaven, that's all I know about it! Angels and trumpets are blowing!"'[172] Religious and spiritual visions like this were not uncommon, but neither were more prosaic hallucinations, such as

[165] *London Medical Gazette* 22 January 1847, p. 168.
[166] *London Medical Gazette* 8 January 1847, p. 85.
[167] 'The Inhalation of Ether in Surgery', *Athenaeum* (30 January 1847), p. 125. See also *London Medical Gazette* 15 January 1847, pp. 129–30.
[168] *London Medical Gazette* 28 January 1848, p. 208.
[169] *Lancet* 49:1220 (16 January 1847), p. 75.
[170] There are innumerable instances of this but for examples see *Lancet* 49:1220 (16 January 1847), p. 78; *London Medical Gazette* 15 January 1847, p. 138.
[171] *London Medical Gazette* 8 January 1847, p. 85.
[172] *Lancet* 49:1222 (30 January 1847), p. 134.

a servant reliving a dispute with his master, or a woman who thought herself in a neighbour's house surrounded by 'several parties' persuading her to submit to the very operation she was then undergoing.[173] These examples manifest the exact same emotional, moral, and physiological idiosyncrasy that, as we saw in Chapter 3, characterised the cultures of pre-anaesthetic surgery. Hence, what patients did or said during and immediately after operations under ether was often thought to offer an insight into their character. It is perhaps unsurprising, given prevailing social prejudices, to learn that many of the most obstreperous and disruptive patients were identified as Irish.[174] Likewise, whereas a correspondent to *The Lancet* thought that being 'at the bar of judgment pleading for mercy' from God was the kind of dream 'which might be expected' from 'an interesting and delicate girl [of] good moral and religious character', a different set of judgements presumably attached to the man who, in 'throw[ing] his arms about', thought himself 'fighting and knocking somebody down in a public-house'.[175]

Another aspect of ether that resembled mesmerism was its erotic connotations and potentialities. In its most extreme form, contemporaries worried that women might be rendered unconscious and sexually assaulted by ethereal assailants.[176] But even within the managed space of the operating theatre, the eroticised gaze might still manifest itself. For example, in a reference to the performance of the celebrated singer Maria Malibran (1808–36) in the aptly titled *La Sonambulista*, J. H. Rogers, acting house surgeon to the Middlesex Hospital, described one young woman, who was having a 'large crop of venereal warts [removed] from the labia' (and who may therefore have been a sex worker), thus: 'The expression of her countenance, her action, and tone of voice, bore a striking resemblance to [...] the character of Amina, in the scene where she awakes and finds herself in the bed-room of the Count'.[177]

Like mesmerism, ether also, at least for a period, offered the disquieting possibility of expanding consciousness beyond conventional bounds, even to the point of madness. Thus, in February 1847, the surgeon Frederick Thomas Wintle (1803–53), medical superintendent to the Warneford Hospital insane asylum in Oxford, wrote a cautionary letter to *The Lancet*, citing the case of a 'talented and intellectual individual' who 'had a strange delusion that he could expand the powers of his mind *ad infinitum*, if he could obtain a free

---

[173] *Lancet* 49:1221 (23 January 1847), p. 106; *London Medical Gazette* 28 May 1847, p. 960.
[174] For example, see *London Medical Gazette* 29 January 1847, pp. 216–17.
[175] *Lancet* 49:1224 (13 February 1847), p. 188; 51:1270 (1 January 1848), p. 26.
[176] Pernick, *Calculus*, pp. 61–2; Snow, *Operations*, pp. 107–8.
[177] *Lancet* 49:1224 (13 February 1847), p. 184. Tellingly, in this scene the Count contemplates taking sexual advantage of Amina's unconscious state.

supply of ether'. Sadly, 'he pursued this delusion so earnestly that his mind became disordered, and, in fact, he suffered paroxysms very nearly allied to delirium tremens'.[178]

As this last observation suggests, ether had potentially problematic associations with 'altered states' other than mesmerism. Many commentators noted the parallels between etherisation and the insensibility produced by excessive alcohol consumption as well as the delirium occasioned by opium use, associations that were only enhanced by the testimony of patients.[179] For example, the unnamed Irishman of the 'sly winks', mentioned above, declared 'let's have another go at the grog' before inhaling ether 'with the greatest avidity', while a female patient at the Stockport Infirmary, when required to take the vapour for the second time, protested 'I wish I had said nothing; you are going to give me some more of that stuff that makes folk drunk'.[180] Likewise, patients recovering from etherisation were often disinclined to be roused from a state that resembled narcotic euphoria. 'Oh! why did you take me from that beautiful place? Let me go back. Oh! how beautiful! It is heaven!' declared a 19-year-old girl after a tooth extraction at the Northern Dispensary, while a young man at the Westminster Hospital was recorded as exhibiting 'a little hysterical sobbing after the operation', The Lancet noting that, in contrast to the terrors of the past, 'a surgical operation has now come to be a source of regret, as an enjoyment too quickly passed away'.[181]

In these last two cases the patients were referred to as hysteric and, indeed, the spectre of hysteria dogged early anaesthesia as much as it did mesmerism. W. H. Hewett was not alone in his claim that 'symptoms of hysteria' were 'a frequent occurrence' of ether 'when administered to females'.[182] In fact, not even the advent of chloroform could entirely eradicate this association and John Snow's case books are full of references to patients exhibiting hysteric symptoms before, during, and after inhaling the vapour.[183] Having said this, whereas the early use of ether had heralded a frenzy of sensational and diverse reports, by the time Snow came to compile his casebooks in the late 1840s and 1850s, much of the plurality of anaesthetic experience had been tamed, thanks in large part to Snow himself.

It is one of the great ironies of early anaesthesia that its profound novelty made patient testimony far more clinically interesting, relevant, and audible than it had been before. As argued in Chapter 3, prior to 1846 the intraoperative experiences of patients were of comparatively little interest to surgeons.

---

[178] Lancet 49:1223 (6 February 1847), pp. 162–3.
[179] For example, see London Medical Gazette 15 January 1847, p. 139.
[180] London Medical Gazette 22 January 1847, p. 168; Lancet 49:1226 (27 February 1847), p. 239.
[181] Lancet 49:1226 (27 February 1847), p. 239; 49:1220 (16 January 1847), p. 79.
[182] Lancet 49:1226 (27 February 1847), p. 239.
[183] Richard H. Ellis (ed.), The Case Books of Dr John Snow (London: Wellcome Institute, 1994).

Pain was, after all, a distressing but entirely predictable consequence of cutting, slicing, and sawing the body of a sentient creature, and one of the functions of the culture of operative fortitude was to make the sufferings of the patient 'more palatable by being refracted through the familiar cultural tropes of pathos and personal self-control'. And yet, if the screaming, writhing patient of the pre-anaesthetic era has been effectively silenced in the historical record, the unconscious patient of early anaesthesia was given remarkable licence to speak, as a returning explorer from the *terra incognita* of ethereal oblivion. But it was not to last. This astonishing flourishing of patient testimony was to continue for little more than a few months before the operative subject was silenced for good.[184] It is not just that, by June 1847, 'the cases had lost all novelty', though they had.[185] It was because, by its very diversity and subjectivity, this testimony highlighted the fundamental idiosyncrasy of anaesthetic experience and conjured uncomfortable associations with the vagaries and uncertainties of mesmerism. Indeed, in the early days of anaesthesia, idiosyncrasy was everywhere. In January 1847, for example, *The Lancet* observed that the 'insensibility produced by etherization appears to be of a peculiar kind, and to vary considerably in different individuals', while the following month, John Adams (1805–77) of the London Hospital thought the action of ether on the blood accounted for 'its power of inducing insensibility [...] according to the idiosyncrasy of the patient'.[186] This was only exacerbated by increasing reports of deaths under ether and, later, chloroform, which raised the disturbing possibility that some patients were physiologically unsuited to the new vapour.[187]

If anaesthesia was going to provide the stable technological solution to the problem of pain that mesmerism had failed to do, such idiosyncrasy had to be eliminated. Chief among the practitioners who attempted to do just this was John Snow. One of Snow's principal characteristics, as perhaps the most active promoter of anaesthesia in England, was his insatiable quest for uniformity and standardisation.[188] As historians have shown, proponents of ether and chloroform were aware that patients might respond differently to them.[189] Snow himself proposed a value-laden hierarchy of influence, suggesting that 'Those persons whose mental faculties are most cultivated appear to retain

[184] Snow, *Operations*, pp. 72–3.   [185] *London Medical Gazette* 26 November 1847, p. 938.
[186] *Lancet* 49:1220 (16 January 1847), p. 75; 49:1226 (27 February 1847), p. 238.
[187] For an excellent discussion of anaesthesia and the negotiation of risk, see Ian Burney, *Bodies of Evidence: Medicine and the Politics of the English Inquest 1830–1926* (Baltimore: Johns Hopkins University Press, 2000), ch. 5; Burney, 'Anaesthesia and the Negotiation of Surgical Risk in Mid-Nineteenth-Century Britain', in Thomas Schlich and Ulrich Tröhler (eds), *The Risks of Medical Innovation: Risk, Perception and Assessment in Historical Context* (London: Routledge, 2006), 38–52.
[188] Snow, *Operations*.   [189] Pernick, *Calculus*, ch. 6.

their consciousness longest', while 'certain navigators and other labourers [...]
having the smallest possible amount of intelligence, often lose their consciousness, and get into a riotous drunken condition, almost as soon as they have
begun to inhale'.[190] Nonetheless, Snow endeavoured to eliminate any doubt
that ether and chloroform were universally applicable. Drawing on his unrivalled experience of its administration, he claimed: 'From what I have seen, I
feel justified in the conclusion that ether may be inhaled for nearly all surgical
operations [...] with safety and without ill consequences, where due care is
taken'.[191] To this end, he rejected all explanations of patient death that suggested the physiological idiosyncrasies of the patient, such as a weak heart,
rendered them unsuitable subjects, suggesting instead that the fault lay in poor
technique, particularly in terms of the dosage administered or the method of
revival employed.[192]

Snow also sought to banish patient-centred subjectivity from anaesthetic
practice. It is notable, for example, that he was a proponent of the use of ether
to detect feigned injury among soldiers, with the idea that it might allow the
surgeon to bypass subjective testimony to reveal an essential bodily truth.[193]
He also had little time for metaphysical debates about the psychology of
patient experience, proposing instead several clearly defined levels of anaesthetic 'narcotism' and suggesting that 'Pain which is not remembered is of
very little consequence, and [...] should not be judged of by the expressions
of the patient'.[194] Likewise, while he acknowledged that the emotions of the
patient might be managed in advance of a procedure, he allowed them no role
in the operation itself, claiming that 'Fear is an affection of the mind, and can
no longer exist when the patient is unconscious'.[195] Moreover, Snow sought to
discipline the space of the operating theatre by quietening the post-operative
patient, putting an end to those elements of etherisation that evoked the popular spectacle of mesmerism. As he wrote in 1847:

If the patient will remain silent during his recovery from the effects of ether, as he generally will, it is better not to trouble him with questions till he has perfectly regained his
faculties, as conversation seems to increase the tendency to excitement of the mind that
sometimes exists for a few minutes as the patient is recovering from the effects of ether.
This kind of inebriation is sometimes amusing, but is not a desirable part of the effects

---

[190] John Snow, *On Chloroform and Other Anaesthetics: Their Actions and Administration*
(London: John Churchill, 1858), p. 36.
[191] John Snow, *On the Inhalation of the Vapours of Ether* (London: Wilson and Ogilvy, 1847), p. 10.
[192] For example, see *London Medical Gazette* 18 February 1848, pp. 283–4.
[193] *Lancet* 49:1239 (29 May 1847), p. 553. This had first been proposed by the French military
surgeon Lucien Jean-Baptiste Baudens (1804–57): *London Medical Gazette* 19 March 1847,
p. 526.
[194] Snow, *Chloroform*, pp. 37–42, 47. See also Snow, *Operations*, p. 73.
[195] Snow, *Chloroform*, p. 77.

of ether, more especially on so grave an occasion as a serious surgical operation; and therefore anything that may prevent or diminish it is worthy of attention.[196]

As Stephanie Snow has demonstrated, perhaps her namesake's most important legacy was his establishment of anaesthesia as a discrete surgical science. From the very early days of etherisation, John Snow had championed the use of specific inhalation apparatus to ensure a safe and controlled administration of vapour. By contrast, James Young Simpson, and many of this followers in Scotland, proposed the use of a simple handkerchief, or other suitable piece of cloth, to administer chloroform to their patients. John Snow opposed this Scottish mode of practice, publishing evidence that the simple infusion of a cloth was associated with a higher fatality rate than his own apparatus. Stephanie Snow locates this disagreement in two contrasting medical cosmologies, one that saw the body as an idiosyncratic entity requiring empirical knowledge, and another that viewed bodies as universal and amendable to predictable laws.[197] There is much truth in this observation, for Snow's universalising drive was certainly calculated to minimise personal subjectivity and bodily idiosyncrasy. But as Stephanie Snow recognises, this disagreement also suggests something about divergent understandings of surgical authority and identity. The use of a simple handkerchief was minimally disruptive and allowed the surgeon to retain much of the old way of doing things, including his own untrammelled authority. By contrast, Snow's apparatus heralded a new era of specialisation and the division of labour.[198] Moreover, whereas there was something quotidian, domestic even, about the use of a handkerchief, Snow's inhalation apparatus, visually reproduced in countless articles and books, provided a prescient vision of surgery as a fundamentally techno-scientific practice (Figure 5.2).

The advent of anaesthesia can certainly be said to have constituted a 'revolution in practice'.[199] However, it is important to recognise that the transformation it brought about was neither immediate nor absolute and that operations without any form of pain relief would continue for many years.[200] In fact, surveying the writings of mid-nineteenth-century surgeons, one could occasionally be forgiven for thinking one had missed something. Remarkably, ether and chloroform warranted no special mention in James Syme's 1853

---

[196] Snow, *Inhalation*, pp. 9–10.   [197] Snow, *Operations*, ch. 3.

[198] Snow, *Operations*, pp. 164–82. The expansion of the surgical team also diffused responsibility for the risks of practice: Claire Brock, 'Risk, Responsibility and Surgery in the 1890s and Early 1900s', *Medical History* 57:3 (2013), 317–37.

[199] Stephanie Snow, 'Surgery and Anaesthesia: Revolutions in Practice', in Thomas Schlich (ed.), *The Palgrave Handbook of the History of Surgery* (London: Palgrave Macmillan, 2018), 195–214.

[200] Pernick, *Calculus*, ch. 6; Snow, *Operations*, pp. 150–1.

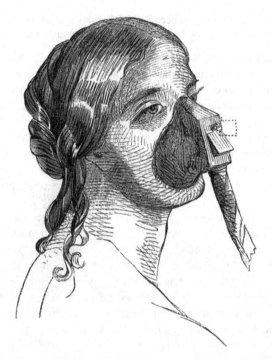

Figure 5.2 John Snow's Apparatus for the Inhalation of Ether and Chloroform, *The Lancet* 51:1276 (12 February 1848), p. 179. Wellcome Collection. Attribution 4.0 International (CC BY 4.0)

account of the improvements that had taken place in surgical practice over his thirty-year career, and only a very brief reference, right at the end, in a similar lecture delivered over a decade later.[201] Meanwhile, in the published version of his introductory address to the surgical pupils of University College London in 1850, John Erichsen (1818–96) relegated chloroform to a couple of footnotes, one of which complicated, if not directly contradicted, his argument about the importance of handling surgical instruments 'with rapidity'.[202] Similarly, if one looks at the major textbooks of the period, one often finds anaesthesia grafted somewhat awkwardly onto long-established

---

[201] James Syme, *On the Improvements Which Have Been Introduced into the Practice of Surgery in Great Britain within the Last Thirty Years* (Edinburgh: Murray and Gibb, 1853); Syme, *Address in Surgery delivered at the Annual Meeting of the British Medical Association, Held at Leamington, August 3, 1865* (Edinburgh: R. Clark, 1865), p. 43.

[202] John Eric Erichsen, *On the Study of Surgery: An Address Introductory to the Course of Surgery Delivered at University College London at the Opening of the Session 1850–1851* (London: Taylor, Walton, and Maberly, 1850), pp. 28–9, 32.

practices. For example, Erichsen threaded chloroform through the text of his 1854 edition of *The Science and Art of Surgery*, but continued to recommend measures, such as covering the instruments with a towel or minimising verbal communication between the surgeon and his assistants, that were of little relevance to a world where the patient was rendered unconscious, perhaps even before they entered the operating theatre.[203] Indeed, it is notable that, by the second edition of 1857, while Erichsen had introduced a whole new section on chloroform, the paragraph on operative preparation and conduct remained unaltered.[204]

Such textual practices serve as a neat exemplar of the more general ways in which anaesthesia was interpolated into established surgical cultures. They also demonstrate that the shift from the emotional regime of Romantic sensibility to one of scientific modernity was gradual and uneven. And yet, there can be little doubt that, ultimately, the introduction of anaesthesia irrevocably transformed the emotional cultures of surgery. As scholars have recognised, anaesthesia did nothing to relieve the pain associated with bodily affliction more generally. Nor did it completely eradicate anxiety and fear at the prospect of surgery.[205] Indeed, anaesthesia could produce its own anxieties. Writing in 1896, Frederick Treves claimed that 'The majority of patients regard the anaesthetic with far greater dread than the operation', for while 'Of the surgeon's work they are assured they will know nothing [...] they do know that they will be horribly conscious of those palpitating moments which precede the onset of the gruesome and unholy sleep'.[206] Treves' description of anaesthetic sleep as 'gruesome and unholy' attests to its continued ambiguity, but it is important to remember that these words were written half a century after the introduction of ether and that the dread of anaesthesia was significant precisely because, by rendering surgery effectively painless, it had removed much of the dread of the operation itself. In this it was truly revolutionary. But that was not all; anaesthesia also reshaped surgical experience and identity in profound and lasting ways. Indeed, it is remarkable how many surgical commentators of the period reflected on the impact that ether and chloroform had upon *them* as much as on their patients. The Edinburgh surgeon James Miller, who was one of the foremost early advocates of anaesthesia, dedicated a whole section of his *Surgical Experience of Chloroform* (1848) to the fact that 'Anaesthesia affords great relief to the operator as well

---

[203] John Eric Erichsen, *The Science and Art of Surgery: A Treatise on Surgical Injuries, Disease and Their Operations* (Philadelphia: Blanchard and Lea, 1854), p. 77.

[204] John Eric Erichsen, *The Science and Art of Surgery: A Treatise on Surgical Injuries, Disease and Their Operations*, 2nd ed. (London: Walton and Maberly, 1857), pp. 5–6.

[205] Snow, *Operations*, pp. 101–5.   [206] Quoted in Burney, *Bodies*, p. 150.

as to the patient'. Reflecting on the emotional burden it had lifted from the shoulders of surgeons, he wrote:

To no ordinarily constituted man is pain otherwise than repugnant; whether it occur in himself or in another. And, hitherto, there can be no doubt that his being compelled to inflict pain, and witness the infliction of it, has always been esteemed by the surgeon as the hardest portion of his professional lot. Now this is gone. He proceeds to operate with a mind wholly unoccupied with regard to the feelings of his patient; for he knows that all the while he will be in unconscious sleep.

By silencing the patient, anaesthesia transformed the sensory landscape of the operating theatre and rendered operative surgery far more palatable. The blood and gore remained, of course, but to Miller this was not the issue. 'Whence was it that students, dressers, and even surgeons grew pale, and sickened, and even fell, in witnessing operations?' he asked:

Not from the mere sight of blood, or of wound; but from the manifestation of pain and agony emitted by the patient. And, now-a-days, this patient—whatever his age, or sex, or however nervous, timid, and apprehensive— gives not one sign of pain, or even discomfort, but lies in happy slumber all the while. A snort is the worst sound that he makes.[207]

For surgeons such as William Fergusson (1808–77), the sensory experience of the operation might now even be actively pleasurable. '[I]nstead of wild outcries or stifled screams and groans coming from the patient under the surgeon's instruments', he suggested, the patient 'may be made to lie as quietly as if in a calm sleep, or [...] he may be mentally engaged in the most pleasing associations of thought, or singing or humming by snatches some favourite air'.[208]

While the somnolence and somniloquy of the anaesthetised patient encouraged metaphors of sleeping and dreaming, the remarkable indifference of the patient to the physical trauma of surgery also invited comparison with the dissected corpse.[209] Reflecting on an early operation under ether to remove a diseased eye, for example, William Lawrence compared the previous patient he had treated for such a condition who 'writhed in agony, not being able to control himself' with his etherised subject who 'lay like a body on a dissecting table, without the slightest manifestation of suffering or even consciousness, without a movement of any part'.[210] Where surgical dissection had once prepared surgeons only incompletely for their operative duties, now the two practices were virtually identical and eradicated the need for surgeons

---

[207] James Miller, *Surgical Experience of Chloroform* (Edinburgh: Sutherland and Knox, 1848), pp. 29–30.
[208] William Fergusson, *A System of Practical Surgery* (London: John Churchill, 1852), p. 22.
[209] Thomas Schlich, 'The History of Anaesthesia and the Patient – Reduced to a Body?', *Lancet* 390:10099 (9–15 September 2017), 1020–1.
[210] *London Medical Gazette* 15 January 1847, pp. 138–9.

to hurry themselves. '[A]s there is no cause or excuse for haste in operating on a dead body stretched on a dissecting-table', Miller wrote, 'so there is as little cause or excuse for haste in operating on an anesthetized body of a living patient'.[211]

This chapter thus comes together in the figure of the quiescent surgical body, for whether the insensible patient was dead, asleep, or somewhere in between, the emotional regime of utilitarian and techno-scientific surgery all but severed the essential intersubjectivity that had shaped the surgical cultures of the Romantic era. In both the dissecting room and the operating theatre, the surgeon might now work 'with a mind wholly unoccupied' by feeling. For some, this was a problem as much as a benefit. As historians have noted, there were a number of contemporaries who believed that pain was a necessary part of surgical operations.[212] Roger Sturley Nunn (1813–82), reflecting on a fatal case under ether at the Essex and Colchester Hospital in February 1847, for example, wrote that 'Pain is doubtless our great safeguard' and 'should be considered as a healthy indication, and an essential concomitant with surgical operations'.[213] Meanwhile, no less an authority than Bransby Cooper stated 'that pain was a premonitory condition' and that 'he should feel averse to the prevention of it'.[214] Such sentiments were given short shrift by James Miller, who, in what was surely a play on Thomas Paine's *Rights of Man* (1791), decried the 'small party', including the notorious vivisector François Magendie (1783–1855), who, in the face of an unalloyed boon for humankind, asserted instead 'the rights of pain'.[215] Indeed, one of the effects of anaesthesia was to divest pain of almost all of its moral value. In a remarkable address to the Hunterian Society in February 1848, for instance, Thomas Blizard Curling (1811–88) declared that the pain caused by the surgeon's knife was unquestionably 'an evil' and that the 'Fortitude displayed under suffering is [...] not always so great as it appears' because it was often a product of a physiological 'incapacity of feeling pain' rather than the expression of 'moral courage'. He even went so far as to suggest that 'monomaniacs' who took a 'morbid pleasure' in pain, such as a woman whose breast was found to be 'full of pins and needles', fully confirmed that there was no inherent nobility in pain.[216]

---

[211] Miller, *Chloroform*, p. 30.   [212] Pernick, *Calculus*, pp. 42–9; Snow, *Operations*, pp. 99–100.

[213] *London Medical Gazette* 5 March 1847, p. 415.

[214] *London Medical Gazette* 30 April 1847, p. 778.

[215] Miller, *Chloroform*, pp. 35–6.

[216] Thomas Blizard Curling, *The Advantages of Ether and Chloroform in Operative Surgery: An Address Delivered to the Hunterian Society on the 9th of February 1848* (London: S. Highley, 1848), pp. 8–12. For more on pain and self-harm in this period, see Lucy Bending, *The Representation of Bodily Harm in Late Nineteenth-Century British Culture* (Oxford: Oxford University Press, 2000), ch. 6; Moscoso, *Pain*, ch. 6; Sarah Chaney, *Psyche on the Skin: A History of Self-Harm* (London: Reaktion, 2017), ch. 2.

But pain was not the only issue. Some surgeons objected to the lack of cooperation that had once been the hallmark of the intraoperative relationship between surgeon and patient, at least in its more idealised forms. Even as late as 1855, William Coulson (1802–77) could ask John Snow whether it was 'always desirable to suspend sensation during surgical operation', suggesting that there were cases, such as lithotrity, 'a delicate operation [...] carried on, as it were, in the dark', where 'the patients' sensations are the chief guide which direct the surgeon when he is going wrong'.[217] Moreover, there were others for whom the haptic qualities of the newly anaesthetised operative subject were deeply unnerving. According to Cooper, 'with the exception of the flow of blood, it was like cutting through dead flesh', and in the case of lithotomy 'the parts fell, as it were, asunder, and the sensations were quite different on passing the finger into the bladder'.[218] Similar sentiments were also expressed by Henry Haynes Walton (1816–89) who, following up on Coulson's questioning, claimed that in the case of cataract, 'the lens did not start so freely after the division of the cornea as when chloroform was not used, but was more like the lens of a dead body'.[219]

If such quibbling from Miller's 'small party' was relatively short-lived (Miller was using the past tense, even in 1848), other concerns took somewhat longer to recede. Anaesthesia had become widespread by the 1860s, but the relative risks of ether and chloroform were still being debated in the 1870s and beyond.[220] Moreover, for some the problem with chloroform lay not in its potential toxicity or its eradication of surgical intersubjectivity, but in the fact that it had opened up a brave but uncertain new world of operative ambition. In 1851 *The Lancet* contemplated the moment, four years earlier, when surgeons no longer had to endure 'the cry of agony issuing from the frail body of some poor nervous, emaciated woman, whose breast was about to be submitted to the knife; nor the scarcely less painful effect of subdued emotion, in the strong frame, while it quivered under the strokes of the scalpel'. 'The surgeon', it remarked, no longer had to 'contend against these calls upon his humanity'. However, it cautioned, 'Like all such blessings [chloroform] has its drawbacks and evils, amongst the more conspicuous of which may be mentioned the facility with which patients are now persuaded to submit to the knife, and the encouragement which it holds out to what are called "promising young men" to "carve their way into practice"'. With the patient unconscious,

---

[217] *Lancet* 66:1677 (20 October 1855), p. 367.
[218] *London Medical Gazette* 30 April 1847, p. 778.
[219] *Lancet* 66:1677 (20 October 1855), p. 367.
[220] For example, see RCSE MS0021/4/1/12, Volume containing William Watson Cheyne's notes on cases in the Royal Infirmary, Edinburgh and Lectures in Clinical Surgery given by [Joseph] Lister 1872–1873, f. 10.

surgeons could now intrude deeper into those cavities of the body that had previously eluded them, continually extending their epistemological empire. Citing the highly controversial practice of ovariotomy as the most 'frightfully illustrative' example of this 'operating mania', it noted that a surgeon might now remove an ovarian tumour 'with as much nonchalance as though it were being removed from the dead body in the dissecting-room'.[221] Looking back to the generation of surgeons immediately before anaesthesia, *his* generation, Wakley remarked that those modern surgeons 'who would vainly aspire to walk in the footsteps of a COOPER or a LISTON' would do well to remember that 'Such men as these did not operate for the sake of cutting: they resorted to the knife only as a substitute, and that, to them, a lamentable one, for other [...] resources of surgery'.[222]

Conclusion

Before long Wakley would pass away, as would the very notion of the pre-anaesthetic era as a model of surgical practice. As we shall see, surgeons of the later nineteenth and early twentieth centuries would solidify the emotional regime of scientific modernity in part through their casting of what had come before as a diabolic counterpart to their own technical and technological sophistication. While surgical innovation could still provoke controversy, the expanding empire of surgery was less a cause for concern than for celebration, mirroring as it did the British state's own increasingly acquisitive territorial ambition.[223] Moreover, where opponents both of anatomical dissection and of anaesthesia had often couched their concerns in terms of the individual patient, the harbingers of a scientific surgical modernity would, by the 1880s at least, appeal less to the individual case than to the statistically demonstrable collective good. Though this shift of emotional focus from the individual to the social would become even more pronounced as the century wore on, this chapter has located its origins in the period between 1820 and 1850 and, in particular, in the cultural and ideological influence of utilitarianism. But it has also shown that this shift was not limited to Benthamites, nor was it without ambiguity or complexity. Emotional intersubjectivity did not disappear overnight, nor, as we shall see, did the language of sentiment. The tone, however, had changed for good. Recalling the visit of the celebrated Scottish divine Thomas Chalmers (1780–1847) to witness one of his first operations under ether, James Miller claimed that it was

---

[221] On ovariotomy, see Frampton, *Belly-Rippers*.
[222] *Lancet* 57:1428–1429 (11 January 1851), p. 54.
[223] Lawrence and Brown, 'Quintessentially Modern'.

one of the early triumphs of Anaesthesia [...] to see that man of large and tender heart witnessing a bloody and severe operation, with composure and serenity; feeling little, because the patient felt not at all; and the little that he himself did feel, far more than compensated by the thought, that a brighter day for that suffering humanity, with which he so closely and continually sympathized, had at length dawned, and that, from henceforth, throughout the domain of surgery, injury and disease were shorn of half their terrors.[224]

[224] Miller, *Chloroform*, pp. 8–9.

6   The 'New World of Surgery'
Sepsis, Sentiment, and Scientific Modernity

Introduction

The Scottish surgeon Alexander Ogston (1844–1929) is significantly less well known than his English contemporary Joseph Lister, the founder of the antiseptic system of surgery. Unlike Lister, he was not ennobled for his contributions to surgery (although he was knighted in 1912) and neither was he memorialised in Westminster Abbey.[1] Nor, unlike Lister, has he been made the subject of innumerable popular biographies.[2] But as the discoverer, in the early 1880s, of what he called *Staphylococcus*, the microorganisms responsible for the infections that produce abscesses, he was in the first rank of British bacteriologists.[3] Indeed, together with his fellow Scot William Watson Cheyne (1852–1932), he was perhaps the only British surgeon of the late nineteenth century truly worthy of that title.[4] Ogston's place in the narrative of antiseptic surgery's rise to prominence is complex. He was a convinced Listerian, whose use of Lister's famous carbolic acid spray was so committed that his students penned comedic verse about it.[5] At the same time, Ogston's claims about the existence of *Staphylococcus* were initially challenged by Lister and

---

[1] Lister was offered burial in Westminster Abbey, but elected instead to be buried beside his wife in Hampstead Cemetery. A memorial plaque to Lister can be found in the north choir aisle.

[2] For example, Rickman John Godlee, *Lord Lister*, 2nd ed. (London: Macmillan, 1918); Hector Charles Cameron, *Joseph Lister: The Friend of Man* (London; Heinemann, 1948); Douglas Guthrie, *Lord Lister: His Life and Doctrine* (Edinburgh: E. & S. Livingstone, 1949); Frederick F. Cartwright, *Joseph Lister, the Man Who Made Surgery Safe* (London: Weidenfeld and Nicholson, 1963); Richard B. Fisher, *Joseph Lister, 1827–1912* (New York: Stein and Day, 1977); Lindsey Fitzharris, *The Butchering Art: Joseph Lister's Quest to Transform the Grisly World of Victorian Medicine* (London: Allen Lane, 2017).

[3] Walter H. Ogston (ed.), *Alexander Ogston K.C.V.O.: Memoirs and Tributes of Relatives, Colleagues and Students, with Some Autobiographical Writings* (Aberdeen: Aberdeen University Press, 1943), pp. 98–100; Alexander G. Ogston, 'Ogston, Alexander (1844–1929)', *ODNB*.

[4] Michael Worboys, *Spreading Germs: Disease Theories and Medical Practice in Britain, 1865–1900* (Cambridge, UK: Cambridge University Press, 2000), pp. 151, 170–1.

[5] T. H. Pennington, 'Listerism, Its Decline and Its Persistence: The Introduction of Aseptic Surgical Techniques in Three British Teaching Hospitals, 1890–99', *Medical History* 39:1 (1995), 35–60, at pp. 43–4.

his 'bulldog', Cheyne, for contradicting their own views on the germlessness of healthy tissue.[6]

Nevertheless, Ogston was responsible for one of the most powerfully symbolic gestures in the history of antisepsis. He trained in Aberdeen and was appointed acting surgeon to the Royal Infirmary in 1870. Years later he wrote: 'How well I remember the old Aberdeen Infirmary before the days of Antiseptic Surgery. The wards, even the very corridors, stunk with the mawkish, manna-like odour of suppuration'. In the staff room, 'there hung a row of old, black coats covered with the dirt of years and encrusted with blood-stains, [...] the dirtier the more venerated'. Round about were hung Christian images, symbols, and scripture, and Ogston recalled the time when, inspired by antiseptic zeal, he entered the operating ward and 'tore down and burned the text in large letters which hung there: "PREPARE TO MEET THY GOD"'.[7]

Ogston's story is perhaps less straightforward than it might initially appear. Firstly, his gesture had as much to do with a distaste for the religious sanctimony of the hospital's lay governors as it did with any improvements in operative surgery brought about by antisepsis. Secondly, and in keeping with a historiography that has emphasised the complexity and mutability of early germ *theories* of disease, his post-hoc reflections on pre-antiseptic surgical practice, notably the reference to dirty coats, seem conditioned by a later, *aseptic* agenda about which Lister and many of his followers were, at least at first, deeply ambivalent, if not actively hostile.[8] Even so, Ogston's removal from the operating ward of this exhortation to eschatological imminence has a profound imaginative appeal and has been deployed by a number of commentators to dramatise the advent of antiseptic surgery.[9] Indeed, if Ogston's story exemplifies anything, it is less the revolutionary impact of germ theory *per se* (Michael Worboys has suggested there was no bacteriological 'revolution') and

---

[6] Ogston (ed.), *Ogston*, p. 100; Worboys, *Spreading Germs*, pp. 172–3.

[7] Ogston (ed.), *Ogston*, p. 93.

[8] This historiography is best exemplified by Lindsay Granshaw, '"Upon This Principle I Have Based a Practice": The Development of Antisepsis in Britain', in John V. Pickstone (ed.), *Medical Innovations in Historical Perspective* (Basingstoke: Palgrave Macmillan, 1992), 17–46; Christopher Lawrence and Richard Dixey, 'Practising on Principle: Joseph Lister and the Germ Theories of Disease', in Christopher Lawrence (ed.), *Medical Theory, Surgical Practice: Studies in the History of Surgery* (London: Routledge, 1992), 153–215; and Worboys, *Spreading Germs*. For two opposed positions on the relationship between antisepsis and asepsis, see Nicholas J. Fox, 'Scientific Theory Choice and Social Structure: The Case of Joseph Lister's Antisepsis, Humoral Theory and Asepsis', *History of Science* 26:4 (1988), 367–97; Worboys, *Spreading Gems*, pp. 186–92.

[9] For example, see Quentin N. Myrvik and Russell S. Weiser, *Fundamentals of Medical Bacteriology and Mycology* (Philadelphia: Lea and Febiger, 1988), p. 141. A version of this story featured on John Green's podcast *The Anthropocene Reviewed* in 2020: www.wnycstudios.org/podcasts/anthropocene-reviewed/episodes/anthropocene-reviewed-staphylococcus-aureus-and-non-denial-denial (accessed 27/07/21).

more the capacity of the Listerian generation for myth-making, for their persistent and unyielding claim that they had effected an epochal transformation in surgical knowledge, practice, and identity, saving humankind through the healing power of science.[10] Writing in 1927, for example, one of Lister's former assistants, John Rudd Leeson (1854–1927), presented antisepsis as a harbinger of techno-scientific modernity, claiming that, like a latter-day Christopher Columbus, Lister had discovered 'a new world of surgery'.[11]

What is also significant about Ogston's story, especially for our purposes, is that it conceived of antisepsis as an emotional, as much as intellectual, watershed: ultimate deliverance from the terrors of operative surgery that had been attenuated, but not entirely eradicated, by the advent of anaesthesia. As Ogston himself put it in an address to the BMA in 1899:

We live in an era that can claim to be one of most exceptional, probably unique, interest. We have witnessed in it the most marvellous and rapid advances the world has ever experienced in the powers of mastering and warding off disease. We have passed through many gloomy years, in which we worked our life's work blindly and in the dark, with dread fastening on the heart as surely as the hand grasped the knife, for ever [sic] trembling before the horrors of surgical pestilence; and now we have been privileged to see the dawn of a new day when septic disease is being robbed of its terrors by the discoveries of Lister, whose great gifts to humanity coming generations will hereafter delight to recall, recognising that whatever we owe to the great surgeons of the past has been but little in comparison with the benefits he has conferred on us and through us on all mankind.[12]

It is perhaps no coincidence that in his memoirs, Ogston's reflections on antisepsis immediately follow those on anaesthesia, wherein he recalls his student days and the surgical practice of William Keith (1802–71), colloquially known as 'Old Danger', who rejected chloroform and implored his patients to '"Put your trust for a minute in Dr Keith and God"'.[13] After all, anaesthesia and antisepsis were often represented in later nineteenth- and early twentieth-century accounts as the twin markers of surgical modernity. But in his 1899 speech, Ogston gave priority to antisepsis and painted the era immediately prior to the advent of germ theory as one of darkness and dread. As Christopher Lawrence has argued, such rhetorical sleights of hand were not uncommon in this period, as Listerian surgeons 'flattened out the brilliant peak of the 1850s from which they had once surveyed the benighted past', consigning even

[10] Worboys, Spreading Germs, pp. 83, 278. Ogston does not fall into the category of the Listerian generation as conceived by Crowther and Dupree, as he was not one of Lister's students. Nonetheless, he was certainly inspired by Lister's work: M. Anne Crowther and Marguerite Dupree, Medical Lives in the Age of Surgical Revolution (Cambridge, UK: Cambridge University Press, 2007), p. 119.
[11] J. R. Leeson, Lister as I Knew Him (London: Ballière, Tindall, and Cox, 1927), p. 170.
[12] Lancet 154:962 (5 August 1899), p. 325.   [13] Ogston (ed.), Ogston, p. 92.

the immediate post-anaesthetic period to the surgical 'dark age'.[14] Indeed, for many surgeons of Ogston's generation, anaesthesia constituted what, to borrow his metaphor, might be called a *false* dawn. In Chapter 5, we explored how anaesthesia transformed the emotional dimensions of surgery, lessening the dread of operations for patient and surgeon alike. By reducing the impact of shock and eliminating the need to operate with haste, it opened up new corporeal horizons for surgical intervention, including such invasive procedures as ovariotomy. However, by the 1860s, a number of practitioners were growing increasingly concerned by rates of post-operative mortality, particularly from septic afflictions such as erysipelas, septicaemia, and pyaemia, and especially among patients in large, urban hospitals. This phenomenon, underscored by broad statistical comparisons between hospitals and between hospital and private practice, was denominated 'hospitalism' by James Young Simpson.[15] This term was subsequently adopted by many surgeons, including John Erichsen, who came to see hospitals themselves, in terms of their management, environment, and even physical structure, as the preeminent problem facing patient recovery and post-operative wound care.[16] Whether there was a *genuine* crisis in post-operative mortality or not is debatable. Some historians have suggested that 'it is entirely plausible that a deterioration in the state of wounds and their contents was coincident with industrialisation and urbanisation'.[17] Others have argued that 'without Simpson there would have been no controversy'.[18] What is certain is that the *perception* of a crisis took something of the shine off anaesthesia, then barely twenty years old, and provoked a heated, protracted, and ultimately hugely significant debate within British surgery.

Joseph Lister's intervention into this debate is so well known as to require no substantial repetition here. Beginning in 1867, Lister, then working at the University of Glasgow, wrote a series of articles in the medical press in which he suggested that sepsis was a chemical process of putrefaction caused by the action of airborne particles or 'germs'. He maintained that these germs might be eliminated by the use of carbolic acid. As historians have pointed out, much of what Lister argued in the late 1860s was relatively uncontentious.[19] It was his reliance on the French chemist Louis Pasteur's (1822–95) germ theory of

---

[14] Christopher Lawrence, 'Democratic, Divine and Heroic: The History and Historiography of Surgery', in Lawrence (ed.), *Medical Theory, Surgical Practice*, 1–47, at p. 10.

[15] James Young Simpson, *Hospitalism: Its Effects on the Results of Surgical Operations* (Edinburgh: Oliver and Boyd, 1869).

[16] John Eric Erichsen, *On Hospitalism and the Causes of Death after Operations* (London: Longmans and Green, 1874).

[17] Worboys, *Spreading Germs*, p. 75.

[18] A. J. Youngston, *The Scientific Revolution in Victorian Medicine* (London: Croom Helm, 1979), p. 220.

[19] Lawrence and Dixey, 'Principle', p. 163; Worboys, *Spreading Germs*, p. 82.

fermentation, together with his exclusive emphasis on the influence of external agents in the production of sepsis, that alienated some of his colleagues. Much of the historiography has contrasted Lister's conception of the action of living germs with the 'cleanliness school' of surgeons who considered a much wider range of environmental factors in the production of post-operative disease. But what is also clear is that Lister's resolute focus on the wound as the principal object of surgical concern, and as the primary site of prophylactic and therapeutic intervention, effectively discounted a whole raft of constitutional factors, including the emotional state of the patient, that had, until then, been central to surgical understandings of patient recovery and, hence, operative success. Lister and his followers would change both their practice and their principles over the succeeding fifteen years, making Listerism something of a conceptual moving target.[20] Nonetheless, as Listerism gained ground, and as bacteriology, in the German mould, came to provide the underlying theoretical rationale for antiseptic practice, the patient, as an idiosyncratic and constitutionally unstable entity, slipped almost entirely from surgical view.

This image, of the surgeon losing sight of the patient through the lens of his microscope, is perhaps *too* seductive, not least because it resonates with Nicholas Jewson's highly influential argument about the 'disappearance of the sick man' from Western medicine.[21] The reality was rather more complicated, for, as Lawrence has shown, British practitioners were generally resistant to German laboratory methods until some way into the twentieth century.[22] Nonetheless, as we shall see in the first part of this chapter, the increasingly materialist and reductionist understandings of the body, and of surgical disease, that came to prominence in the last three decades of the nineteenth century, and were not seriously questioned until the emergence of holism in the 1920s, had profound implications for the emotional cultures of surgery.[23] They completed that shift away from the patient as an emotionally agentive individual that had been initiated by the advent of anaesthesia, and concluded the transition from an emotional regime of Romantic sensibility to one of scientific modernity.

As the second part of this chapter will demonstrate, however, the place of emotions within modern antiseptic surgery was somewhat more complex than

---

[20] Lawrence and Dixey, 'Principle'.
[21] Nicholas D. Jewson, 'The Disappearance of the Sick Man from Medical Cosmology, 1770–1870', *Sociology* 10 (1976), 225–44.
[22] Christopher Lawrence, 'Incommunicable Knowledge: Science, Technology and the Clinical Art in Britain, 1850–1914', *Journal of Contemporary History* 20:4 (1985), 503–20. For a counterpoint, see Rosemary Wall, *Bacteria in Britain, 1880–1939* (London: Pickering and Chatto, 2013), pt. I.
[23] Christopher Lawrence and George Weisz (eds), *Greater Than the Parts: Holism in Biomedicine, 1920–1950* (Oxford: Oxford University Press, 1998).

simple erasure, for if the *ontology* of emotions in surgical practice certainly diminished to the point of insignificance, their *rhetorical* deployment by Lister and his acolytes positively flourished. As we shall see, Lister was frequently portrayed by his supporters and hagiographers as an almost preternaturally compassionate man whose care of, and attention to, his patients was unsurpassed. Indeed, emotions played a vital part in the mythologising of antisepsis as an almost divine deliverance from human suffering. And yet, while Lister was something of a transitional figure in terms of the emotional regime of surgery, a man who had one foot in the cultures of Romantic sensibility, this chapter argues that his emotional disposition was more akin to a performative politesse than to the ideals of Romantic intersubjectivity. It likewise asserts that the rhetorical deployment of emotion by his supporters was part of a wider strategy by which sentimentalised ideas of medical virtue were used to counter growing popular anxiety about medical morality in relation to such issues as vivisection and the women's movement. Indeed, despite such images of surgery being presented to the public, Lister can be said to have ushered in a new model of surgical identity, based on varied notions of *detachment*, that would come to form the basis for the professional ideal in the twentieth century.

'A Different Thing Altogether': Emotions, Ontology, and Antiseptic Surgery

In October 1867, between the publication of the first and second of his *Lancet* articles outlining the antiseptic system of surgery, Joseph Lister wrote to his father, Joseph Jackson Lister (1786–1869), claiming that 'I now perform an operation for the removal of a tumour, etc., with a totally different feeling from what I used to have; in fact, surgery is becoming a different thing altogether'.[24] That phrase 'a different thing altogether' clearly evokes the fundamental break that Lister thought he had made with the 'old world' of surgery. That Lister referred to performing operations with a 'totally different *feeling*' also suggests the phenomenological and affective dimensions of that transformation. We shall consider Lister's emotional disposition in due course. Firstly, however, we must determine what was distinct about his approach and what exactly it was different *from*. While Lister's talk of disjuncture was amplified by his supporters into a rhetoric of revolution, the historiography has demonstrated that the emergence of antisepsis was a messy, complex, and contested affair that was not truly settled until at least the mid-1880s.[25] And yet, even if there was no revolution, the surgery of the early 1890s looked quite different

---

[24] Godlee, *Lister*, p. 198.
[25] Granshaw, '"Upon This Principle"'; Lawrence and Dixey, 'Principle'; Worboys, *Spreading Germs*.

to that of the early 1860s. While the literature has tended to focus on the environmental dimensions of antiseptic and aseptic surgery, and the tensions between germ theory and hospitalism, another major object of contemporary contention, which has received less attention in the scholarship, was the role of the patient's constitution, including their emotional and mental state, in post-operative recovery. This section addresses that oversight, demonstrating that Listerian antisepsis had transformative implications for the place of emotion within British surgery.

In order to understand how this transformation was effected, and indeed resisted, we need to understand the place of emotion in surgery in the early 1860s, in the years immediately before Lister's work on wounds. Chapter 3 demonstrates that the pre-anaesthetic surgical patient was characterised by an ontological 'messiness' in which their reaction to, and recovery from, operative surgery was dependent upon a 'complex melding of constitutional, nervous, and emotional factors'. Thus, according to surgeons such as Astley Cooper and John Abernethy, a patient might bring about their own demise through overwhelming feelings of dread and despair, might sink under mental despondency during their recovery, or might die, delirious, under the influence of a post-operative hectic fever. This was particularly true of complex, 'capital' operations but, so powerful was the impact of emotions on patient recovery, even relatively minor procedures might be attended with dire consequences if the patient was not of the right mind.

The advent of anaesthesia transformed this situation, eliminating the pain of operative surgery and mitigating some of the dread experienced by patients at the prospect of a procedure. And yet, revolutionary though it was, anaesthesia did not signal an immediate end to the role of the patient's emotions in determining the outcome of an operation. For one thing, and as we saw in the previous chapter, anaesthesia produced its own anxieties. In 1870, for example, *The Lancet* expressed concern about the popular reporting of deaths under chloroform, stating that 'they serve to alarm patients and their friends, to surround the idea of an operation with unnecessary anticipations of evil, and possibly, in some cases, to *modify through the emotions the ultimate results of treatment*'.[26] For another, in terms of patient subjectivity, surgical case reports from the early 1860s could exhibit a remarkable continuity with the pre-anaesthetic past. Take, for instance, the following description by Cornelius Black (1822–86) of a patient undergoing ovariotomy in 1863:

The state of the patient's mind was placid, cheerful, and of confident hope in the result. She had long contemplated the operation, and she felt a satisfaction when the day for it arrived. In speaking of it she never betrayed the slightest apprehension as to the result.

[26] *Lancet* 95:2420 (15 January 1870), p. 90. Emphasis added.

She slept more soundly the night before the operation than she had slept for a long time before. She took a hearty breakfast on the following morning; and when the hour for testing her courage came, she walked to the operating table without evincing the least fear of the issue which awaited her. Few will doubt that this state of mind conduced to her recovery.[27]

A good way to gauge the place of emotions within the surgery of the early 1860s is to look at the lectures of two surgeons who came to play an ambivalent role in the reception of antisepsis. The first of these men was James Paget (1814–99), who would receive Lister's ideas with cautious curiosity, before ultimately rejecting them. In 1862, he delivered the 'Address in Surgery' to the Edinburgh meeting of the BMA, in which he spoke about the effect of nervous shock on a patient's recovery from surgery. 'If we include under this heading only those in which patients die without ever rallying from the depression into which the operation has cast them', he stated, 'then they are very rare [...] and my impression is that they are made rarer than they used to be [...] by the use of anaesthetics'. 'Yet such deaths do happen', he maintained, for the 'mental state of dread or grief, the loss of blood; the anaesthetic; the violent impression on the nervous centres [...] is reflected from these centres, not upon the heart alone, but upon all the organs of organic life'. Indeed, he continued, 'My impression is that the tendency of the present day is to attribute too much to the loss of blood, and too little to the impression on the nervous system, which being, through anaesthetics, not consciously perceived, is apt to be forgotten'.[28] The second man was Paget's St Bartholomew's Hospital colleague, William Savory (1826–95), who would become one of Lister's most outspoken and implacable critics. In a series of lectures on 'life and death' delivered to the Royal Institution in 1862, Savory spoke of the impact of the emotions on the functioning of the heart. The heart, he argued, 'may be arrested by causes which operate through the nervous system'. 'It is quite true', he affirmed, 'that the heart will leap from joy, or sink from fear, and emotions in still stronger degree may check its action to an extent sufficient to produce death'.[29]

As can be seen, the action of the emotions on the body was often absorbed into a concept of nervous shock, and was part of more general ideas about the constitutional idiosyncrasies of the patient inherited from the pre-anaesthetic era. But such ideas were not static. Indeed, reading Paget's lectures across the 1860s, it is possible to detect a subtle shift away from the idea that emotional states were an unambiguous determinant of operative outcomes, even before the advent of antisepsis. Speaking to his students on the 'Various Risks

[27] *Lancet* 82:2081 (18 July 1863), p. 63.
[28] *British Medical Journal* 2:85 (16 August 1862), p. 157.
[29] William Savory, *On Life and Death: Four Lectures Delivered at the Royal Institution of Great Britain* (London: Smith and Elder, 1863), p. 167.

of Operations' in the summer of 1867, Paget argued that statistical tables of hospital mortality could not 'tell the several or united influences of differences of constitution, of sound or unsound health, of diseases of internal organs, of race and temper and habits of life. Yet the question of the safety of an operation may turn on these very things'.[30] However, he was equivocal about how much could be predicted from a patient's temperament:

The healthiest nervous system, in so far as it may be judged of by the mind, is that in which a patient faces an operation quietly, and with a courage which is not too demonstrative. Cases are told, and some of them, probably, are true, and I have seen confirmations of them, which would make it very probable that an abiding gloom, or fear of death, or a foretelling of death, or an utter indifference to the result of the operation, are very bad states. But, after all, your estimate of the risks on any such grounds as these must be a vague one. A better sign is the capacity for sleep.[31]

Worboys has called these broadly constitutionalist approaches to surgical recovery, which represented the intellectual *status quo* in 1865, 'physiological', in that they conceptualised disease as 'disturbances in normal functioning that resulted from a patient's predisposition interacting with a configuration of environmental influences'.[32] Such models often had a residual humoralist aspect, for as John Rudd Leeson recalled of his time at St Thomas' Hospital in the early 1870s: 'A great deal was said about "temperaments": if high fever followed an operation it was due to a "sanguineous temperament"; if luckily the patient escaped a gross infection, the beneficent possession of a "phlegmatic temperament" was assumed'.[33] Shortly, however, they would be challenged by Lister's 'ontological' conception of disease, which 'made diseases "things" or entities that were separate from the patient'.[34]

Lister's first public intervention into the issue of wound management was concerned with compound fractures, a condition whose unpredictable, though often dire, resolution had long vexed surgeons, and had led John Abernethy to proclaim that only God knew why some of his patients died and others did not.[35] Indeed, Lister opened his article by stating that the 'frequency of disastrous consequences in compound fracture, contrasted with the complete immunity from danger to life or limb in simple fracture, is one of the most striking as well as melancholy facts in surgical practice'.[36] Most surgeons of the period

[30] *Lancet* 90:2288 (6 July 1867), p. 1.
[31] *Lancet* 90:2295 (24 August 1867), p. 220.
[32] Worboys, *Spreading Germs*, pp. 4–5.
[33] Leeson, *Lister*, pp. 9–10.
[34] Worboys, *Spreading Germs*, p. 5.
[35] RCSE, MS0232/1/1, John Flint South, 'Lectures on the Principles of Surgery delivered by John Abernethy Esq. FRS in the Anatomical Theatre at St Bartholomew's Hospital in the years 1818 and 1819', f. 241.
[36] Joseph Lister, *The Collected Papers of Joseph Lister*, vol. 2 (Oxford: Clarendon Press, 1909), p. 1.

would doubtless have agreed. Where many demurred was Lister's explanation for this phenomenon. Lister had been introduced to the theories of the French chemist Louis Pasteur around 1865 and was persuaded by Pasteur's argument that the 'atmosphere produces decomposition of organic substances', not due to the action of oxygen 'or any of its gaseous constituents', but because of 'minute particles suspended in it, which are the germs of various low forms of life [...] regarded as merely accidental concomitants of putrescence, but now shown [...] to be its essential cause'.[37] For Lister, these germs were deposited on the dead tissue of wounds, such as those produced by compound fractures, giving rise to a process of putrefaction, or sepsis, that poisoned the patient, often fatally. As Lister famously declared to the BMA Annual Meeting in August 1867, 'Upon this principle I have based a practice'.[38] This practice involved the application of a chemical substance, carbolic acid (or German creosote as it was popularly known), in order to kill these germs, or at least inhibit their entry into the wound. At first, Lister employed carbolic-infused putty laid upon the wound, but he shortly abandoned this in favour of a complicated multi-layered dressing that provided a chemical barrier without allowing the acid, which was highly irritating, to come into direct contact with the skin and produce 'carbolic induced suppuration'.[39] In 1871, Lister also introduced a steam-powered spray to diffuse carbolic acid over the patient during surgery. This spray became the most iconic symbol of Lister's technique. However, it ultimately proved of dubious value and, after little more than a decade, it was increasingly marginalised, although not entirely abandoned until 1887.[40]

What is important about Lister's technique, and what made it different from what had come before, was its singular focus upon the condition of the wound. In his early writings, Lister made reference to the state of his surgical wards at the Glasgow Royal Infirmary, including their proximity to a 'foul drain' and their having been built just above 'a multitude of coffins, which had been placed there at the time of the cholera epidemic of 1849'. However, he cited these factors not in support of an environmentalist explanation for post-operative mortality, but rather in order to disprove their significance, his rates of mortality having declined precipitously in spite of these conditions. It was, he maintained, the implementation of his antiseptic system that had effected this dramatic change.[41] Likewise, while Lister attended to the post-operative 'comfort' of his patients, he showed little or no interest in

---

[37] Godlee, *Lister*, p. 162; Lister, *Papers*, vol. 2, p. 2.
[38] Lister, *Papers*, vol. 2, p. 37.
[39] Lawrence and Dixey, 'Principle', pp. 165, 169.
[40] Godlee, *Lister*, p. 286; Worboys, *Spreading Germs*, pp. 95, 170. Lawrence and Dixey, 'Principle', p. 191.
[41] Lister, *Papers*, vol. 2, pp. 45, 124–5.

their general physical condition, or the specifics of their diet, at least when compared to his ever-watchful contemporaries. Leeson arrived in Edinburgh (to where Lister had returned in 1869 as Professor of Clinical Surgery) from St Thomas', which, following hospitalist concerns, had been entirely rebuilt to Florence Nightingale's (1820–1910) 'pavilion principle' in 1871. He was therefore somewhat surprised by what he found on Lister's wards. '[N]o medicine was ordered', he observed, 'a strange thing in those days, and everyone seemed to be on the same diet':

I seemed to have been in a dream where everything was topsy-turvy and all that I had been taught to consider essential seemed non-essential; the costly buildings, the spacious wards, the indispensable "Nightingales" [nurses] and the bottles of medicines, so far as the well-being of the patient was concerned, appeared superfluous.[42]

Lister evidently relished overturning established wisdom about post-operative patient care. In marked contrast to the views of the cleanliness school, he 'seemed to revel in the "dirty" conditions of his wards' in a manner that was positively provocative.[43] For Lister, the condition of the wound was all that mattered. But even here, appearances could be deceptive. In 1875, for example, he famously rejected conventional notions of cleanliness *in toto*. 'If we take cleanliness in any other sense than antiseptic cleanliness', he claimed, 'my patients have the dirtiest wounds and sores in the world. I often keep on the dressings for a week at a time, during which the discharges accumulate and undergo chemical alteration', which 'conveys [...] both to the eye and to the nose an idea of anything rather than cleanliness'. 'Aesthetically they are dirty', he maintained, 'though surgically clean'.[44] It was as if antisepsis not only provided a new logic for explaining post-operative infection, but severed the very connection between surgical pathology and observable reality.

Lister's contemporaries challenged his ideas on a number of grounds. For some, such as the Glasgow surgeon John Reid (1809–81), they went against everything that surgeons had come to believe about 'natural' healing. 'The atmosphere, which from their earliest years they were accustomed to regard as their best friend', he exclaimed, 'must now be looked on as their worst enemy. Instead of breathing a pure mixture of oxygen and nitrogen, they were really swallowing myriads of living animalcule. The idea was too absurd to be soberly entertained'.[45] Others refused to countenance the existence not only of germs, but even of sepsis itself. As late as 1880, the surgeon Thomas Darby (c.1809–86) of Bray in Ireland told the BMA Annual Meeting that he 'entirely disbelieved

---

[42] Leeson, *Lister*, p. 19.
[43] Christopher Lawrence, 'Lister, Joseph (1827–1912)', *ODNB*.
[44] Lister, *Papers*, vol. 2, p. 254.
[45] *Glasgow Medical Journal* 2:1 (November 1869), p. 135.

the germ-theory', and that 'there was no such thing, properly speaking, as anti-septic treatment, seeing there was no such thing as septicaemia'.[46]

However, perhaps the most consistent grounds for opposing Lister's theory was that it completely neglected what Reid called 'the state of the system of the patient'.[47] Such objections were forcibly outlined in a series of addresses to the BMA Annual Meeting in the later 1860s and 1870s. One of the first of these was given by the Leeds surgeon Thomas Nunneley (1809–70), who referred to the 'fashionable [...] method of treating wounds by what has been called "antiseptic treatment"' in which 'the sound physiological and pathological doc-trines and practice of the last generation of British surgeons are unheeded, and in danger of being [...] forgotten'. For Nunneley, the *truly* antiseptic measures of the past were applied 'to the constitutional condition, and not to extrinsic circumstances as now'. Compared to the holistic practice of his generation, Lister's system took 'No account [...] of the constitution of the patient, his hab-its of life, his strength or his weakness, the condition of his digestive organs, the state of his blood, his temperament, diathesis, hereditary disposition, age or sex, [or] his state of mind'. Instead, 'Surgical science and medical knowledge are reduced to the one plain rule of, *in full faith* – for that is as essential as the acid itself – plentifully imbruing the part with carbolic acid'.[48]

Similar views were expressed almost exactly a decade later by William Savory, in what has been described as 'perhaps the last set-piece attack on [Lister's] system by an elite metropolitan surgeon'.[49] Savory did not reject germ theory *per se*, but he was concerned that 'what is called "antiseptic surgery", fixes the surgeon's attention too exclusively on the dressing of the wound, to the exclusion of other matters of at least equal importance'.[50] Like Nunneley, Savory thought that too little scrutiny was being paid to the consti-tutional condition of the patient and too much to external factors, or, as he put it, 'I venture to think that of late the [...] error has prevailed, of regarding only the conditions under which the poison is formed, and losing sight altogether of the conditions under which it affects the blood'. Quoting William Roberts (1830–99), whose words were, he claimed, 'some of the wisest which have been spoken' on the subject of post-operative sepsis, Savory concluded that the 'essence of the principle [...] is not exactly to protect the wound from the septic organisms, but to *defend the patient against the septic poison*'.[51]

In the eyes of his critics, Lister's myopic focus on the condition of the wound, which came at the expense of the whole patient, was epitomised by

---

[46] *British Medical Journal* 2:1026 (28 August 1880), p. 342.
[47] *Glasgow Medical Journal* 2:1 (November 1869), p. 135.
[48] *British Medical Journal* 2:449 (7 August 1869), pp. 152–3. Emphasis in original.
[49] Worboys, *Spreading Germs*, p. 161.
[50] *British Medical Journal* 2:971 (9 August 1879), p. 232.
[51] *British Medical Journal* 2:971 (9 August 1879), pp. 211, 216. Emphasis in original.

his elaborate system of carbolic-infused dressings. For Savory, the practice of dressing wounds had to be shaped by patient subjectivity as much as pathological observation. 'I am guided', he claimed, 'by the state of the patient; whether spare or full-bodied; his sense of local and general comfort, freedom from or complaint of pain; and the season or temperature'. Indeed, in recommending a simple bread poultice, Savory explicitly appealed to the patient's general sense of well-being. This 'homely article', he claimed, 'far more frequently draws from the patient the word "comfort" than any other form of dressing. "Yes, that is comfortable", is a familiar expression after the application of a poultice'.[52] For another of Lister's high-profile opponents, the Birmingham surgeon Sampson Gamgee (1828–86), a regular and highly technical re-dressing of the wound also undermined one of the most important aspects of post-operative care:

A system of treatment which requires that whenever discharge is seen to come through the dressings, these are to be changed under the carbolic spray, is opposed to the great principle of local and constitutional rest, subjecting the patient to a great deal of pain and the surgeon to a great deal of trouble.[53]

What lay behind this powerful resistance to Lister's shift from the constitutional to the local and the subjective to the objective? Lister's supporters generally framed opposition to antisepsis in terms of age. For example, Lister's nephew and biographer, Rickman John Godlee (1849–1925), pointedly referred to John Erichsen's 1874 lectures on hospitalism as demonstrating 'the mental aspect of the middle-aged London surgeon at that time towards the whole question'.[54] There is an element of truth in these claims; Reid, Darby, and Nunneley were all around 58 when Lister first mooted his theory of antisepsis in 1867, while Nunneley's constant reference to John Hunter as his intellectual Pole Star suggests that he was a surgeon of the 'old school'.[55] But such explanations can only go so far. After all, Erichsen was only nine years older than Lister. Moreover, despite Godlee's claims that Savory's 1879 address 'warmed and comforted the soul of many a middle-aged man, who had begun to feel the discomforts of an undermined faith', Savory was actually less than five months older than Lister, while Gamgee, who had been a classmate of Lister's at University College London, was almost exactly a year *younger*.[56]

Perhaps a more important continuity between antiseptic sceptics can be found in their rejection of what they saw as Lister's universalist understanding of sepsis, wherein an exposure to germs was, in and of itself, sufficient to

---

[52] *British Medical Journal* 2:971 (9 August 1879), pp. 213–14.
[53] *Lancet* 112:2886 (21 December 1878), p. 870.
[54] Godlee, *Lister*, p. 131.
[55] *British Medical Journal* 2:449 (7 August 1869), pp. 143–56.
[56] Godlee, *Lister*, p. 323.

produce disease. 'If the germ-theory [...] contained the truth, the whole truth, and nothing but the truth', Savory asked, 'what possible explanation is to be given of that which is witnessed daily and hourly – the kindly repair of exposed wounds?' An adherent of germ theory 'would inevitably come to the conclusion that to expose any wound unguarded to the atmosphere would be to seal the fate of the patient', when this was clearly not the case.[57] For Savory, recovery was, rather, a highly contingent and idiosyncratic process that required delicate surgical judgement.

Another objection to Lister's approach stemmed from his tendency towards theoretical abstraction over an experiential knowledge of individual bodies, constitutions, and temperaments. This is not to say that Lister did not produce case histories; he did. However, these generally failed to satisfy his critics, as did his hesitancy, at least before the 1880s, to publish consistent statistical data.[58] Rather, in explicating his theory, Lister regularly employed experimental and demonstrative methods that were more in keeping with chemistry than surgery, and which confused and antagonised some of his contemporaries. This difference in method was most clearly exemplified by his beloved flasks. These, which were a modification of Pasteur's famous experiments from the early 1860s, contained boiled urine, one with an open neck, another 'lightly plugged with cotton wool' and a third exposed to the air, but with a curved neck. Within days, the open necked-flask was 'turbid and putrid' while the other two, even after six months, were 'clear and perfectly "sweet"'. Given that the urine in the curved-neck flask was as exposed to the atmosphere as that in the straight-necked one, its unaltered state suggested that some particulate entity had been prevented from reaching the urine and that the 'cause of putrefaction was therefore something *in* the air and not of the air itself'.[59] When Leeson was first shown these flasks, he remembered 'thinking it was strange that so eminent a surgeon should be interested in such an unusual subject and could find time to study such irrelevant and out-of-the-way matters'. And yet they were 'the most precious of the Professor's possessions', which, when Lister was appointed Professor of Surgery at King's College London in 1877, were the cause of much 'concern and anxiety' as he and his wife Agnes (1834–93) carried them on their laps, in a first-class railway compartment, all the way from Edinburgh to London, lest any misfortune should befall them.[60]

[57] *British Medical Journal* 2:971 (9 August 1879), p. 210.
[58] Savory was one of Lister's most vocal critics on this point: Ulrich Tröhler, 'Statistics and the British Controversy about the Effects of Joseph Lister's System of Antisepsis for Surgery, 1867–1890', *Journal of the Royal Society of Medicine* 108:7 (2015), 280–7; Thomas Schlich, 'No Time for Statistics: Joseph Lister's Antisepsis and Types of Knowledge in Nineteenth-Century British Surgery', *Bulletin of the History of Medicine* 94:3 (2020), 394–422.
[59] Leeson, *Lister*, pp. 94–5. See also Godlee, *Lister*, pp. 224–5.
[60] Leeson, *Lister*, pp. 24, 94.

For Lister's critics, his attachment to these flasks was indicative of his detachment from the complexities of quotidian surgical experience. Thus, while Gamgee confessed that he was 'quite willing to admit the facts of the flasks', he asked: 'What do the facts amount to in their *surgical application*? Is not the whole history of physiology and surgery full of examples, to prove the fallacy of arguing from the demeanour of organic parts *removed from the body*, to what occurs in the living system?'[61] Similarly, when Lister gave his opening lecture of the winter session at King's College London and chose to speak on the fermentation of milk by what he called '*Bacillus lactis*', Cheyne remembered that the 'expression on the faces of the audience was very interesting and rather amusing; the majority of the surgeons present could not understand what the lactic fermentation of milk had to do with surgery'.[62] Where once the patient had been a complex, messy, and idiosyncratic entity, now they were akin to a urine- or milk-filled flask, subject to a chemical process of putrefaction. As Godlee explained, for a Listerian surgeon treating an abscess was 'comparatively simple'. All he had to do was 'open the abscess—so to say, to uncork the bottle full of putrescible material—and to keep its contents from decomposing in spite of the admission of air'.[63]

In accounting for the response to that first King's lecture, Cheyne recalled that 'Those were the days of the "practical surgeon" as opposed to the "scientific surgeon"'.[64] This was a distinction that had been made by Erichsen in 1873, and it warrants some consideration.[65] In Chapter 1, we saw how Romantic surgeons harnessed the legacy of John Hunter to claim that *theirs* was the generation of the 'scientific' surgeon. Such claims exemplify the changing meanings of the word 'science'. For surgeons of the early nineteenth century, scientific surgery connoted something more than manual craft: it suggested a thorough knowledge of anatomy and physiology. During the course of the nineteenth century, however, the notion of science as applied to surgery expanded to include pathology, experimental physiology, and biochemistry.[66] While Leeson recalled that, during his time at Edinburgh, 'we never saw a microscope [...], nor did we ever seen Lister use one', surgical science would, as the 1880s dawned, also increasingly include microbiology and, of course, bacteriology.[67] Even so, there were many surgeons in the later

[61] Sampson Gamgee, *On the Treatment of Wounds: Clinical Lectures* (London: J. & A. Churchill, 1878), pp. 132 3. Emphasis added.
[62] William Watson Cheyne, *Lister and His Achievement* (London: Longmans and Green, 1925), p. 33.
[63] Godlee, *Lister*, p. 188.   [64] Cheyne, *Lister*, pp. 3–4.
[65] John Eric Erichsen, *Modern Surgery, Its Progress and Tendencies* (London: H. K. Lewis, 1873), p. 4.
[66] William F. Bynum, *Science and the Practice of Medicine in the Nineteenth Century* (Cambridge, UK: Cambridge University Press, 1994).
[67] Leeson, *Lister*, p. 92.

decades of the nineteenth century who classed themselves as 'practical' men. Nunneley framed his 1869 Address in precisely those terms, while, even as late as 1908, the Edinburgh surgeon John Chiene (1843–1923) could decry what he regarded as an overemphasis on laboratory work, reminding his audience that the 'most important elements' of human life 'are beyond the reach of the knife and the penetration of the microscope'.[68] The practical surgeons of the late nineteenth century prided themselves on their clinical skill and on an exquisite judgement honed by long experience. Theirs was surgery in the 'real world'. By contrast, they were generally suspicious of what they saw as the abstract, theoretical approaches of men like Lister. It has often been said that Lister's ideas met with more approval in Germany than in his native land, and there was a definite view among some surgeons that scientific surgery was a foreign import. Commenting on Savory's 1879 address, for example, the *British Medical Journal* wrote:

[T]hose who are tempted to give in to the fashionable folly of national self-depreciation, and to believe that every thing of value in science must be imported from somewhere, and by preference from Germany, may be brought to a sounder mind when they see, by this address, how far in advance the English surgeons are of their foreign compeers in that essential of the art: the saving of human life.[69]

It would be a crude oversimplification to reduce late nineteenth-century British surgery to a practical/scientific binary, and to align the former with Lister's opponents and the latter with his supporters. Such binaries certainly had rhetorical force, and men like Cheyne were not averse to claiming that the days of the practical surgeon were past.[70] But even Erichsen acknowledged that he did not 'for one moment wish it to be supposed that I consider them as being absolutely separated by a hard and fast line'.[71] Nor would it be accurate to suggest that a sensitivity to the emotional and mental state of a patient was intrinsically incompatible with a Listerian approach. Indeed, it is possible to find examples, at least in the later 1860s and early 1870s, of surgeons who combined constitutionalist and antiseptic principles.[72]

Moreover, it is important to recognise that the persistence of emotion as an ontological category within post-operative patient care varied according to surgical specialism. It may perhaps come as no surprise, given what we heard in Chapter 5 about the gendering of emotion in surgery from the 1840s onwards, that it was in the field of gynaecology and obstetrics, as well as in the

---

[68] *British Medical Journal* 2:449 (7 August 1869), p. 144; John Chiene, *Looking Back 1907–1860* (Edinburgh: Darien Press, 1908), p. 6.
[69] *British Medical Journal* 2:971 (9 August 1879), p. 233.
[70] Cheyne, *Lister*, p. 34.   [71] Erichsen, *Modern Surgery*, p. 4.
[72] For example, see *Lancet* 96:2461 (29 October 1870), pp. 604–7.

treatment of women more generally, that emotion retained its greatest explanatory force for the longest time. At the height of antiseptic disputation in the mid-1870s, the Obstetrical Society of London hosted a series of debates on puerperal fever, a septic condition afflicting postpartum women. As Worboys points out, the contagiousness of puerperal fever had long been contested, but the issue was 'sharpened' in 1875 by the prosecution of two midwives for 'manslaughter by infection'.[73] What is notable about these debates, at least for our purposes, is the sheer ubiquity of emotion as a causal agent. For example, William Newman (1833–1903) of Stamford asserted that 'one should take into consideration [...] the mental conditions which not uncommonly associate themselves with pregnancy', claiming that, of the cases of puerperal fever he had encountered, 'a good number of them' involved 'elements of distinct mental disturbance'. Newman was not talking here about 'insanity' but rather 'the distressing circumstances, of the condition of pregnancy', which, he alleged, played 'a material part [...] in predisposing the system to the virulent development of septic poisons'. Newman's comments were echoed by John Braxton Hicks (1823–97), who claimed that it 'is evident that mental emotions have the power in some way, directly or indirectly, of bringing about a state of things which we term puerperal fever'.[74] Elsewhere, in 1877, the aural surgeon William Bartlett Dalby (1840–1918) stated: 'that emotional causes exercise a very decided influence on the function of hearing cannot fail to be observed by those who are in the habit of paying attention to affections [sic] of the ear' and 'because women are, more than men, mastered by their emotions, it is far more frequently in their case that such causes appear to exercise an influence in this direction'.[75] Of course, this is to say nothing of non-surgical conditions such as hysteria, in which 'mental emotion' and gender remained inextricably intertwined.

And yet, caveats aside, there is little doubt that the triumph of antisepsis brought about the end of emotion as an ontological category within surgical practice and that, in so doing, it extinguished the dying embers of an emotional regime of Romantic sensibility and signalled the hegemony of modern techno-scientific surgery. As the historiography has clearly shown, Lister's ideas were highly flexible, and were often reconfigured to accommodate new challenges. Hence, he was able to quell a certain amount of opposition by moving away from a purely exogenous understanding of sepsis towards a 'seed and soil' model.[76] Even so, his epistemology allowed little, if any, room for what he called the 'philosophical investigation of "constitutional conditions"'. At the 1879 International Congress of Medical Science in Amsterdam, for example,

---

[73] Worboys, *Spreading Germs*, p. 104.   [74] *Lancet* 105:2694 (17 April 1875), p. 541.
[75] *Lancet* 110:2815 (11 August 1877), p. 200.   [76] Worboys, *Spreading Germs*, pp. 161–4.

he was compelled to answer some objections to his theories based on the fact that they discounted such issues as diathesis (predisposition):

Mr. Lister said that it was one of the glories of antiseptic surgery that it set the patient so free from what were formerly known as the "surgical risks" of operation [...] that it was only in quite exceptional cases and conditions that the operator had to ask himself any question of the kind. The questions of diathesis were not so much neglected by the antiseptic surgeon; they were rather removed out of the way by the antiseptic method, and taken into another category.[77]

A good example of the broader impact of this shift away from the constitutional, the psychological, and the emotional in understandings of operative surgery can be found in the multi-volume *System of Surgery*, edited by Frederick Treves and published in 1895. One of the essays in this collection, as comprehensive an insight into British surgical thought at the turn of the twentieth century as can be found, was titled 'The Influence of Constitutional Conditions upon Injuries' and was written by Treves himself. For the most part, Treves' chapter is concerned with factors such as age, sex, weight, and so on. Nonetheless, there is one very brief section dedicated to 'Affections [*sic*] of the nervous system', in which Treves declares that the 'mental state of a healthy patient as expressed by the terms "nervous", "neurotic", "excitable", "apathetic", has little definite effect upon the result of an operation or injury'. Immediately below this, however, is a brief coda to the following effect: 'The least favourable frame of mind is that marked by gloom and utter apathy, and by a morbid, stoical indifference, difficult to dispose of'.[78] These two passages appear to contradict each other, and it might therefore be best to think of this coda as a vestigial, almost folkloric, relic of a previous emotional regime, one that no longer possessed a substantive ontological referent.

Needless to say, the disappearance of emotion, and of subjectivity more generally, from late nineteenth-century surgical ontology had its most profound impact on the patient, who, in marked contrast to the Romantic surgical era, no longer exercised a meaningful emotional agency, either within or without the operating theatre. But it also had significant and far-reaching implications for surgeons too. One of the most important of these concerned ideas of *responsibility*. As we saw in Chapter 2, Romantic surgical culture was steeped in a pathos that derived from the frequently tragic outcome of surgical intervention. While early nineteenth-century surgeons often gave expression to feelings of personal responsibility concerning operative failure, the sheer unpredictability of events meant that virtually nothing was guaranteed. As such, men like John Abernethy reassured their students that they could

---

[77] *British Medical Journal* 2:977 (20 September 1879), p. 454.
[78] Frederick Treves (ed.), *A System of Surgery*, vol. 1 (London: Cassell, 1895), p. 268.

not be blamed if a patient died due to circumstances outside of their control (which, beyond active incompetence, covered most things). As we saw in the previous chapter, the advent of anaesthesia relieved many of the emotional burdens on surgeons, and markedly reduced the frequency of intraoperative or immediate post-operative death. But the high mortality from post-operative infections that characterised (or was said to characterise) the 1850s and 1860s meant that, in this regard at least, the experience of post-anaesthetic surgeons was not so different from that of their pre-anaesthetic forebears. Thus, in his 1869 address, Thomas Nunneley appealed to chance in a way that would have been eminently recognisable to Abernethy and his contemporaries when he asserted that, beyond all the other constitutional variables involved, there was a 'general law affecting all' surgeons, namely that 'At one time, all his operations do well; he hardly loses a case, whatever the operation may be [...] while, at another time, precisely similar cases do as badly, so that even very trivial wounds and operations are followed by death'.[79] This concept of 'runs of luck' was often remarked upon by post-antiseptic surgeons reflecting on the past. Lister's house surgeon and close personal friend Hector Clare Cameron (1843–1928) told his audience:

In the absence of any certain knowledge of the real mode of causation of these wound-begotten diseases [...] the surgeon felt no real personal responsibility regarding them, whatever grief and disappointment he might experience when his best efforts repeatedly ended in disaster and failure. When his patients were decimated and his heart was well-nigh broken by those terrible visitants [...] he received the sympathy of his friends and pupils. He had done his work well, and a hail in harvest had come to destroy it. He was in no way to blame. He was a man beset by misfortune.[80]

However, by establishing an ontological framework within which the hitherto unpredictable occurrence of sepsis might be explained and, ultimately, prevented, Listerian antisepsis transformed notions of personal responsibility in surgery. This was no accident. It was, in fact, a central component of Listerian ideology. Thus, Leeson remembered attending to the dressing of an abscess on the surgical ward of the Edinburgh Royal Infirmary when Lister 'made a surprise visit, accompanied by two foreign professors'. Pausing at the foot of the bed, Lister allegedly explained to his guests 'in a most impressive voice' that '"If this gentlemen dares to let a single germ enter this wound he will be as culpable as though he took his scalpel and plunged it into the patient's carotid"'. 'It was not a light matter working under such responsibility', Leeson explained, 'but this was the spirit in which all the work was done;

[79] *British Medical Journal* 2:449 (7 August 1869), p. 156.
[80] Hector Clare Cameron, *Lord Lister, 1827–1912: An Oration* (Glasgow: James MacLehose and Son, 1914), pp. 12–13.

we knew that Lister relied upon us not to fail him'.[81] By making the surgeon what *The Lancet* called 'the custodian of the wound', antisepsis had ushered in a surgical modernity that promised ever greater control and perfection, but also demanded ever greater certainty and accountability.[82] In the second part of this chapter, we shall therefore consider the ways in which such factors shaped professional identities and laid the groundwork for the modern surgical ideal.

'One Cannot Consult with a Deity!' Emotions, Performance, and the Modern Surgeon

As a young man, the English poet William Ernest Henley (1849–1903) was blighted by ill-health and in 1868–9 was forced to spend nine months in St Bartholomew's Hospital, during which time his left leg was amputated below the knee. Shortly thereafter his right foot was similarly afflicted, and he spent some time at the Royal Sea-Bathing Hospital in Margate. The doctors there recommended amputation, but Henley declined, opting instead to make the long journey to Edinburgh to seek treatment under Joseph Lister.[83] During his two-year-long stay at the Edinburgh Royal Infirmary, Henley penned a number of poems, which first appeared in the *Cornhill Magazine* in 1875 and later as the collection *In Hospital* (1903). One of these poems, initially entitled 'A Surgeon' and subsequently retitled 'The Chief', is a portrait of Lister himself. As its final stanza reads: 'His wise, rare smile is sweet with certainties, / And seems in all his patients to compel / Such love and faith as failure cannot quell. / They hold him for another Herakles, / Warring with Custom, Prejudice, Disease, / As once the son of Zeus with Death and Hell'.[84] Lister's acolytes would quote Henley's poem routinely, to the point of ubiquity, as evidence of his compassionate character.[85] Meanwhile, subsequent historical research has suggested that as a patient, Henley was not alone in his positive estimation of Lister.[86] But what is notable about this poem is the relative emotional distance at which Lister resides from the narrator. Lister is a man who 'compels' 'love and faith' through his 'wise, rare smile' and his demeanour of certainty, but he

---

[81] Leeson, *Lister*, pp. 144–5; Claire Brock, 'Risk, Responsibility and Surgery in the 1890s and Early 1900s', *Medical History* 57:3 (2013), 317–37.

[82] *Lancet* 106:2725 (20 November 1875), p. 744. For a later reflection on this transformation, see Cameron, *Joseph Lister*, pp. 174–5.

[83] Ernest Mehew, 'Henley, William Ernest (1849–1903)', *ODNB*.

[84] *Cornhill Magazine* 32:187 (July 1875), pp. 124–5. Intriguingly, in the later version, the 'they' becomes 'we': William Ernest Henley, *In Hospital* (Portland: Thomas Mosher, 1903), p. 21.

[85] For example, see Godlee, *Lister*, pp. 160–1; RCSE, MS0021/1/15, St Clair Thomson, *Lister, 1827–1912: A House Surgeon's Memories* (1937), p. 28.

[86] For an account of Lister's relationships with his patients, see Mary Wilson Carpenter, 'Lister's Relationships with Patients: "A Successful Case"', *Notes and Records of the Royal Society* 67:3 (2003), 231–44.

is also a god-like hero, a largely unapproachable figure, engaged in intellectual and moral battles on a far higher plane.

As we have seen, Lister's system of antiseptic surgery, which, in various modified forms, was effectively axiomatic by the 1890s, had hugely significant implications for the role of emotions in surgical practice, notably in the conceptualisation of surgical disease and the management of surgical cases. Surgeons were no longer required, as they had been in the Romantic era, to effect an intersubjective engagement with their patients, to monitor their mood and watch for signs of despondency or dejection. Instead, all they had to do was follow Lister's system, keep the wound free of germs, and all would be well. But if emotions no longer possessed a meaningful surgical *function*, that does not mean that they disappeared from surgical culture altogether. Rather, as this section demonstrates, they underwent something of a transmutation, which originated with anaesthesia and was completed by antisepsis, from the highly wrought and profoundly intersubjective qualities of Romantic sensibility to the more performative, rhetorical, and detached cultures of scientific modernity. This does not mean that Romantic surgical emotions were not performative, for we have seen that they were and, as Reddy's concept of the emotive suggests, all forms of emotional expression are both outwardly directed and inwardly felt. Neither should 'detachment' necessarily be taken to suggest a cooling of emotional tone and tenor, for the rhetoric of Listerian surgery was often characterised by the highest forms of sentimentality. What is undoubtedly true, however, is that during the course of the later nineteenth century, the emotional identity of the British surgeon shifted from that of the man of feeling, fighting to save his individual patient from an unseen and largely unknowable enemy, to that of a heroic miracle worker whose achievements were emblematic of the triumphs of techno-scientific modernity.

Perhaps the best way of understanding this process of transmutation is to consider the emotional identity of Lister himself. Now, lest it appear that this chapter is advancing a 'great man' understanding of history that gives undue weight to the influence of an individual, it is important to clarify that Lister was not alone in exemplifying this change, nor was he singularly responsible for it. At the risk of indulging in counterfactuals, it seems entirely plausible, given the contemporaneous developments in later nineteenth-century European and North American medical science, that this shift would have happened even without him. And yet, Lister presents a particularly important and valuable case study for two reasons. Firstly, as we shall see, he is something of a transitional figure, who clearly demonstrates the shifts in surgical rhetoric, performance, and representation across the second half of the nineteenth century. Secondly, he attained a uniquely exalted position in the pantheon of late nineteenth-century surgery, not only in Britain but also abroad, meaning that his character and demeanour were readily translated into a broader professional ideal.

Joseph Lister was educated at University College London in the mid to late 1840s, the precise moment at which anaesthesia was first introduced. Indeed, he was present at Robert Liston's first operative use of ether on 21 December 1846, albeit as an arts student, as he did not begin his medical course until the winter of 1848.[87] Lister was therefore initiated into what was effectively a pre-anaesthetic surgical culture, one that had yet to fully absorb the practical and emotional implications of the shift from operative subject to operative object. That Lister owed much of his early influence to the crepuscular cultures of Romantic sensibility is powerfully evident in the first lecture he ever gave. This was an 1855 introduction to a course of surgery at Edinburgh, where Lister had moved two years earlier in order to work under James Syme.[88] As was common for introductory addresses in this period, this lecture sought to inculcate students in what were called surgical 'morals', namely the values and behaviour deemed appropriate to the office of surgeon. Lister's text, which survives in both draft and manuscript forms, is saturated with a language of love, something that was undoubtedly shaped by his Quaker upbringing.[89] Thus, he told his students that it would be a 'delightful reflection to any man of rightly constituted mind' that his studies would allow him to gain 'so much additional power of benefitting your fellow creatures' and help him to fulfil his 'grand duty to his fellow man, that of loving his neighbour as himself'. Lister represented surgical education as a divinely ordained process of transformation, stating that it was 'in the dissecting room that the medical student first discerns the spell which the holy object of our profession casts over all that is intimately connected with it, changing as if by enchantment things previously offensive and loathsome into objects of intense interest or even of affection'.[90] But what is perhaps most remarkable about this lecture was the ways in which it invoked the emotional cultures of Romantic surgery, even in its points of reference. Thus, despite the advent of anaesthesia nearly a decade earlier, Lister spoke as if that transformation had never taken place:

> if there be among you any who feel that they have warm, tender, and anxious hearts, and fear that they will never be able sufficiently to steel their breast against the 'dint of pity', wilfully to inflict pain on man, woman and child, and perform the most torturing operations, deaf to the tears, groans and entreaties of their patients, to such I would say

[87] Lister, *Papers*, vol. 2, p. 491; Godlee, *Lister*, pp. 15–18; Lawrence, 'Lister'.
[88] See Godlee, *Lister*, p. 43.
[89] Lister was raised a Quaker, but left the Society of Friends on his marriage to Syme's daughter, Agnes, in 1856. He later joined the Episcopalian Church.
[90] RCSE, MS0021/4/1/2 [folder 13], Draft and manuscript of Lister's introductory lecture to new students at his surgery lectures at Edinburgh University, 1855, manuscript, pp. 1–2.

be not at all discouraged. It is indeed a very prevalent notion [among the public] that a good surgeon must necessarily be hard hearted, callous and indifferent to the welfare of his patients; but there cannot possibly be a greater mistake.[91]

In support of these claims about the affinity between surgery and emotional sensitivity, Lister gave the example of the early eighteenth-century surgeon William Cheselden, who felt 'sickness and moral anxiety' in advance of an operation, as well as that of the recently deceased Liston who, despite being 'renowned over the whole world as a bold and most skilful operator', once declared "'I wish to God I might never touch the knife again"; so anxious had he been made by a Case in private practice'.[92] As Lister concluded: 'Be assured Gentlemen, that it is for the better for you to possess a somewhat over sensitive and over anxious temperament than the contrary; and that you are rather called upon to foster rather than to repress the generous and refined feelings of your nature'.[93]

Such emotional elements would continue to feature in Lister's lectures in the early 1860s, although by that time they would occupy significantly less space. For example, his introductory lecture to the medical students of Glasgow, delivered on 1 November 1864, was more concerned with such matters as 'the vitality of cells', 'inflammation', and the 'classification of surgical diseases' than with surgical morals. And yet, at the very end, he assured them, in terms reminiscent of his earlier talk, that:

I would not have any gentlemen to think himself too tender-hearted or too loving in his disposition. It is only the general public who suppose that cruelty is essential to a surgeon: the truth is that the more feeling and love for his fellow creatures he has, the better it will be.[94]

By the late 1860s, however, the emotional dimensions of surgery had completely disappeared from his lectures, which were now dominated by the scientific theory and technical application of antisepsis. This was the case with his first talk as Professor of Clinical Surgery at Edinburgh in 1869, which was entirely concerned with the management of wounds.[95] Nor would these emotional or moral elements ever reappear in his public presentations. On opening

---

[91] RCSE, MS0021/4/1/2, manuscript, p. 15. The text in square brackets was inserted above the original wording, suggesting that Lister was keen to clarify that this was a public misapprehension, not a professional ideal.

[92] RCSE, MS0021/4/1/2, manuscript, p. 15.

[93] RCSE, MS0021/4/1/2, manuscript, pp. 16–17.

[94] RCSE, MS0021/4/1/9, Volume containing notes of lectures on surgery delivered by Lister at Glasgow University 1–21 November 1864, p. 8.

[95] RCSE, MS0021/4/1/10, Published copy of the Introductory Lecture given by Lister to students at the University of Edinburgh, 8 November 1869 [Folder 36]. One of Lister's students estimated that he spent 75 per cent of his teaching time on the topic of dressings: Crowther and Dupree, *Medical Lives*, p. 105.

his inaugural lecture to the staff and students of King's College London in October 1877, Lister suggested that he had two options. The first was 'to convey to the student some of the exalted privileges and correspondingly high responsibilities of the beneficent calling to which he proposes to devote himself'. The second was 'to treat of some special subject, in the hope that I might say something which may have interest [and] instruction'. Tellingly, he announced that the 'latter is the course which I have decided to follow', and he spent the rest of the lecture, as we have heard, talking about the fermentation of milk, much to the confusion of his audience.[96]

Such developments may provide only a crude measure of Lister's personal emotional disposition. Nonetheless, they tell us a great deal about the relative value that he ascribed to the emotional dimensions of surgery over the course of his career and, as such, they provide a useful way to track the ideological shift from one emotional regime to another. We can, moreover, gain a greater insight into Lister's emotional identity from his private correspondence. In 1853, shortly after arriving in Edinburgh, he wrote:

> If the love of surgery is a proof of a person's being adapted for it, then certainly I am fitted to be a surgeon: for thou canst hardly conceive what a high degree of enjoyment I am from day to day experiencing in this bloody and butcherly department of the healing art. I am more and more delighted with my profession, and sometimes almost question whether it is possible such a delightful pursuit can continue. My only wonder is that persons who really love Surgery for its own sake are rare.[97]

What is striking about this statement is how markedly it contrasts with the sentiments of Romantic surgeons like Henry Robert Oswald, John Abernethy, or Charles Bell. As we saw in Chapter 2, these men often reflected on the intense anxiety engendered by the practice of operative surgery, and on the profound misery occasioned by their frequent exposure to the sufferings and deaths of their patients.[98] Lister, on the other hand, expresses nothing but joy at his experiences and marvels that more people do not share his love of surgery. No doubt this change in tone owed a great deal to the introduction of anaesthesia, and the reduction of pain and distress that it brought about. It would also be unreasonable to judge Lister's emotional disposition from such statements alone, not least because this letter coincides with the period of his career when he was still deploying the cultural tropes of Romantic sensibility. Nonetheless, it is clear that, in terms of his personal reflection on

---

[96] RCSE, MS0021/4/2/2 [folder 53], Address delivered by Lord Lister at the opening of the Medical Session of 1877 at King's College, Strand, 1 October 1877, p. 2.
[97] Godlee, *Lister*, p. 35.
[98] See also Michael Brown, 'Wounds and Wonder: Emotion, Imagination and War in the Cultures of Romantic Surgery', *Journal for Eighteenth Century Studies* 43:2 (2020), 239–59.

the surgeon's art, his sentiments lack the agonised introspection that was so characteristic of his pre-anaesthetic forebears.

This is not to say that emotions do not feature in Lister's private papers or his publications, because they do. He did write to his father about the anxiety he felt during an operation, though this feeling was swiftly eclipsed by 'a greater thrill of surgical joy than I ever before experienced'.[99] In his early work on antisepsis, he also wrote about the 'sickening and often heartrending' experience of losing his patients to post-operative infection.[100] Moreover, much of Lister's correspondence is underwritten by a religious faith, which, as in his first lecture, was expressed in terms of a love for humanity. Thus, in March 1857, he told his sister that 'I trust I may be enabled in the treatment of patients always to act with a single eye to their good, and therefore to the glory of our Heavenly Father'. 'If a man is able to act in this spirit', he continued, 'and is favoured to feel something of the sustaining love of God in his work, truly the practice of surgery is a glorious occupation'.[101]

Lister was, furthermore, widely noted for the tenderness and care that he displayed towards his patients. As Leeson recalled of his first impressions of the man, 'I had never witnessed such personal care bestowed upon a case, nor ever remember a surgeon who seemed to be working under such a sense of anxious responsibility over a dressing'. In fact, he described Lister's care as 'almost womanly'.[102] Leeson, like Henley, also remembered Lister's 'sweet and assuring smile', which, he claimed, cast everything else about him 'into shadow'. 'It went to the patient's heart and nerved him with strength', he rhapsodised; 'It flooded his mind with confidence and hope; he felt that his was no mere "case" but the supreme concern of a friend as well as of a supreme healer'.[103] As to the patients themselves, Leeson maintained that '[t]heir confidence in him was absolute and their reverence boundless'.[104]

Leeson's comments are fulsome in the extreme, but they are mirrored by other accounts, such as that of St Clair Thomson (1859–1943), who was Lister's house surgeon at King's College Hospital in the 1880s. Like Leeson, he remembered Lister's 'great gentleness and sympathy' with even the 'humblest or roughest of his hospital patients'. Like Leeson, he also remarked upon Lister's tendency to refer to his patients in 'such kindly terms as "this poor fellow", or "this good woman" or "this little chap"'.[105] There is, moreover, ample evidence of Lister using such terms in his correspondence. For example, in a letter he sent in February 1891 to Lionel Vernon Cargill (1866–1955), another of his house surgeons at King's, he wrote:

[99] Godlee, *Lister*, p. 98.   [100] Lister, *Papers*, vol. 2, p. 124.   [101] Godlee, *Lister*, p. 62.
[102] Leeson, *Lister*, pp. 19, 120.   [103] Leeson, *Lister*, pp. 51, 86.   [104] Leeson, *Lister*, p. 159.
[105] RCSE, MS0021/1/15, p. 25; Leeson, *Lister*, pp. 63, 67–8, 103.

I have to go out today, and cannot visit the Hospital. It seems a pity the poor woman with erysipelas should not have the benefit of the [iodine trichloride] if it really is of use to her. Accordingly I send by the bearer a bottle of 1:20 carb[olic] solution, which is that which I used before.[106]

Likewise, in another letter to Cargill, possibly about the same case, Lister wrote: 'Poor woman, she was the victim of a series of unhappy circumstances. The very fact of our having special means, young and not so much explained, to look after her, prevented perhaps the due care in guarding against bed sore'.[107]

Ostensibly, then, Lister might appear to be a man of emotional sensitivity and compassion, very much in the mould of his Romantic forebears. But what comes across from his writings and, in particular, his ubiquitous use of the phrase 'this poor man' or 'this poor woman' is less a sense of deep emotional communion than a rigid formalism, a kind of paternalistic politesse in which the rhetoric of care takes precedence over a substantive intersubjectivity. This is not to imply that Lister did not care for his patients, or that he was not, in a norma-tive, clinical way, *kind* to them. Nor is it to suggest that all Romantic surgeons were, in practice, the men of feeling that authors like John Bell maintained they should be. But it is notable that, even for the most generous observers like Leeson, the principal manifestations of Lister's care were a concern over the state of his patients' dressings (the centrepiece of his antiseptic system) and a customarily polite form of address. Again, this does not mean that Lister did not listen to his patients, because their testimony suggests that he did.[108] But when one looks for the *substance* of Lister's emotional engagement with those under his care, at least within the sources available to us, one is apt to come up short.

And yet, at the same time, it is remarkable to what extent the *myth* of Lister, shaped as it was by the hagiographic accounts of men like Godlee, Leeson, Cheyne, and Thomson, was underpinned by a rhetoric of emotion. Leeson's book in particular is characterised by a lavish language of sentiment, which adorns virtually every other page. So powerful was this apparent desire to pres-ent Lister as a man of deep feeling that some authors chose to read emotions onto him, even when there was no evidence for them. This is particularly true of Godlee's canonical biography, published in 1917, five years after Lister's death. For instance, in relation to Lister's early exposure to the 'sad calling' of surgery in the sepsis-ridden wards of University College Hospital, Godlee remarks:

Amidst such surroundings Lister had his first introduction to surgery, and its sadder side made a deep impression upon him. But there is little or no reference to this in his letters. Medical students have not much time, as a rule, for letter-writing, and are not apt to indulge in moralizing.[109]

[106] RCSE, MS0021/1/2/4, Cargill, Lionel Vernon, Lister to Cargill, 12 February 1891.
[107] RCSE, MS0021/1/2/4, Lister to Cargill, 20 April 1891.
[108] Carpenter, 'Lister's Relationships'.   [109] Godlee, *Lister*, p. 20.

Likewise, in relation to the loss of Lister's patients from post-operative infection in the years immediately prior to his development of the antiseptic system, Godlee writes:

But, so far, his correspondence contains hardly one reference to this gloomy subject. This can only be explained by supposing that he looked upon it as the common lot, and did not allow himself to be so much depressed by it as to lose interest in the improvement of the science to which he had devoted his life. Possibly he did not like to burden his father with accounts of the melancholy side of what he was constantly holding up as the noblest and happiest of callings.[110]

Another striking aspect of the mythic portrayal of Lister is the way in which emotions are presented as perhaps the *primary* motivation for his development of the antiseptic system. Like Godlee, Leeson asserts that Lister's first encounters with post-operative sepsis made a profound impact on him. He even claims that the very mention of the words 'hospital gangrene' would induce Lister's head to fall and his speech to falter 'under the emotion that its memory evoked'.[111] However, whereas Godlee's biography states that this 'dismal aspect of surgery' was forced 'into the background' by 'the interest of the work', Leeson maintains that it 'orientated his life', for he was 'so distressed [...] by its ravages that it kindled that fire to unravel these mysteries which burnt henceforth on the altar of his heart'.[112] Indeed, Leeson repeatedly suggests that this 'overwhelming sense of responsibility [...] took its full toll of anxiety and care, and clothed him with a garment of sadness which he seldom seemed able to discard'.[113]

Such hagiographic narratives also tend to instrumentalise emotions. In almost all the Whiggish historical accounts written by his acolytes in the early twentieth century, the positive emotions of sympathy and compassion are arraigned on the side of Lister and his associates, while their opponents are represented as blinkered, officious, and cold-hearted. This is particularly conspicuous with regard to the opposition that Lister encountered on his arrival at King's College London. We have already heard about the scepticism with which his inaugural lecture was received, and this response was also characteristic of those charged with implementing his system, namely the nursing staff. In his biography, Godlee quotes extensively from Lister's former student, John Stewart (1848–1933), on this point. Stewart recalled the case of a young boy with osteomyelitis of the femur whose removal from the ward to the operating theatre was checked by the sister, who stated that patients could not be moved without a permit from the Hospital Secretary. Stewart proceeded, in defiance of both official protocol and the 'menacing' demeanour of the nurses,

110 Godlee, *Lister*, p. 124. 111 Leeson, *Lister*, p. 41.
112 Godlee, *Lister*, p. 20; Leeson, *Lister*, p. 31. 113 Leeson, *Lister*, pp. 58–60.

to 'wrap the unconscious boy in his bed-clothes' and take him to his surgery. 'To us coming from the Royal infirmary [of Edinburgh] with its simple, kindly, common sense routine, in which the patients' welfare and comfort were the first consideration, this cold machine-like system was intolerable', Stewart reflected.[114] Godlee, meanwhile, perceived the insidious implications of such resistance:

This lack of sympathy and absence of enthusiasm amongst the sisters were unheard of in Lister's previous experience. He could hardly believe such a state of mind to be possible. It created an unpleasant atmosphere in the wards. But it did more. The success of his new treatment depended largely on the local assistance of the nursing staff in carrying out details which it was almost impossible for him personally to supervise. Their indifference or veiled opposition was therefore a source of real danger to his patients.[115]

Such accounts beg the question of why Lister and his antiseptic system were so frequently configured in emotive terms. In answering this question, it is important to note that such framing was not simply the product of early twentieth-century retrospection. Rather, the groundwork for this mythos was laid in the later nineteenth century, including by Lister himself.[116] And indeed, the impetus behind these highly emotionalised representations derived from a set of circumstances that straddled both the late nineteenth and early twentieth centuries and concerned the wider social and cultural identity of medicine and surgery in late Victorian and Edwardian Britain.

The shift away from a holistic and constitutional understanding of disease towards the laboratory-based microbiological and biochemical approaches of modern medicine and surgery had not gone unnoticed by the public. As early as 1879, the *British Medical Journal* noted:

In more than one place lately, outside critics have discussed the bearing and manner of physicians towards their patients, and have developed a somewhat unexpected thesis. Medical men of the present day, we are told [...], are too apt to assume an abrupt and cold manner, and to treat their patients rather as impersonal elements in a scientific problem, than as individuals whose feelings and conditions are all-important to themselves.[117]

The *Journal* vigorously refuted the accusation that modern medical practitioners displayed a 'tendency either to hardness, coldness or severity of demeanour', as well as the claim that they dealt with their patients as

---

[114] Godlee, *Lister*, pp. 409–10.
[115] Godlee, *Lister*, p. 412. On the relationship of nursing staff to antiseptic practice, see Claire L. Jones, Marguerite Dupree, Iain Hutchison, Susan Gardiner, and Anne Marie Rafferty, 'Personalities, Preferences and Practicalities: Educating Nurses in Wound Sepsis in the British Hospital, 1870–1920', *Social History of Medicine* 31:3 (2018), 577–604.
[116] For example, see his defence of his 'enthusiasm' for antisepsis: *Lancet* 114:2336 (6 December 1879), p. 854.
[117] *British Medical Journal* 2:980 (11 October 1879), p. 583.

'pathological specimens, rather than as human beings self-contained and differentiated by their moral and mental conditions no less than their physical suffering'.[118] Nonetheless, the charge was a serious one and it stuck as closely to surgeons as to physicians.

Neither were such concerns solely restricted to the general public. In 1895, Lister's colleague at King's College Hospital, the physician Isaac Burney Yeo (1835–1914), penned an essay for the influential monthly periodical *The Nineteenth Century* in which he claimed that increased specialisation and a narrowing of the clinical gaze had a negative impact on the patient–practitioner relationship. When a practitioner has 'the care of the whole complex organisation of his patient', Yeo maintained, 'he feels an interest in his charge altogether different from that experienced by the man who looks after a small portion of it only'. 'It is impossible', he alleged, 'to feel the same kind of interest in such a fractional part of the patient as in the whole man' and he was 'convinced that this modern tendency to extreme specialisation detracts from the wholesome and legitimate influence which the profession of medicine should exercise on society'. Compared to the healers of old, he concluded, the modern physician and surgeon were looked upon as 'more mercenary and less disinterested than they were wont to be'.[119]

Such suggestions of clinical coldness and self-interest were only the most moderate manifestation of a contemporary anxiety about medical and surgical science, which, at its more extreme end, could lead to far more damaging accusations of medical immorality. The advent of anaesthesia and antisepsis may have allowed the surgeon to reach hitherto unimaginable heights of public approbation, and even to trump the physician in the imagined hierarchy of medicine's 'golden age', but the last quarter of the nineteenth century also saw the emergence of perhaps the most powerful and coordinated opposition movement that medicine and surgery had yet faced. This opposition was all the more significant for Lister and his followers, in that it centred on several related issues in which he was deeply implicated.

The first, and most important, of these issues was vivisection. Lister was a vocal proponent of physiological experiments on living animals and was an active member of the Association for the Advancement of Medicine by Research (AAMR), founded in 1882.[120] As Rob Boddice has demonstrated, debates around vivisection in this period were framed by contested understandings and representations of emotion. Opponents of vivisection presented

---

[118] *British Medical Journal* 2:980 (11 October 1879), p. 583.
[119] J. [*sic*] Burney Yeo, 'Medicine and Society', *Nineteenth Century* 38:226 (December 1895), 1025–40, at pp. 1026–7.
[120] Rob Boddice, *The Humane Professions: The Defence of Experimental Medicine, 1876–1914* (Cambridge, UK: Cambridge University Press, 2020), pp. 42–3.

it as a cruel, barbaric act that brutalised those who practised it. Meanwhile, supporters of physiological research sought to discriminate between the alleged sentimentalism of their adversaries, focused as it was on the sufferings of the individual animal, and the higher emotional object of their own endeavours, namely the good of humankind.[121] Lister's interventions into this debate conformed precisely with this latter approach. In 1875, Queen Victoria (1819–1901) wrote to Lister requesting that he make a public statement opposing vivisection in advance of a Royal Commission on the issue. Lister politely declined, explaining his reasons for doing so. He contrasted vivisection with the hunting of animals, stating that the former was 'justified by far nobler and higher objects', namely 'devising [the] means [...] for procuring the health of mankind, the greatest of earthly blessings, and prolonging of human life'. Countering the charge of cruelty levelled at men like himself, he suggested that 'the term cruelty seems to me altogether misapplied in the discussion of this question. An act is cruel or otherwise, not according to the pain which it involves, but according to the mind and object of the actor'. Unlike the huntsman, the vivisector did not relish the immediate consequences of his actions. Rather, he performed experiments 'at great sacrifice to his own feelings and with every care to render the pain as slight as is compatible with the high object in view'.[122]

The emotional politics of vivisection were shaped by the fact that many of its leading opponents, including Frances Power Cobbe (1822–1904), were women. Many of these individuals, Cobbe included, were also prominent members of the late nineteenth-century women's movement, which sought greater rights and freedoms for women, including the right to vote and the freedom to pursue the career of their choice.[123] One of the key issues that galvanised the early women's movement in Britain was the passage of the Contagious Diseases Acts (CDAs) between 1864 and 1869. These Acts infamously sought to reduce the incidence of venereal disease among members of the armed forces by allowing suspected sex workers to be forcibly detained, subject to medical examination, and potentially confined to a lock hospital. For many first-wave feminists there was an intrinsic connection between violence towards women (both in general and in the specific context of sexual exploitation) and cruelty towards animals, given that both groups nominally

---

[121] Rob Boddice, *The Science of Sympathy: Morality, Evolution and Victorian Civilization* (Urbana: University of Illinois Press, 2016), chs. 3 and 4; Boddice, *Humane Professions*.

[122] Godlee, *Lister*, pp. 377–80.

[123] Carol Lansbury, *The Old Brown Dog: Women, Workers, and Vivisection in Edwardian England* (Madison: University of Wisconsin Press, 1985); Diana Donald, *Women against Cruelty: Protection of Animals in Nineteenth-Century Britain* (Manchester: Manchester University Press, 2019), ch. 5.

came under the social and legal 'protection' of men. Furthermore, both involved the exercise of a state-sanctioned medical authority.[124] Lister was not as outspoken on the CDAs as he was on the issue of vivisection, but he was certainly supportive of them; as late as 1897, more than a decade after their repeal, he aroused some disquiet in the House of Lords when he stated that 'he had no objection in principle to the Contagious Diseases Act; that he thought it a most beneficent Act and that he hoped, at no distant time, to see it re-enforced in this country'.[125] Lister was, moreover, no friend to the wider women's movement and vigorously opposed female entry into the medical profession. Not only did he ban women from his own classes, but in 1878 he even pressured the BMA to redraft its constitution to exclude women and demanded that it expel its two existing female members, Elizabeth Garrett Anderson (1836–1917) and Frances Hoggan (1843–1927).[126]

By the early twentieth century, Lister's strident opposition to female medical graduates was something of an embarrassment and was generally dismissed, fudged, or ignored altogether. Godlee mentions it in the most fleeting manner imaginable, while Leeson inaccurately claims that Lister was 'mildly inclined' to grant women the right to practise medicine and maintains he was 'not aware that [Lister] took any part in the matter'.[127] In the late nineteenth century, however, the combined issues of vivisection and women's rights made for a potent challenge to surgical authority. This is perhaps most clearly exemplified by Cobbe's influential 1881 *Monthly Review* article 'The Medical Profession and Its Morality'. Herein, Cobbe addresses the medical profession's treatment of women and animals, claiming that their involvement with the CDAs derived from their 'gross materialism' and 'utter disregard for human souls when lodged in the bodies of the despised and wretched'. Long after these Acts were repealed, she argued, 'the memory of them will make the hearts of all women burn with indignation against the profession'.[128]

Cobbe had a specific political agenda, of course, but she situated this agenda within a broader critique of medical science and emotional authenticity that, as the editorial commentary on her article suggests, tapped into wider anxieties.[129] It was, she claimed, the 'misfortune of the Medical profession that the performance of its ordinary duties involves the *appearance of human feelings*, which may or may not be present [...], but which the patient and his

[124] Anne L. Scott, 'Physical Purity Feminism and State Medicine in Late Nineteenth-Century England', *Women's History Review* 8:4 (1999), 625–53.
[125] Godlee, *Lister*, p. 545.   [126] Crowther and Dupree, *Medical Lives*, pp. 152–4.
[127] Godlee, *Lister*, p. 476; Leeson, *Lister*, pp. 174–5.
[128] [Frances Power Cobbe], 'The Medical Profession and Its Morality', *Modern Review* (April 1881), 296–328, at pp. 321–22.
[129] [Cobbe], 'Medical Profession', p. 326.

friends will usually expect to see exhibited, and the doctor be almost *driven to simulate*.[130] The apparent 'kindness' of the profession was, she maintained, illusory: 'a patient is to a doctor what a rock is to a geologist, or a flower to a botanist – the much coveted *subject of his studies*':

The impression may be false, and is necessarily vague, but it is extremely strong and widespread that the primary beneficent object of the profession, its only ostensible object – namely, Healing, – is daily more and more subordinated to the secondary object, namely Scientific Investigation; in short, that the means have become the end, and the end the means.[131]

Cobbe's comments reflect her intense distrust of the medical profession, a distrust that derived from her identity as a feminist and anti-vivisectionist. But her critique was not an isolated one and clearly resonates with George Bernard Shaw's (1856–1950) later excoriation of medical morality, contained in his famous 1909 'Preface on Doctors' to *The Doctor's Dilemma* (1906).[132] Such criticisms presented modern medical and surgical science as self-interested, cruel, and remote from the patient, concerned only with narrow technical detail. And they provide an essential context for understanding why Lister's early twentieth-century biographers sought to present him and, by association, modern scientific surgery in such profusely sentimental terms. Take, for example, the following episode recounted by Leeson. This was what he called the 'delightful doll story', which supposedly took place on Lister's wards in Glasgow. A 'little girl' was suffering from an abscess of the knee, which Lister proceeded to dress:

When all was finished she produced her doll which had lost a leg; a fumble under her pillow brought out the limb, and holding dolly in one hand and the leg in the other, gravely handed them to Lister. With seriousness and concern he received the case, shook his head ominously, for it was very serious, fitted them together, asked for a needle and cotton, and carefully and securely stitched on the limb, and with quiet delight handed her back to her mother. Her large brown eyes spoke endless gratitude but neither uttered a word.[133]

This story is accompanied by an illustration (Figure 6.1), presumably commissioned for the occasion. It is historically inaccurate, for the surgeon in the foreground is shown holding a carbolic acid sprayer, which Lister did not invent until after he had left Glasgow. But accuracy is not the point here. Like the story itself, it is a highly sentimentalised allegory about Lister's loving care for the most vulnerable, and about the essential humanity behind the austere

[130] Cobbe], 'Medical Profession', p. 302, Emphasis added.
[131] [Cobbe], 'Medical Profession', pp. 302, 310. Emphasis in original.
[132] George Bernard Shaw, *The Doctor's Dilemma, Getting Married, and The Shewing-up of Blanco Posnet* (London: Constable, 1921), pp. xiii–xciv.
[133] Leeson, *Lister*, p. 160.

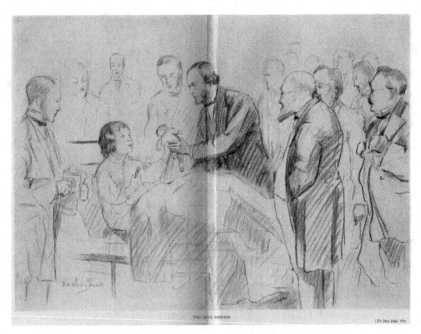

Figure 6.1 'The Doll Episode' from J. R. Leeson, *Lister as I Knew Him* (1927). Author's photograph.

façade of scientific surgery. Indeed, in contrast to the story, the illustration dispenses with the figure of the mother, emphasising the direct emotional connection between Lister and the girl, while the juxtaposition of the carbolic acid sprayer and the tender exchange between the two suggests a congruity between the technical dimensions and emotional implications of antiseptic surgery. But what is also interesting about this image is that it includes a large audience to witness the 'delightful' scene. Lister's compassion is, then, a performance, a rhetorical device with which to counter accusations of cruelty, self-interest, and narrow technical specialism.

In this sense, 'The Doll Episode' is reminiscent of that most iconic representation of late nineteenth-century medical humanitarianism, Luke Fildes' *The Doctor* (1891) (Figure 6.2). As Barry Milligan has shown, Fildes' work, which depicts a doctor anxiously watching over a sick young girl in the cottage of a poor family, was only the most successful of a raft of late nineteenth-century genre paintings that combined the medical and the domestic.[134] Fildes' image was unusual, however, in focusing so squarely on the figure of the doctor. As

[134] Barry Milligan, 'Luke Fildes' *The Doctor*, Narrative Painting, and the Selfless Professional Ideal', *Victorian Literature and Culture* 44:3 (2016), 641–68, at pp. 642–54.

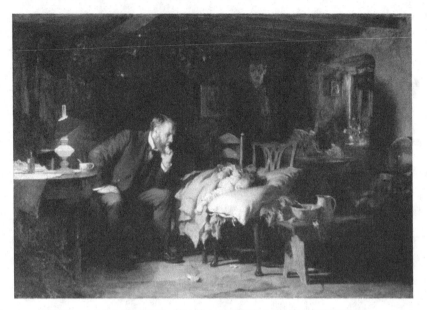

Figure 6.2 Luke Fildes, *The Doctor* (1891). Item No. N01522. Tate.

Fildes himself remarked, 'He should be *the* actor in the little drama I had conceived – father, mother, child should only help to show *him* to better advantage'.[135] As with 'The Doll Episode', here the child's parents (and even the
child herself) serve merely as witnesses to professional compassion and self-
lessness. Moreover, as a number of commentators have pointed out, by focusing on the supposedly timeless relationship between doctor and patient, Fildes'
painting presented a vision of professional practice that was, in many ways,
antithetical to the reality of modern medicine.[136] Indeed, in the United States,
The Doctor functioned for many decades as a palatably homely means to assert
the moral value of an individualised, free-market form of healthcare in the face
of more bureaucratic and statist models.[137] Within the context of late nine-
teenth- and early twentieth-century Britain, however, it represented an attempt
to reconcile the triumphs of techno-scientific medical modernity with popular
sentimentalism and established notions of care.

Such considerations bring us back to where we began with William Henley,
for if these attempts to meet accusations of medical and surgical immorality

---

[135] Quoted in Milligan, '*The Doctor*', p. 655. Emphasis in original.
[136] Milligan, '*The Doctor*', pp. 656–7.
[137] John Harley Warner, 'The Aesthetic Grounding of Modern Medicine', *Bulletin of the History
of Medicine* 88:1 (2014), 1–47, at pp. 32–45.

presented the practitioner as compassionate, they also served to elevate him to a level of heroism that rendered him remote. This was certainly the case for Lister who, as even his supporters averred, was an emotionally distant figure. Though possessed of a 'scrupulous politeness' there was, Leeson claimed, 'an atmosphere of indescribable distance which enveloped Lister' that 'forbade familiar approach and which neither time could bridge nor custom abate'.[138] Lister always referred to his dressers as 'Mr', rather than by their surname alone, was not easy in company, and, as Leeson recalled, if he had friends 'we never saw them'.[139] Thomson concurred in this estimation. 'His manner had a certain aloofness in it', which 'encouraged no familiarity'. 'I, myself, always felt that his soul "was like a star and dwelt apart"', he wrote.[140]

This remoteness underpinned Lister's heroic identity, presenting the image of a man who operated on a different plane to the rest of humanity. Cheyne reached for a medieval analogy, writing: 'I like to think of Lister, with his courtly manners and indomitable courage, as one of the knights of olden times sallying out single-handed to find and destroy a formidable enemy'.[141] But for most of his acolytes, Lister was more than this: he was a saint or, more accurately, a god. As has been argued elsewhere, despite the ostensibly secularising tendencies of modernity, late nineteenth-century surgical heroism was often couched in religious terms, with the achievements of modern techno-scientific surgery presented as a miraculous salvation from suffering.[142] In this sense, the deification of Lister was in keeping with broader cultural currents. Nevertheless, as the man often referred to as the 'father' of modern, scientific surgery, he was, perhaps, its ultimate expression.[143] Leeson, for example, marked out Lister's very birth as a near-divine deliverance from 'the pestilence that walketh in darkness' and claimed that just as 'Jesus never wrote a line [...] no text-book or treatise upon antiseptic appeared from Lister's pen'. Instead, the task of spreading Lister's 'gospel' fell to his 'disciples'.[144] And yet, although a class apart, readily identified by their hands, roughened and coarsened by the effects of carbolic acid, theirs was a drone-like existence compared to their master, for, as a patient once remarked, '"When the Professor [Lister] enters the wards I feel as though God Almighty Himself has come in"'.[145]

[138] Leeson, *Lister*, pp. 51, 60. [139] Leeson, *Lister*, pp. 61, 142.
[140] RCSE, MS0021/1/15, pp. 22, 23. [141] Cheyne, *Lister*, p. 13.
[142] Christopher Lawrence and Michael Brown, 'Quintessentially Modern Heroes: Surgeons, Explorers, and Empire, c.1840–1914', *Journal of Social History* 50:1 (2016), 148–78, at pp. 169–70.
[143] For example, see Rhoda Traux, *Joseph Lister: The Father of Modern Surgery* (New York: Bobbs-Merrill, 1944).
[144] Leeson, *Lister*, pp. 99, 183, 190, 196. St Clair Thomson referred to Lister's 'evangel': RCSE, MS0021/1/15, p. 19.
[145] Leeson, *Lister*, pp. 50, 54–5.

Historians and medical ethicists alike have often sought to locate the origins of modern 'clinical detachment' in the writings of the Canadian physician William Osler (1849–1919), notably his 1889 address to the medical students of the University of Pennsylvania on 'Aequanimitas'.[146] This speech, in which he advocates the values of emotional self-control, of equanimity and imperturbability, in clinical practice, is perhaps more complex than the 'conscious callousness' it has sometimes been taken for, as Osler was careful to warn against 'hardening "the human heart by which we live"'.[147] Nonetheless, it is remarkable for the ways in which Osler sought to inject a self-conscious, scientific objectivity into the psychic management of the patient.[148] However, when it comes to the emotional disposition, and cultural identity, of the *surgeon*, a strong case can be made for Joseph Lister providing the blueprint for the modern professional ideal. Lister was the epitome of the emotional regime of scientific surgical modernity with whose legacy we continue to grapple. He was a man who, while effectively denuding emotional intersubjectivity of clinical meaning, reconfigured that emotion into the professional performance of a compassionate and selfless dedication to a higher calling. In this sense, he might be called 'emotionally detached'. But he was also detached in the sense of being set apart from his patients. Unlike Romantic surgeons, whose failures made them all too human, the achievements of antiseptic surgery rendered Lister virtually unimpeachable, in the eyes of his patients as much as his hagiographers. And in so doing, it set the template for the modern surgeon as a god among (wo)men, one whose authority, for good or ill, brooks no argument. After all, as Leeson put it: 'One cannot consult with a deity!'[149]

Conclusion

The deification of Lister and the celebration of modern techno-scientific surgery were, as we have seen, frequently couched in terms of human salvation. While appeals had long been made to medicine and surgery's 'benefit to mankind', such claims were, at least prior to the second quarter of the nineteenth century, largely figurative or symbolic. By the last quarter of the nineteenth century, on the other hand, the notion of surgery's social utility was increasingly conceived of as substantive. At one level, this is because it was now statistically demonstrable. But just as importantly, it was because the object of care was no longer simply an amorphous humanity but was increasingly figured as being co-extensive with a discrete bio-political entity in the form of the imperial nation state. As we saw

[146] Jodi Halpern, *From Detached Concern to Empathy: Humanizing Medical Practice* (Oxford: Oxford University Press, 2001), pp. 22–5; Boddice, *Science of Sympathy*, pp. 49–50.
[147] Boddice, *Humane Professions*, p. 3; William Osler, *Aequanimitas: With Other Addresses to Medical Students, Nurses and Practitioners of Medicine* (London: H. K. Lewis, 1904), p. 5.
[148] Halpern, *Detached Concern*, p. 23.   [149] Leeson, *Lister*, p. 65.

in Chapter 5, promoters of the Anatomy Act often made a connection between surgery and war as equivalent forms of national service and, from the 1830s onwards, war and imperial conquest would become perhaps the dominant conceptual framework through which the medical profession conceived of its relationship with the state.[150] These tendencies would only intensify in the latter decades of the nineteenth century when, as the focus of surgical emotion moved from the individual patient to the collective social good, that good was conceived in increasingly nationalistic, imperialistic, and militaristic terms.[151]

In 1898, an elderly Lister returned to Edinburgh in order to accept the freedom of that city. Also there to collect his honour was Sir Garnet Wolseley (1833–1913), the celebrated imperial officer and Commander-in-Chief of the British Army. In his speech, Lister drew an association between their two different forms of heroism:

> The work of a general of the very highest rank, like Lord Wolseley, has certain analogies to that of the ideal surgeon. For the cure of ills in the body-politic he performs operations – bloody, painful, dangerous. But he executes his task with the least possible expenditure of human life and of human suffering, and he addresses himself to his work in the spirit of self-denying, of self-sacrificing devotion.[152]

There was a certain irony in this juxtaposition, given both Lister's pacifist upbringing and Wolseley's general contempt for doctors.[153] But if Lister was only an uncertain exemplar of this trend (he was, after all, the only one of seven resident surgeons at Edinburgh who did *not* volunteer to serve in the Crimea), then many of his colleagues demonstrated a far closer affinity for the military-imperial project of late Victorian and Edwardian Britain.[154] Such values were inculcated in the student through introductory lectures that, as the century wore on, became increasingly bellicose in tone, and drew ever closer links between Britain's perceived imperial glories and what the Orientalist poet Edwin Arnold (1832–1904), speaking to the students of St Thomas' in 1895, called 'a march of constantly augmenting conquests, over that strange fascinating waste of twilight and wondering exploration which is called "science"'.[155] Others signalled their active investment by volunteering for military service. Alexander Ogston, for example, served in three military campaigns, namely the Suakin Expedition (1885), the South African War (1899–1902),

---

[150] Michael Brown, '"Like a Devoted Army": Medicine, Heroic Masculinity, and the Military Paradigm in Victorian Britain', *Journal of British Studies* 49:3 (2010), 592–622.

[151] Lawrence and Brown, 'Quintessentially Modern'.   [152] Godlee, *Lister*, p. 552.

[153] For example, see Jessica Meyer, *An Equal Burden: The Men of the Royal Army Medical Corps in the First World War* (Oxford: Oxford University Press, 2019), p. 25.

[154] John Shepherd, 'The Civil Hospitals in the Crimea (1855–1856)', *Proceedings of the Royal Society of Medicine* 59:3 (1966), 199–204, at p. 199.

[155] *Lancet* 146:3762 (5 October 1895), p. 827. Military volunteer organisations were also popular among students: see Leeson, *Lister*, p. 145.

and the First World War (1914–18).[156] Meanwhile, when Frederick Treves embarked at Waterloo station on the first leg of his journey to South Africa in November 1899, the 'hero of the day' was carried shoulder high through a crowd of over 400 cheering medical students in a manner that reminded *The Times* of 'a rush of forwards on the football field'.[157]

There were complexities here of course, not least because the later nineteenth century also saw the flowering of a culture of medical and surgical internationalism, epitomised by the International Congress of Medical Science, an event at which Lister was frequently fêted and at which, in 1881, he even managed to get the Frenchman Louis Pasteur and the German Robert Koch (1843–1910) to shake hands, despite the bitterness caused by the Franco-Prussian War.[158] Even so, in the context of the fraught, social-Darwinist tensions of international relations in the late nineteenth and early twentieth centuries, surgery was as much a vehicle for nationalism and militarism as for international cooperation.[159] And when the Great War finally came, it led many surgeons, including Alexander Ogston, to rewrite their personal memories of that most German of sciences, bacteriology, and induced the *British Journal of Surgery* to claim, in defiance of all evidence, that Germany's contribution to surgery had been negligible.[160]

If the outbreak of the First World War encouraged British practitioners to write Germany out of the history of modern scientific surgery, then a move to rewrite the broader history of surgery had already been underway for some time. As we have heard, antiseptic surgeons of the Listerian and post-Listerian generations tended to present the surgery of the past, even sometimes the mid-century achievements of anaesthesia, as part of an undifferentiated surgical 'dark age' that served merely to amplify the greater glories of techno-scientific surgical modernity. Often this contrast was expressed in emotive terms, the pre-antiseptic age being one of almost inconceivable pain, misery, and distress. In the Epilogue, we shall consider how such historical narratives have laid the groundwork for contemporary perceptions of the pre-anaesthetic era and have contributed to our long-standing neglect of that period's deep emotional richness and complexity.

---

[156] Alexander Ogston, *Reminiscences of Three Campaigns* (London: Hodder and Stoughton, 1919).

[157] *Times* 13 November 1899, p. 12; Lawrence and Brown, 'Quintessentially Modern', p. 156.

[158] Godlee, *Lister*, p. 445. On the culture of surgical internationalism, see Thomas Schlich, '"One and the Same the World Over": The International Culture of Surgical Exchange in an Age of Globalization, 1870–1914', *Journal of the History of Medicine and Allied Sciences* 71:3 (2016), 247–70.

[159] See Osler, *Aequanimitas*, pp. 277–306 for complaints about 'chauvinism' and 'nationalism' in medicine.

[160] Ogston (ed.), *Ogston*, pp. 86–91; *British Journal of Surgery* 3:9 (January 1915), pp. 1–2. See also M. Anne Crowther, 'Lister at Home and Abroad: A Continuing Legacy', *Notes and Records of the Royal Society* 67:3 (2013), 281–94, at p. 288.

Epilogue
New Pasts, New Futures

In September 1879, Joseph Lister arrived in Amsterdam for the International Congress of Medical Science as something like a conquering hero. According to the *British Medical Journal*, the public address he gave there was received 'with an enthusiasm which knew no bounds'. As Lister approached the lectern, 'the whole assembly rose to their feet [...] with deafening and repeated rounds of cheers'. After five full minutes, this scene, which the *Journal* thought 'unprecedented [...] in the history of medical science', was interrupted by the President of the Congress, Franciscus Donders (1818–89), who announced: '"Professor Lister, it is not only our admiration which we offer to you; it is our gratitude, and that of the nations to which we belong"'.[1]

The adulation did not end there. Three days later, the evening's entertainment consisted of a series of short theatrical performances, including two 'artistically dressed tableaux *vivants*'. The first of these was based upon a 'well-known print' of the pioneering sixteenth-century surgeon Ambroise Paré, 'dressing a wounded man on the field of battle'. However, in place of Paré was 'a similitude of Lister', and 'in the foreground an immense *foyer* of carbolic acid'.[2] 'The idea', the *British Medical Journal* reported, 'was immediately seized, and from the whole theatre there rose such an universal acclamation, with continuous ovation to the name of Lister, that it was only after Mr Lister had, under compulsion, bowed his acknowledgments from his place [...] that the enthusiasm subsided'.[3]

This 'idea', it might be imagined, was that Lister had rewritten the history of surgery, that he had supplanted the achievements of the past by his own revolutionary discovery. Paré was said to have been one of Lister's personal heroes and he would frequently quote the Frenchman's famous dictum concerning the patient: 'I dressed him, God cured him'.[4] Now, however, Lister stood, quite

---

[1] *British Medical Journal* 2:977 (20 September 1879), p. 453.
[2] The meaning of the term 'foyer' here is uncertain, though it could be taken to imply a visual centrepiece. Either that or it was simply at the front of the stage.
[3] *British Medical Journal* 2:977 (20 September 1879), p. 454.
[4] Rickman John Godlee, *Lord Lister*, 2nd ed. (London: Macmillan, 1918), pp. 91, 566–7.

literally, in Paré's place, usurping his oft-acknowledged position as 'the father of surgery' and suggesting that there was, in essence, no *true* surgery before Lister. As St Clair Thomson wrote nearly sixty years later:

Lister, this genius, created anew the ancient art of healing. He did more for surgery and mankind in his life-time than all the surgeons of all the ages have been able to effect since the time of Hippocrates [...] The history of our world is divided into the two periods, before and since the coming of Christ – BC and AD. The history of Medicine and Surgery, and of human bodily suffering, will always be divided into the time before and after Lister.[5]

As we saw at the beginning of Chapter 1, each generation of surgeons had rehearsed its place in the history of surgery, casting itself as the pinnacle of achievement and presenting those who came before as, at best, stepping stones on the way to greatness or, at worst, unenlightened butchers labouring in darkness. And, in turn, each of these narratives was overwritten by the one that succeeded it.[6] All generations were guilty of the same presumption in this regard. But what is remarkable about the Listerian myth of the birth of modern surgery is how durable it has been. So much about surgery has changed since Lister's time, yet no surgeon has usurped his place at the summit of the surgical pantheon in the way that he can be said to have displaced those, like Ambroise Paré or John Hunter, who came before him.

The Listerian myth is thus still with us and it has served to shape popular and professional perceptions of the history of surgery in profound ways, not least in terms of its emotional dimensions. Such perceptions are founded upon a fundamental disjuncture in historical continuity established by commentators like Thomson. In the first half of the twentieth century, most surgical history was written by surgeons, and these surgeons were, almost exclusively, supporters of the antiseptic system. Many of them, such as Thomson, Godlee, or John Rudd Leeson, were either relatives or former colleagues of Lister. But even beyond the realm of hagiography and reminiscence, there were attempts to craft a historical narrative that set Listerian surgery apart from all that had preceded it. In the very early twentieth century, the popular science and technology writer F. M. Holmes (b. 1851) penned a paean to surgical modernity entitled *Surgeons and Their Wonderful Discoveries* in which the story of antisepsis was told almost entirely in Lister's own words.[7] Meanwhile in 1912,

---

[5] RCSE, MS0021/1/15, St Clair Thomson, *Lister, 1827–1912: A House Surgeon's Memories* (1937), pp. 27–8.

[6] See also Christopher Lawrence, 'Democratic, Divine and Heroic: The History and Historiography of Surgery', in Christopher Lawrence (ed.), *Medical Theory, Surgical Practice: Studies in the History of Surgery* (London: Routledge, 1992), 1–47; Lawrence, 'Surgery and Its Histories: Purposes and Contexts', in Thomas Schlich (ed.), *The Palgrave Handbook of the History of Surgery* (London: Palgrave Macmillan, 2018), 27–48.

[7] F. M. Holmes, *Surgeons and Their Wonderful Discoveries* (London: S. W. Partridge, c.1901).

the year of Lister's death, the eugenicist physician Caleb Williams Saleeby (1878–1940) published *Surgery and Society: A Tribute to Listerism*, which, he claimed, answered the 'lack [...] of any book devoted to the most beneficent achievement in the entire record of science'. While Saleeby acknowledged that 'Surgery of some kind is doubtless almost as old as the human race', he maintained that 'its history, until the second quarter of the nineteenth century, scarcely needs writing'.[8] Such sentiments were commonplace. In his popular biography of Lister, published in 1948, Hector Charles Cameron (1878–1958), son of Lister's friend Hector Clare Cameron, wrote that 'modern surgery began' in 1865 when Joseph Lister 'stepped from his carriage at the gates of the Royal Infirmary Glasgow' holding 'the first crude sample of carbolic acid'.[9] For others, however, there was at least some value in a longer historical perspective, if only to better reflect the achievements of techno-scientific modernity. In 1925, for example, a correspondent to *The Lancet* wrote of the challenges involved in 'enabl[ing] the present generation to realise the state of affairs that existed' before Lister. 'Even those who experienced something of the fringe of its horrors are apt sometimes to forget the advantages we enjoy to-day', he opined. He therefore recommended that 'All students ought to read the story of "Rab and His Friends", by Dr John Brown' wherein 'they will find in beautiful language an accurate description of an old-time operation for removal of the breast'. But, in terms of a general understanding of the pre-Listerian past, 'we require an exact description with some detail as much for educational as for historical purposes'. 'It would', he claimed, 'supply a real want'.[10]

These early histories of surgical modernity smoothed out the complexities of the recent past in order to present a seamless narrative of triumphant discovery. Thus, despite the ambiguous relationship between antiseptic and aseptic surgery, many accorded with the view propounded by Lister's closest allies that asepsis, which had become the dominant mode of surgical cleanliness by the early twentieth century, was merely 'Listerism perfected'.[11] Meanwhile, other authors sought to subordinate the earlier discovery of anaesthesia to a narrative of Listerian triumph. They did this either by rolling the two together (Lister's presence at the first operation under ether in Britain was useful here, his antagonistic relationship with James Young Simpson, the pioneer of chloroform, less so), or by diminishing the relative importance of anaesthesia when compared to antisepsis. According to Saleeby, anaesthesia did not fully conquer

---

[8] C. W. Saleeby, *Surgery and Society: A Tribute to Listerism* (New York: Moffat and Yard, 1912), pp. 1, 28.

[9] Hector Charles Cameron, *Joseph Lister: The Friend of Man* (London; Heinemann, 1948), p. 1.

[10] *Lancet* 206:5319 (8 August 1925), p. 302.

[11] Harvey Graham, *The Story of Surgery* (New York: Doubleday, 1939), p. 365. See also Holmes, *Surgeons*, ch. 3.

surgical pain, for while post-anaesthetic operations may have constituted 'an utterly different spectacle and an utterly different experience for the patient, [...] surgical fever supervened in practically every case'. Hence, pre-Listerian surgery remained 'eminently painful surgery, for inflammation was its normal sequel, and though anaesthesia was a mighty boon, the worst was always yet to come'.[12] In a similar vein, the Leeds surgeon Berkeley Moynihan (1865–1936) claimed that 'Before Lister came' surgical operations were characterised not only by 'heavy mortality', but also by an 'almost insupportable burden of terror and of suffering' that even chloroform could not alleviate.[13]

Moynihan's words highlight perhaps the most important and enduring way in which such early accounts configured the history of surgery, as the physical agonies and emotional terrors of the pre-modern past came to dominate popular representation. Almost all early histories of surgical modernity presented the pre-Listerian and pre-anaesthetic era in deeply emotive terms. In opening his chapter on the origins of antisepsis, for example, F. M. Holmes chose to imagine the following pre-Listerian dialogue:

'Dead! my brother dead! But you said the amputation was proceeding favourably?'
'So it was, but erysipelas set in, and, I am sorry to say, it has proved fatal.'
To this sorrowful announcement no more could be added, and sick and faint with the sudden news of death, instead of the cheering intelligence of progress, the inquirer staggered away to bear the crushing blow as best he might.[14]

As this passage suggests, such emotive qualities were most closely attached to the experiences of patients and their loved ones. These experiences were often condensed into endlessly recycled parables. For example, Thomson wrote of how, in the days before Lister, the public 'shrank and shuddered at the suggestion of entering a hospital', the surgical ward being perceived as little more than 'the entrance to the valley of the shadow of death'. To exemplify his point, he recounted an anecdote from Frederick Treves who, as a house surgeon at Whitechapel's London Hospital in the mid-1870s, was called upon to secure the consent of 'an East-End mother' for 'some trifling operation' on her daughter. '"That's all right" said the patient, "it's easy enough to give my consent, but what I want to know is: who's going to pay for the poor girl's funeral?"'[15]

This emphasis upon the emotional, mental, and physical trials of the pre-modern patient served to communicate the misery from which humankind had been delivered by the heroic triumphs of modern surgery. There was an element of truth in this, of course, for the pre-anaesthetic past was indeed

---

[12] Saleeby, *Surgery*, pp. 31, 37.   [13] *Lancet* 209:5406 (9 April 1927), p. 746.
[14] Holmes, *Surgeons*, p. 35.
[15] RCSE, MS0021/1/15, pp. 18–19. This story appears in a number of histories, including Graham, *Story*, p. 336.

characterised by great suffering and profound anxiety on the part of surgical patients. However, what such accounts also did was to establish a stereotype of the pre-anaesthetic *practitioner* that was fundamentally at odds with the image that Romantic surgeons had sought to craft of themselves. To be sure, popular satires of the late eighteenth and early nineteenth centuries had often carica-tured surgeons as heartless butchers, just as they had depicted medical practi-tioners more generally as self-interested and lacking in compassion.[16] But, as we have seen in Chapters 1 and 2, Romantic surgeons challenged this cliché by emphasising their heartfelt sensibility, commitment to care, and deep emo-tional connection to their patients. By contrast, in consigning the pre-modern past to a dark age of ignorance and agony, and by presenting modern surgery as both uniquely curative *and* uniquely compassionate, early twentieth-century commentators overemphasised pre-anaesthetic surgical dispassion, often to the extent of alleging a passive cruelty in their forebears. As Frederick Treves claimed in 1900:

It is little wonder if the older surgeon became rough and stern, if his sense of feeling became dulled, and if the sympathetic side of his nature suffered some suppression. Indeed, contemporary accounts are apt to represent the operator of pre-anaesthetic times as rough almost to brutality and as coarse both in his conduct and in his utterances.

Compressing anaesthesia and antisepsis into a simultaneous surgical revolution, he continued:

Within the compass of some thirty years the whole state of affairs has changed. Consid-eration for the patient and for the patient's sensibilities have become a matter of the first moment and the operator has learnt that his work is best done if done with gentleness and tact, and that haste and bluster, coarseness and coarse handling are out of place around the operating table.[17]

It is hardly surprising, perhaps, that the nuance and complexity of the pre-anaesthetic past were obscured by the shining light of surgical modernity. And it is important to note that such accounts often acknowledged the achievements of surgeons like John Hunter, Astley Cooper, and Charles Bell. Even so, by emphasising the professional beneficence of their own era, early twentieth-century surgeons and surgical historians levelled the emotional landscape of the period that had immediately preceded them. Indeed, they rendered the emotional regime of Romantic surgery virtually unintelligible. Some commen-tators acknowledged the emotions experienced and expressed by surgeons of the earlier era, but these served merely to exemplify what Berkeley Moynihan

[16] Fiona Haslam, *From Hogarth to Rowlandson: Medicine in Art in Eighteenth-Century Britain* (Liverpool: Liverpool University Press, 1996); Roy Porter, *Bodies Politic: Death, Disease and the Doctors in Britain, 1650–1900* (London: Reaktion, 2001).
[17] *Lancet* 156:4014 (4 August 1900), p. 314.

called 'the full horror of the old days'. Speaking to the Royal College of Surgeons on the centenary of Lister's birth in 1927, he stated:

It is startling to read that when in the year 1821 Astley Cooper operated upon George IV for a small sebaceous cyst on the head, so tortured was he by anxiety lest erysipelas or pyaemia might develop that he sought to put upon others the responsibility of the operation, on Cline, on Everard Home, on anybody but himself. He speaks of the operation in terms which to us now appear absurd, fearing that 'it might by possibility be followed by fatal consequences'. He says, 'I saw that the operation if it were followed by erysipelas would destroy all my happiness and blast my reputation', and 'I felt giddy at the idea of my fate hanging upon such an event' [...] It is hard to believe that a surgeon eminent enough to be chosen for service to the King should be so deeply moved at the prospect of what was to him, as to us, technically the simplest of operations. The exercise of the art of surgery brought terror then where it now brings joy, to surgeon no less than to patient.[18]

Cooper's expression of intense emotion, once so culturally resonant, was, by the early twentieth century, merely an 'absurd' relic of pre-modern misery and professional impotence.

This emphasis on the horrors of the past, on its capricious and callous cruelties, continues to structure popular perceptions of the pre-anaesthetic era. The bifurcation of surgical history into a glorious modernity and a benighted past is perhaps most neatly exemplified by Guy Williams' two-volume popular history of medicine and surgery, *The Age of Agony* (1975) and *The Age of Miracles* (1981). Chronology plays a somewhat confused, yet highly suggestive, role in Williams' account. The *Age of Agony* is ostensibly concerned with the 'Art of Healing' between 1700 and 1800, whereas the *Age of Miracles* explores the period from 1800 to 1900. But in reality, the late eighteenth and early nineteenth centuries are fractured across both books. When used to illustrate the horrors of the pre-modern, early nineteenth-century surgeons like Astley Cooper are consigned to the 'age of agony'.[19] When harnessed to a narrative of progress, meanwhile, eighteenth-century practitioners like John Hunter find themselves alongside anaesthesia and antisepsis in the 'age of miracles'.[20] The message is clear. As Williams writes in his brief introduction to the first book: 'Do we realize sufficiently what we have escaped by being alive in the twentieth century, not the eighteenth century? The following pages will tell'.[21]

---

[18] *Lancet* 209:5406 (9 April 1927), pp. 746–7. The original account is taken from Bransby Blake Cooper, *The Life of Sir Astley Cooper, Bart.*, vol. 2 (London: John W. Parker, 1843), pp. 229, 233.
[19] Guy Williams, *The Age of Agony: The Art of Healing, c.1700–1800* (Chicago: Academy Chicago Publishers, 1986 [1975]), pp. 113–14.
[20] Guy Williams, *The Age of Miracles: Medicine and Surgery in the Nineteenth Century* (Chicago: Academy Chicago Publishers, 1987 [1981]), ch. 2.
[21] Williams, *Agony*, p. 2.

For much of the twentieth century, Astley Cooper served as the touchstone for the 'old world' of surgery, something that doubtless owed much to the legacy of his nephew's biography. Since the late 1970s and early 1980s, however, it has been Robert Liston, conceived as a muscular mixture of bravura and brutality, who has come to most powerfully embody the supposed contradictions of the pre-anaesthetic age. As we saw in Chapter 1, Lister's modern reputation is founded, at least in part, on factually unstable ground. Thus, in his curiously influential book *Great Medical Disasters* (1983), Richard Gordon alleges that Liston amputated a leg in two-and-a-half minutes 'but in his enthusiasm [removed] the patient's testicles as well'. Meanwhile in another instance, Gordon maintains that Liston amputated the leg of a patient (who later died of gangrene) and, in his haste, severed two fingers from his 'young assistant' (who likewise died of gangrene), as well as slicing the coattails of a 'distinguished surgical spectator, who was so terrified that the knife had pierced his vitals he dropped dead from fright'. It was, Gordon claims, a 'triple knockout', 'the only operation in history with a 300 percent mortality'.[22]

Gordon's account is a specious mélange of half-truths and outright fiction. There is no evidence for the death of a surgical spectator in this manner (and hence no basis to the 300 per cent mortality claim). Likewise, his story about Liston accidentally severing the fingers of his assistant, as well as the testes of his patient, can be traced back no more than five years to *The Rise of Surgery* (1978) by Owen and Sarah Wangensteen.[23] In this book, Owen Wangensteen recalls a 'Very likely apocryphal [...] anecdote' told to him by his 'former physiology professor, Frederick H. Scott, who as a student of [Ernest Henry] Starling in London heard that a surgeon of the *Liston era* [note: not Liston himself], in his hurry to amputate a thigh "included two fingers of his assistant and both testes of his patient"'.[24]

Regardless of their dubious veracity, these stories about Liston have worked their way into countless popular histories and have served to underscore the horrors of the surgical past. For example, Richard Hollingham's *Blood and Guts* (2008), produced as a tie-in to a BBC television series of the same name, features Liston prominently in its first chapter, tellingly entitled 'Bloody Beginnings'. Alongside a number of questionable statements and outright

---

[22] Richard Gordon, *Great Medical Disasters* (New York: Stein and Day, 1983), pp. 19–21.

[23] At least two other near-contemporary texts contain a version of this story: Elisabeth Bennion, *Antique Medical Instruments* (London: Sotheby Parke Bernet, 1979), p. 55, Steven Lehrer, *Explorers of the Body: Dramatic Breakthroughs in Medicine from Ancient Times to Modern Science* (New York: Doubleday, 1979), p. 92.

[24] Owen D. Wangensteen and Sarah D. Wangensteen, *The Rise of Surgery: From Empiric Craft to Scientific Discipline* (Minneapolis: University of Minnesota Press, 1978), pp. 36, 38. Emphasis added. The fact that, in his version of this story, Gordon separates the severing of the testes from the severing of the fingers raises further questions about its historical veracity.

factual errors (including the bizarre suggestion that Liston died in a sailing accident), Hollingham repeats the claim about Liston's 300 per cent operative mortality.[25] He constructs Liston as a man approaching the cusp of modernity, yet one who remained firmly rooted in the 'messy, bloody and traumatic' world of the pre-modern, an operator who prioritised skill over sympathy but who, because he washed his hands and wore a clean apron, somehow perceived, albeit dimly, the distant light of surgical redemption.[26] As with Williams, there is a clear moral to the story: 'If you need an operation, just be grateful that you are alive today and not 170 years ago – the next patient on Robert Liston's operating schedule'.[27]

Liston also appears in the early pages of Lindsey Fitzharris' best-selling popular history of surgery, *The Butchering Art* (2017). Fitzharris' book is a good place to conclude this synopsis of surgical myth-making, not only because it constitutes the apotheosis of the literary genre, but also because it is functionally indistinguishable from the Listerian hagiographies of the early twentieth century, thus bringing us full circle. Fitzharris' book is a lively, if oddly truncated, biography of Joseph Lister that draws heavily, and uncritically, on earlier accounts written by his relatives, friends, and associates. As such, it recounts a tale of heroic individualism in which, as Christopher Lawrence notes, the 'mythic aspects of Lister's work' reach 'Arthurian dimensions'.[28] Like so much of its source material, Fitzharris' book glosses over the complexities of contemporary germ theory and avoids substantive reference to Lister's vociferous support for vivisection, or his vehement opposition to female medical education. It likewise presents the history of antiseptic surgery as a near-miraculous redemption from suffering. Pre-antiseptic and pre-anaesthetic surgery are, as ever, the straw man of history, an 'age of agony' in which 'savagery, sawing and gangrene' rule the day.[29] Fitzharris deploys the customary clichés about Liston, 'one of the profession's last great butchers', and even suggests that the social status of early nineteenth-century surgeons was so low that 'many were illiterate' and that they were viewed 'much like a key cutter or a plumber today', something that would, no doubt, have come as a surprise to Sir Astley Cooper, Sir Everard Home, or Sir Charles Bell.[30]

---

[25] Richard Hollingham, *Blood and Guts: A History of Surgery* (New York: Thomas Dunne Books, 2008), pp. 41–2, 65.

[26] Hollingham, *Blood*, pp. 40, 42.   [27] Hollingham, *Blood*, p. 298.

[28] Christopher Lawrence, 'Blood and Guts: Victorian Achievements in Surgery', *Times Literary Supplement* (4 May 2018), 28–9.

[29] Lindsey Fitzharris, *The Butchering Art: Joseph Lister's Quest to Transform the Grisly World of Victorian Medicine* (London: Allen Lane, 2017), prologue. The line about 'savagery, sawing and gangrene' appears on the front flap of the dust jacket of this edition.

[30] Fitzharris, *Butchering*, pp. 9, 10, 18, 22. She does, however, acknowledge that the 'triple-knockout' story might be apocryphal.

The Butchering Art is a conventionally Whiggish tale of the triumphs of scientific modernity. But it is also part of a broader culture of contemporary popular history that mines the pre-anaesthetic past for gruesome stories and gory 'thrills'. Indeed, the period even finds itself the subject of grisly humour, as evidenced by numerous blogs, podcasts, and the BBC television comedy series *Quacks* (2017). One cannot help but think that such ghoulish frisson motivates a not insignificant number of visitors to sites such as the Old Operating Theatre of St Thomas' Hospital, or to the museums of the Royal Colleges of Surgeons in Edinburgh and London. Of course, public history is a vital, perhaps *the* vital, mechanism for enhancing our understanding of, and engagement with, the past, and museums in particular do an immensely valuable job in this regard. However, public preconceptions are hard to shift, especially when many popular histories tend to reiterate the myths of surgical modernity rather than challenge them.

A question could be posed as to why any of this matters. Why is it important that, within the popular mythology of scientific modernity, the pre-anaesthetic past seems destined to remain an age of ignorance, butchery, and brutality, dominated by caricature and cliché? Well, at the most obvious level, it matters historiographically, for such narratives present us with a flatly two-dimensional picture of surgery in the pre-anaesthetic period, one that diminishes that era's emotional richness and complexity. It is not simply a question of refuting the idea that all early nineteenth-century surgeons were rough sawbones or heartless butchers, any more than it is a matter of proposing that they were uniformly men of deep and heartfelt sensibility. Rather, by simplifying or stereotyping the place of emotions within pre-modern surgery, we miss the opportunity to explore the vitally important cultural and political work that emotions performed, in surgery as much as in any other area of human history. My experience with the Surgery & Emotion project has convinced me that the public are open to having their preconceptions challenged by new insights. I remember when, having delivered a paper on the place of emotions in the life and work of John and Charles Bell, a member of the audience told me that they had previously thought that all surgeons in the past were ignorant and cruel, or words to that effect. It was one of those moments that seemed almost calculated to answer the 'impact agenda' of modern historical research.

Yet there is, I would propose, even more at stake than this, for the myths that underwrite the narrative of surgical modernity not only condition public perceptions, but also sustain an emotional regime that continues to shape *surgical* practice and identity to this day. This book has presented something of a history in reverse. Whereas most conventional accounts of nineteenth-century surgery tell a story of unalloyed progress, a journey from darkness into light, this book has been concerned with the ways in which emotions and emotional expression were marginalised within surgical culture. This is not to suggest that it is an anti-progressive narrative *per se*, for it would be ludicrous to claim that being a surgeon or a patient in the pre-anaesthetic era was, in any conceivable way, *better* than being a surgeon or a patient today. But it is, perhaps, a counterintuitive narrative, one that provokes us to think about what has been lost as much as what has been gained. As we have seen, emotions played an important role in early nineteenth-century surgery, in part because the practical conditions of that period meant there was more occasion for the experience and expression of such feelings as anxiety, dread, pity, and sympathy. But their presence in surgery also owed a great deal to the fact that the sensation and expression of feeling were valued within the cultural conventions of Romantic sensibility. By the same token, the relative decline in the importance of emotions within later nineteenth-century surgery, in terms of ontology, intersubjectivity, and reflexivity, derived from the fact that patients and surgeons were increasingly relieved of the emotional burdens of operative surgery, as well as from the fact that modern surgeons were shaping new professional identities that emphasised techno-scientific rationality and biopolitical authority over reflective introspection, affective engagement, or emotional self-fashioning.

As we saw Chapter 6, modern surgeons like Joseph Lister laid the ground-work for a professional surgical ideal in which claims to compassion were mediated through a scientific and intellectual authority, as well as through forms of social, cultural, and political prestige, that rendered them increasingly remote and 'god-like'. These tendencies would only be exacerbated as the twentieth century progressed and as surgery, like medicine in general, became increasingly bound up with the political functions of the nation state. This was especially true of the United Kingdom, where, from 1948 onwards, the bulk of healthcare provision was assimilated into the state-run National Health Service (NHS), a body that, as much as it is threatened by the forces of neoliberalism, currently enjoys a mythic status within the British popular consciousness. And yet, however much the NHS may generate profound expressions of popular emotion, notably gratitude, and however much, like Lister's patients, we may feel (or think we feel) the operations of a detached yet inherently compassionate largesse, the practice of surgery itself, in its idealised forms at least, is an emotions-free zone. Within contemporary surgical culture, emotions are generally seen as something dangerous, a contaminant of the professional persona and a threat to rational decision-making.[31] Anthropological and medical studies have shown that surgeons, the vast

[31] Jodi Halpern, *From Detached Concern to Empathy: Humanizing Medical Practice* (Oxford: Oxford University Press, 2001); Daniel Ofri, *What Doctors Feel: How Emotions Affect the Practice of Medicine* (Boston: Beacon Press, 2013).

majority of whom are male, tend to internalise a model of heroic individualism, seeing themselves as 'problem-fixers' rather than as caring for patients
as whole human entities.[32] And in so doing, they have little space, or cause,
for intersubjective engagement or emotional introspection. The high-profile
former cardiac surgeon Stephen Westaby may have framed his 2019 memoir
The Knife's Edge: The Heart and Mind of a Cardiac Surgeon largely in terms
of emotions, but it is notable that, in a 2017 interview with the *Financial
Times*, he claimed: 'You've got to have the characteristics of a psychopath to
make a good surgeon'.[33]

It should be noted that Westaby's fellow interviewee in this instance, the
former neurosurgeon Henry Marsh, disagreed with his colleague's assessment,
claiming instead that 'when surgeons talk about themselves as psychopaths,
what they're talking about is this awkward problem of how you are both compassionate and professionally detached at the same time'.[34] Psychopathy might
seem an odd balance to strike between compassion and detachment, but even
so, it is remarkable that two eminent surgeons should be talking about emotions at all, let alone making them the structuring device for their memoirs,
as both Marsh and Westaby have done.[35] It could be argued that Marsh and
Westaby, as retired, white, male consultants, are in a peculiarly privileged
position to reflect on their careers with apparent emotional honesty, and that
such licence is unlikely to be granted to more junior practitioners, or those of a
different gender or ethnicity, especially in a profession where clinical detachment remains the norm. But in my work with the Surgery & Emotion project I
have been struck by the extent to which surgeons, or a distinct sub-set of them
at least, are increasingly prepared to talk about the place of emotions in their
work. In my experience, this increased sensitivity to the importance of emotion
is generally practitioner centred, focusing on such issues as stress, burnout,

[32] Joan Cassell, 'Dismembering the Image of God: Surgeons, Heroes, Wimps and Miracles',
Anthropology Today 2:2 (April 1986), 13–15; Pearl Katz, *The Scalpel's Edge: The Culture
of Surgeons* (Needham Heights, MA: Allyn & Bacon, 1999); Rachel Prentice, *Bodies in
Formation: An Ethnography of Anatomy and Surgery Education* (Durham, NC: Duke University
Press, 2013); Kim Peters and Michelle Ryan, 'Machismo in Surgery Is Harming the Specialty',
BMJ 348 (2014), g3034, https://doi.org/10.1136/bmj.g3034 (accessed 26/08/21); Kirsty Foster
and Chris Roberts, 'The Heroic and the Villainous: A Qualitative Study Characterising the
Role Models That Shaped Senior Doctors' Professional Identity', *BMC Medical Education*
16:206 (2016), https://bmcmededuc.biomedcentral.com/articles/10.1186/s12909-016-0731-0
(accessed 18/10/2021).
[33] *Financial Times* 8 September 2017, www.ft.com/content/d53f2422-9314-11e7-a9e6-11d2f0ebb7f0
(accessed 26/08/21).
[34] *Financial Times* 8 September 2017.
[35] Henry Marsh, *Do No Harm: Stories of Life, Death and Brain Surgery* (London: Weidenfeld &
Nicolson, 2014); Stephen Westaby, *The Knife's Edge: The Heart and Mind of a Cardiac
Surgeon* (London: HarperCollins, 2019).

responses to grief, and relations with colleagues.[36] In general, it is less overtly concerned with the intersubjective emotional relations between surgeons and their patients and the ways in which better emotional interactions and more emotionally sensitive communication might improve healthcare outcomes. Many surgeons still tend to assume that *care* is a natural function of their work, rather than something that needs to be cultivated.[37]

History, I would argue, has a vital role to play in this process of professional self-reflection. The persistence of emotional detachment as a professional ideal is the result of socialisation and education rather than the inherent nature of surgical practice.[38] Surgeons structure their emotional relationships with patients and with each other in ways that are expected of them, and these expectations are often predicated on historical assumptions about the way it has 'always been'. Both the stereotypes of surgical modernity, with the surgeon as hyper-rational fixer of bodies, and those of surgical pre-modernity, with the surgeon as hardened butcher, sustain the idea that emotional detachment or dispassion is the timeless quality of the practitioner confronted by difficult decisions and emotionally challenging experiences. However, as this book has shown, this is not the way it has 'always been'. Detachment is not the eternal emotional disposition of the surgical operator. Quite the contrary, in fact. At a time when surgery was perhaps at its most dangerous and challenging, in the decades immediately preceding the introduction of anaesthesia, surgeons shaped professional identities that placed emotions at the heart of the doctor–patient relationship and that took them seriously as a vital element in the regulation of health and well-being. Likewise, if the emotional regime of scientific modernity provides few spaces of 'emotional refuge' for surgeons to divest themselves of the onerous burden of professional responsibility and to ward off burnout or 'compassion fatigue' (short of resorting to psychopathy), then the relative emotional introspection and freedom of emotional expression experienced by Romantic surgeons confronted

---

[36] For example, see Uttam Shiralkar, *Surgeon Heal Thyself: Optimising Surgical Performance by Managing Stress* (Boca Raton, FL: CRC Press, 2017); A. Pinto, O. Faiz, C. Bicknell, and C. Vincent, 'Surgical Complications and Their Implications for Surgeons' Well-being', *British Journal of Surgery*, 100:13 (2013), 1748–55; S. C. Zambrano, A. Chur-Hansen, and G. B. Crawford, 'How Do Surgeons Experience and Cope with the Death and Dying of Their Patients? A Qualitative Study in the Context of Life-Limiting Illnesses', *World Journal of Surgery*, 37:5 (2013), 935–4; M. Orri, A. Revah-Lévy, and O. Farges, 'Surgeons' Emotional Experience of Their Everyday Practice – a Qualitative Study', *PLoS ONE*, 10:11 (2015), https://doi.org/10.1371/journal.pone.0143763 (accessed 7/5/2022); Erin Dean, 'Burnout and Surgeons', *Bulletin* [Royal College of Surgeons of England] 101:4 (May 2019), 134–6.
[37] Much of the impetus to think about the role of emotions in improving care comes from non-professional bodies like the Point of Care Foundation: www.pointofcarefoundation.org.uk (accessed 26/08/21).
[38] Prentice, *Bodies*; Foster and Roberts, 'Heroic'.

by equally profound challenges might provide an interesting counterpoint.[39] This is not to argue for a naïvely instrumentalist approach to medical history where, as in the early days of the discipline, the past functions as little more than a storehouse for professional instruction or inspiration.[40] As we have seen in this book, emotions also played a deeply political role in shaping the identity of an inchoate and aspirational professional body. And yet, the very existence of such an identity allows us to challenge both historical preconceptions and professional ones, and forces us to think not only about how we do history, but also about how we might do surgery.

---

[39] For the concept of 'emotional refuge', see William Reddy, *The Navigation of Feeling: A Framework for the History of Emotions* (Cambridge, UK: Cambridge University Press, 2001), pp. 128–9. For an excellent discussion of the concept of 'compassion fatigue', see Bertrand Taithe, 'Compassion Fatigue: The Changing Nature of Humanitarian Emotions', in Dolores Martín Moruno and Beatriz Pichel (eds), *Emotional Bodies: The Historical Performativity of Emotions* (Urbana: University of Illinois Press, 2019), 242–62.

[40] Elisabeth Fee and Theodore M. Brown, 'Using Medical History to Shape a Profession: The Ideals of William Osler and Henry E. Sigerist', in Frank Huisman and John Harley Warner (eds), *Locating Medical History: The Stories and Their Meanings* (Baltimore: Johns Hopkins University Press, 2004), 139–65.

Select Bibliography

Primary Sources

Archives

Cumbria Archives Service, Carlisle
- D HUD 17/90, Correspondence between Andrew Whelpdale and John de Whelpdale.

National Archives, London
- PROB 11/1609/366, Will of William Forbes, Surgeon of Camberwell, Surrey (29 October 1818).
- PROB 11/1885/81, Will of Reverend George Chamberlaine, Clerk, Rector of Wyke Regis and Weymouth, Dorset (31 October 1837).

National Library of Scotland, Edinburgh
- MS 9003, Diary of H. R. Oswald Snr, describing his first six months as surgeon to the 4th Duke of Atholl, Governor General of the Isle of Man (1812–13).

Royal College of Surgeons of Edinburgh
- GD82, Bell family archive.

Royal College of Surgeons of England, London
- MS0008, Papers of Sir Astley Paston Cooper.
- MS0021, Papers of Sir Joseph Lister.
- MS0232, Papers of John Flint South.
- MS0276, Papers of Benjamin Travers.
- MS0470/1/2, Lectures of Sir Benjamin Brodie.

Wellcome Library, London
- MS.1860, William Hamilton Brown Ross, 'Lectures on Surgery by Mr A. A. Cooper [sic]' (1815).
- MS.5604, Lawrence W. Brown, 'Notes on Twelve Lectures by Everard Home on the Principal Operations of Surgery' (1811–12).
- MSS.6084-6094, Original letters from [Robert] Liston to [James] Miller.

Books and Pamphlets

Abernethy, John, *The Hunterian Oration for the Year 1819* (London: Longman, Hurst, Rees, Orme, and Brown, 1819).

Abernethy, John, *Surgical Observations on Tumours and on Lumbar Abscesses*, 3rd ed. (London: Longman, Hurst, Rees, Orme, and Brown, 1822).

[Anon.], *Letters of Sir Charles Bell* (London: John Murray, 1870).

[Anon.], *The London Dissector; or, a System of Dissection Practised in the Hospitals and Lecture Rooms of the Metropolis*, 3rd ed. (London: John Murray, 1811).

Bell, Charles, *Illustrations of the Great Operations of Surgery* (London: Longman, Hurst, Rees, Orme, and Brown, 1821).

Bell, Charles, *Surgical Observations* (London: Longman, Hurst, Rees, Orme, and Brown, 1816).

Bell, John, *Answer for the Junior Members of the Royal College of Surgeons of Edinburgh to the Memorial of Dr James Gregory* (Edinburgh: Peter Hill, 1800).

Bell, John, *Discourses on the Nature and Cure of Wounds* (Edinburgh: Bell and Bradfute, 1795).

Bell, John, *Engravings Explaining the Anatomy of the Bones, Muscles and Joints* (Edinburgh: John Patterson, 1794).

Bell, John, *Letters on Professional Character and Manners: On the Education of a Surgeon, and the Duties and Qualifications of a Physician* (Edinburgh: John Moir, 1810).

Bell, John, *The Principles of Surgery* (Edinburgh: T. Cadell Jr and W. Davies, 1801).

Bentham, Jeremy, *An Introduction to the Principles of Morals and Legislation* (London: T. Payne and Son, 1789).

Brown, John, *Rab and His Friends*, 8th ed. (Boston: Colonial Press, 1906).

Cameron, Hector Charles, *Joseph Lister: The Friend of Man* (London: Heinemann, 1948).

Cameron, Hector Clare, *Lord Lister, 1827–1912: An Oration* (Glasgow: James MacLehose and Son, 1914).

Campbell, Robert, *The London Tradesman: Being an Historical Account of All the Trades, Professions, Arts, Both Liberal and Mechanic*, 3rd ed. (London: T. Gardner, 1747).

Cheyne, William Watson, *Lister and His Achievement* (London: Longmans and Green, 1925).

Chiene, John, *Looking Back 1907–1860* (Edinburgh: Darien Press, 1908).

Clarke, James Fernandez, *Autobiographical Recollections of the Medical Profession* (London: J. and A. Churchill, 1874).

Cockburn, Henry, *Memorials of His Time* (New York: D. Appleton, 1856).

Cooper, Astley, *Illustrations of the Diseases of the Breast*, vol. 1 (London: Longman, Rees, Orme, Brown, and Green, 1829).

Cooper, Astley, and Travers, Benjamin, *Surgical Essays*, Part 1 (London: Cox and Son, 1818).

Cooper, Bransby Blake, *The Life of Sir Astley Cooper, Bart.*, 2 vols (London: John W. Parker, 1843).

Curling, Thomas Blizard, *The Advantages of Ether and Chloroform in Operative Surgery: An Address Delivered to the Hunterian Society on the 9th of February 1848* (London: S. Highley, 1848).

Davy, Humphry, *Researches Chemical and Philosophical, Chiefly Concerning Nitrous Oxide or Dephlogisticated Nitrous Air and Its Respiration* (London: J. Johnson, 1800).

Dawplucker, Jonathan [Bell, John], *Number Second, Being Remarks on the First Volume of Mr Benjamin Bell's System of Surgery* (London: 1799).

Elliotson, John, *The Harveian Oration, Delivered before the Royal College of Physicians, London, June 27 1846* (London: H. Baillière, 1846).

Ellis, Sarah Stickney, *The Daughters of England: Their Position in Society, Character and Responsibilities* (London: Fisher and Son, 1842).

Erichsen, John Eric, *Modern Surgery, Its Progress and Tendencies* (London: H. K. Lewis, 1873).

Erichsen, John Eric, *On Hospitalism and the Causes of Death after Operations* (London: Longmans and Green, 1874).

Erichsen, John Eric, *On the Study of Surgery: An Address Introductory to the Course of Surgery Delivered at University College London at the Opening of the Session 1850–1851* (London: Taylor, Walton, and Maberly, 1850).

Erichsen, John Eric, *The Science and Art of Surgery: A Treatise on Surgical Injuries, Disease and Their Operations* (Philadelphia: Blanchard and Lea, 1854).

Erichsen, John Eric, *The Science and Art of Surgery: A Treatise on Surgical Injuries, Disease and Their Operations*, 2nd ed. (London: Walton and Maberly, 1857).

Fergusson, William, *A System of Practical Surgery* (London: John Churchill, 1852).

Gamgee, Sampson, *On the Treatment of Wounds: Clinical Lectures* (London: J. & A. Churchill, 1878).

Godlee, Rickman John, *Lord Lister*, 2nd ed. (London: Macmillan, 1918).

Graham, Harvey, *The Story of Surgery* (New York: Doubleday, 1939).

Henley, William Ernest, *In Hospital* (Portland: Thomas Mosher, 1903).

Holmes, F. M., *Surgeons and Their Wonderful Discoveries* (London: S. W. Partridge, c.1901).

Home, Everard, *Observations on Cancer Connected with Histories of the Disease* (London: J. Johnson, 1805).

Hume, David, *A Treatise of Human Nature*, vol. 3 (London: Thomas Longman, 1740).

Laycock, Thomas, *A Treatise on the Nervous Diseases of Women* (London: Longman, Orme, Brown, Green, and Longmans, 1840).

Leeson, J. R., *Lister as I Knew Him* (London: Ballière, Tindall, and Cox, 1927).

Lister, Joseph, *The Collected Papers of Joseph Lister*, 2 vols (Oxford: Clarendon Press, 1909).

Liston, Robert, *Elements of Surgery*, vol. 1 (London: Longman, Orme, Brown, and Green, 1831).

Liston, Robert, *Practical Surgery* (London: John Churchill, 1837).

Lizars, John, *A System of Anatomical Plates ... Part II. Blood Vessels and Nerves of the Head and Trunk* (Edinburgh: Daniel Lizars, 1823).

Lizars, John, *A System of Anatomical Plates ... Part IV. The Muscles of the Trunk* (Edinburgh: Daniel Lizars, 1824).

Macilwain, George, *Memoirs of John Abernethy*, 2 vols, 2nd ed. (London: Hurst and Blackett, 1854).

Mackenzie, William, *An Appeal to the Public and the Legislature on the Necessity of Affording Dead Bodies to the Schools of Anatomy, by Legislative Enactment* (Glasgow: Robertson and Atkinson, 1824).

Miller, James, *Surgical Experience of Chloroform* (Edinburgh: Sutherland and Knox, 1848).

Norris, William, *The Hunterian Oration Delivered Before the Royal College of Surgeons* (London: T. Cadell and W. Davies, 1817).

Ogston, Alexander, *Reminiscences of Three Campaigns* (London: Hodder and Stoughton, 1919).

Ogston, Walter H. (ed.), *Alexander Ogston K.C.V.O.: Memoirs and Tributes of Relatives, Colleagues and Students, with Some Autobiographical Writings* (Aberdeen: Aberdeen University Press, 1943).

Osler, William, *Aequanimitas: With Other Addresses to Medical Students, Nurses and Practitioners of Medicine* (London: H. K. Lewis, 1904).

Palmer, James F. (ed.), *The Works of John Hunter, F.R.S.*, vol. 1 (London: Longman, Orme, Brown, Green, and Longman, 1835).

Paterson, Robert, *Memorial of the Life of James Syme* (Edinburgh: Edmonston and Douglas, 1874).

Reynolds, John Russell, *Essays and Addresses* (London: Macmillan, 1896).

Saleeby, C. W. *Surgery and Society: A Tribute to Listerism* (New York: Moffat and Yard, 1912).

Savory, William, *On Life and Death: Four Lectures Delivered at the Royal Institution of Great Britain* (London: Smith and Elder, 1863).

Simpson, James Young, *Acupressure: A New Method of Arresting Surgical Haemorrhage* (Edinburgh: Adam and Charles Black, 1864).

Simpson, James Young, *Hospitalism: Its Effects on the Results of Surgical Operations* (Edinburgh: Oliver and Boyd, 1869).

Skey, Frederic, *Operative Surgery* (London: John Churchill, 1850).

Smith, Adam, *The Theory of Moral Sentiments* (London: A. Miller, 1759).

Smith, Thomas Southwood, *A Lecture Delivered over the Remains of Jeremy Bentham Esq.* (London: Effingham Wilson, 1832).

Snow, John, *On the Inhalation of the Vapours of Ether* (London: Wilson and Ogilvy, 1847).

Snow, John, *On Chloroform and Other Anaesthetics: Their Actions and Administration* (London: John Churchill, 1858).

South, John Flint, *Memorials of John Flint South* (London: John Murray, 1884).

Southey, Robert, *A Vision of Judgement* (London: Longman, Hurst, Rees, Orme, and Brown, 1821).

Sprigge, Samuel Squire, *The Life and Times of Thomas Wakley* (London: Longmans and Green, 1897).

Struthers, John, *Historical Sketch of the Edinburgh Anatomical School* (Edinburgh: Maclachlan and Stewart, 1867).

Syme, James, *Address in Surgery delivered at the Annual Meeting of the British Medical Association, Held at Leamington, August 3, 1865* (Edinburgh: R. Clark, 1865).

Syme, James, *On the Improvements Which Have Been Introduced into the Practice of Surgery in Great Britain within the Last Thirty Years* (Edinburgh: Murray and Gibb, 1853).

Travers, Benjamin, *An Inquiry Concerning That Disturbed State of the Vital Functions Usually Denominated Constitutional Irritation* (London: Longman, Rees, Orme, Brown, and Green, 1827).

Treves, Frederick (ed.), *A System of Surgery*, vol. 1 (London: Cassell, 1895).

Wakley, Thomas, *A Report of the Trial of Cooper v. Wakley for an Alleged Libel* (London: 1829).

Newspapers and Periodicals

Athenaeum
Blackwood's Edinburgh Magazine
British Journal of Surgery
British Medical Journal
Cobbett's Weekly Register
Contemporary Review
Cornhill Magazine
Critic
Edinburgh Medical and Surgical Journal
Examiner
Fortnightly Review
Fraser's Magazine
Gentleman's Magazine
Glasgow Medical Journal
Imperial Magazine
Kaleidoscope, or Literary and Scientific Mirror
Lancet
Lion
London Medical Gazette
Medico-Chirurgical Review
Medico-Chirurgical Transactions
Mirror
Modern Review
Monthly Magazine
Morning Chronicle
Nineteenth Century
North British Review
Penny Satirist
Saturday Magazine
Times
University College Hospital Magazine
Westminster Review

Official Publications

Hansard
Report from the Select Committee on Anatomy (1828)

Secondary Sources

Ackerknecht, Erwin, *Medicine at the Paris Hospital, 1794–1848* (Baltimore: Johns Hopkins Press, 1967).
Andrew, Donna, *Philanthropy and Police: London Charity in the Eighteenth Century* (Princeton: Princeton University Press, 1989).

Arnold-Forster, Agnes, *The Cancer Problem: Malignancy in Nineteenth-Century Britain* (Oxford: Oxford University Press, 2021).

Bailey, Joanne, 'Masculinity and Fatherhood in England c.1760–1830', in John H. Arnold and Sean Brody (eds), *What Is Masculinity? Historical Dynamics from Antiquity to the Contemporary World* (Basingstoke: Palgrave, 2011), 167–86.

Bailey, Joanne, *Parenting in England, 1760–1850: Emotion, Identity and Generation* (Oxford: Oxford University Press, 2012).

Bailey, Joanne, '"Think Wot a Mother Must Feel": Parenting in English Pauper Letters c. 1760–1834', *Family and Community History* 13:1 (2010), 5–19.

Bailey, Joanne, 'A Very Sensible Man: Imagining Fatherhood in England c.1750–1830', *History* 95:319 (2010), 267–92.

Bailey, Joanne, 'Voices in Court: Lawyers or Litigants?', *Historical Research* 74:186 (2011), 392–408.

Barclay, Katie, *Caritas: Neighbourly Love and the Early Modern Self* (Oxford: Oxford University Press, 2021).

Barclay, Katie, *Men on Trial: Performing Emotion, Embodiment and Identity in Ireland, 1800–45* (Manchester: Manchester University Press, 2018).

Barclay, Katie, 'Performing Emotion and Reading the Male Body in the Irish Court, c.1800–1845', *Journal of Social History* 51:2 (2017), 293–312.

Barker-Benfield, G. J., *The Culture of Sensibility: Sex and Society in Eighteenth-Century Britain* (Chicago: Chicago University Press, 1992).

Begiato, Joanne, 'Between Poise and Power: Embodied Manliness in Eighteenth- and Nineteenth-Century British Culture', *Transactions of the Royal Historical Society* 26 (2016), 125–47.

Begiato, Joanne, '"Breeding" a "Little Stranger": Managing Uncertainty in Pregnancy in Later Georgian England', in Jennifer Evans and Ciara Meehan (eds), *Perceptions of Pregnancy from the Seventeenth to the Twentieth Century* (Basingstoke: Palgrave Macmillan, 2017), 13–33.

Begiato, Joanne, *Manliness in Britain, 1760–1900: Bodies, Emotion, and Material Culture* (Manchester: Manchester University Press, 2020).

Begiato, Joanne, 'Punishing the Unregulated Manly Body and Emotions in Early Victorian England', in Joanne Ella Parsons and Ruth Heholt (eds), *The Victorian Male Body* (Edinburgh: Edinburgh University Press, 2018), 46–64.

Begiato, Joanne, 'Selfhood and "Nostalgia": Sensory and Material Memories of the Childhood Home in Late Georgian Britain', *Journal for Eighteenth-Century Studies* 42:2 (2019), 229–46.

Berkowitz, Carin, *Charles Bell and the Anatomy of Reform* (Chicago: Chicago University Press, 2015).

Boddice, Rob, *The History of Emotions* (Manchester: Manchester University Press, 2018).

Boddice, Rob, *A History of Feelings* (London: Reaktion, 2019).

Boddice, Rob, *The Humane Professions: The Defence of Experimental Medicine, 1876–1914* (Cambridge, UK: Cambridge University Press, 2020).

Boddice, Rob (ed.), *Pain and Emotion in Modern History* (Basingstoke: Palgrave Macmillan, 2014).

Boddice, Rob, *The Science of Sympathy: Morality, Evolution and Victorian Civilization* (Urbana: University of Illinois Press, 2016).

Bostetter, Mary, 'The Journalism of Thomas Wakley', in Joel H. Wiener (ed.), *Innovators and Preachers: The Role of the Editor in Victorian England* (London: Greenwood Press, 1985).

Bound Alberti, Fay, 'Bodies, Hearts, and Minds: Why Emotions Matter to Historians of Science and Medicine', *Isis* 100:4 (2009), 798–810.

Bound Alberti, Fay, *Matters of the Heart: History, Medicine and Emotion* (Oxford: Oxford University Press, 2010).

Bound Alberti, Fay (ed.), *Medicine, Emotion and Disease, 1700–1950* (Basingstoke: Palgrave Macmillan, 2006).

Bourdieu, Pierre, *The Logic of Practice* (Cambridge, UK: Polity Press, 1990).

Bourke, Joanna, *The Story of Pain: From Prayers to Painkillers* (Oxford: Oxford University Press, 2014).

Brock, Claire, *British Women Surgeons and Their Patients, 1860–1918* (Cambridge, UK: Cambridge University Press, 2017).

Brock, Claire, 'Risk, Responsibility and Surgery in the 1890s and Early 1900s', *Medical History* 57:3 (2013), 317–37.

Brooks, Peter, *The Melodramatic Imagination: Balzac, Henry James, Melodrama and the Mode of Excess*, 2nd ed. (New Haven: Yale University Press, 1995).

Brown, Michael, '"Bats, Rats and Barristers": *The Lancet*, Libel and the Radical Stylistics of Early Nineteenth-Century English Medicine', *Social History* 39:2 (2014), 182–209.

Brown, Michael, '"Like a Devoted Army": Medicine, Heroic Masculinity, and the Military Paradigm in Victorian Britain', *Journal of British Studies* 49:3 (2010), 592–622.

Brown, Michael, 'Medicine, Reform and the "End" of Charity in Early Nineteenth-Century England', *English Historical Review* 124:511 (2009), 1353–88.

Brown, Michael, *Performing Medicine: Medical Culture and Identity in Provincial England* (Manchester: Manchester University Press, 2011).

Brown, Michael, 'Redeeming Mr Sawbone: Compassion and Care in the Cultures of Nineteenth-Century Surgery', *Journal of Compassionate Healthcare* 4:13 (2017), https://doi.org/10.1186/s40639-017-0042-2.

Brown, Michael, 'Rethinking Early Nineteenth-Century Asylum Reform', *Historical Journal* 49:2 (2006), 435–52.

Brown, Michael, 'Surgery and Emotion: The Era before Anaesthesia', in Thomas Schlich (ed.), *Handbook of the History of Surgery* (London: Palgrave Macmillan, 2018), 327–48.

Brown, Michael, 'Surgery, Identity and Embodied Emotion: John Bell, James Gregory and the Edinburgh "Medical War"', *History* 104:359 (2019), 19–41.

Brown, Michael, 'Wounds and Wonder: Emotion, Imagination, and War in the Cultures of Romantic Surgery', *Journal for Eighteenth-Century Studies* 43:2 (2020), 239–59.

Burney, Ian, 'Anaesthesia and the negotiation of surgical risk in mid-nineteenth-century Britain', in Thomas Schlich and Ulrich Tröhler (eds), *The Risks of Medical Innovation: Risk, Perception and Assessment in Historical Context* (London: Routledge, 2006), 38–52.

Burney, Ian, *Bodies of Evidence: Medicine and the Politics of the English Inquest 1830–1926* (Baltimore: Johns Hopkins University Press, 2000).

Burney, Ian, 'Medicine in the Age of Reform', in Arthur Burns and Joanna Innes (eds), *Rethinking the Age of Reform: Britain, 1780–1850* (Cambridge, UK: Cambridge University Press, 2003), 163–81.

Bynum, William F., *Science and the Practice of Medicine in the Nineteenth Century* (Cambridge, UK: Cambridge University Press, 1994).

Bynum, William F., Lock, Stephen, and Porter, Roy (eds), *Medical Journals and Medical Knowledge: Historical Essays* (London: Routledge, 1992).

Carpenter, Mary Wilson, 'Lister's Relationships with Patients: "A Successful Case"', *Notes and Records of the Royal Society* 67:3 (2003), 231–44.

Carpenter, Mary Wilson, 'The Patient's Pain in Her Own Words: Margaret Mathewson's "Sketch of Eight Months a Patient in the Royal Infirmary of Edinburgh AD 1877"', *19: Interdisciplinary Studies in the Long Nineteenth Century* 15 (2012), http://doi.org/10.16995/ntn.636.

Condrau, Flurin, 'The Patient's View Meets the Clinical Gaze', *Social History of Medicine* 20:3 (2007), 525–40.

Crowther, M. Anne, 'Lister at Home and Abroad: A Continuing Legacy', *Notes and Records of the Royal Society* 67:3 (2013), 281–94.

Crowther, M. Anne, and Dupree, Marguerite, *Medical Lives in the Age of Surgical Revolution* (Cambridge, UK: Cambridge University Press, 2007).

Csengei, Ildiko, *Sympathy, Sensibility and the Literature of Feeling in the Eighteenth Century* (Basingstoke: Palgrave Macmillan, 2012).

Cunningham, Andrew, and Jardine, Nicholas (eds), *Romanticism and the Sciences* (Cambridge, UK: Cambridge University Press, 1990).

Davison, Lee, Hitchcock, Tim, Keirn, Tim, and Shoemaker, Robert (eds), *Stilling the Grumbling Hive: The Response to Social and Economic Problems in England, 1689–1750* (New York: St Martin's Press, 1992).

Desmond, Adrian, *The Politics of Evolution: Morphology, Medicine, and Reform in Radical London* (Chicago: University of Chicago Press, 1992).

Dixon, Thomas, '"Emotion": The History of a Keyword in Crisis', *Emotion Review* 4:4 (2012), 338–44.

Dixon, Thomas, *From Passions to Emotions: The Creation of a Secular Psychological Category* (Cambridge, UK: Cambridge University Press, 2003).

Dixon, Thomas, 'The Tears of Mr Justice Willes', *Journal of Victorian Culture* 17:1 (2012), 1–23.

Dixon, Thomas, *Weeping Britannia: Portrait of a Nation in Tears* (Oxford: Oxford University Press, 2015).

Dodman, Thomas, *What Nostalgia Was: War, Empire, and the Time of a Deadly Emotion* (Chicago: University of Chicago Press, 2018).

Donald, Diana, *Women against Cruelty: Protection of Animals in Nineteenth-Century Britain* (Manchester: Manchester University Press, 2019).

Downes, Stephanie, Holloway, Sally, and Randles, Sarah (eds), *Feeling Things: Objects and Emotions through History* (Oxford: Oxford University Press, 2018).

Ellis, Markman, *The Politics of Sensibility: Race, Gender and Commerce in the Sentimental Novel* (Cambridge, UK: Cambridge University Press, 1996).

Ellis, Richard H. (ed.), *The Case Books of Dr John Snow* (London: Wellcome Institute, 1994).

Epstein, James, *Radical Expression: Political Language, Ritual and Symbol in England, 1790–1850* (Oxford: Oxford University Press, 1994).

Faflak, Joel, and Wright, Julia M. (eds), *A Handbook of Romanticism Studies* (Chichester: Wiley, 2012).

Fairclough, Mary, *The Romantic Crowd: Sympathy, Controversy and Print Culture* (Cambridge, UK: Cambridge University Press, 2013).

Fissell, Mary E., 'The Disappearance of the Patient's Narrative and the Invention of Hospital Medicine', in Roger French and Andrew Wear (eds), *British Medicine in an Age of Reform* (London: Routledge, 1992), 92–109.

Fitzharris, Lindsey, *The Butchering Art: Joseph Lister's Quest to Transform the Grisly World of Victorian Medicine* (London: Allen Lane, 2017).

Foucault, Michel, *The Birth of the Clinic: An Archaeology of Medical Perception*, trans. A. M. Sheridan (London: Tavistock, 1973).

Fox, Nicholas J., 'Scientific Theory Choice and Social Structure: The Case of Joseph Lister's Antisepsis, Humoral Theory and Asepsis', *History of Science* 26:4 (1988), 367–97.

Frampton, Sally, *Belly-Rippers, Surgical Innovation and the Ovariotomy Controversy* (London: Palgrave Macmillan, 2018).

Frampton, Sally, and Wallis, Jennifer (eds), *Reading the Nineteenth-Century Medical Journal* (London: Routledge, 2021).

Gilmartin, Kevin, *Print Politics: The Press and Radical Opposition in Early Nineteenth-Century England* (Cambridge, UK: Cambridge University Press, 1996).

Gordon, Richard, *Great Medical Disasters* (New York: Stein and Day, 1983).

Granshaw, Lindsay, '"Upon This Principle I Have Based a Practice": The Development of Antisepsis in Britain', in John. V. Pickstone (ed.), *Medical Innovations in Historical Perspective* (Basingstoke: Palgrave Macmillan, 1992), 17–46.

Habermas, Jürgen, *The Structural Transformation of the Public Sphere: An Inquiry into a Category of Bourgeois Society*, trans Thomas Burger (Cambridge, UK: Polity Press, 1989).

Hadley, Elaine, *Melodramatic Tactics: Theatricalized Dissent in the English Marketplace, 1800–1885* (Stanford: Stanford University Press, 1995).

Halpern, Jodi, *From Detached Concern to Empathy: Humanizing Medical Practice* (Oxford: Oxford University Press, 2001).

Hanley, Anne, and Meyer, Jessica (eds), *Patient Voices in Britain, 1840–1948* (Manchester: Manchester University Press, 2021).

Harrison, Debbie, 'All the Lancet's Men: Reactionary Gentleman Physicians vs. Radical General Practitioners in the *Lancet*, 1823–1832', *Nineteenth-Century Gender Studies* 5:2 (2009), www.ncgsjournal.com/issue52/harrison.html.

Haslam, Fiona, *From Hogarth to Rowlandson: Medicine in Art in Eighteenth-Century Britain* (Liverpool: Liverpool University Press, 1996).

Hitchcock, Tim, King, Peter, and Sharpe, Pamela (eds), *Chronicling Poverty: The Voices and Strategies of the English Poor, 1640–1840* (New York: St. Martin's Press, 1997).

Hochschild, Arlie Russell, 'Emotion Work, Feeling Rules, and Social Structure', *American Journal of Sociology* 85:3 (1979), 551–75.

Hochschild, Arlie Russell, *The Managed Heart: Commercialization of Human Feeling* (Berkeley: University of California Press, 1983).

Hogarth, Stuart, 'Joseph Townend and the Manchester Infirmary: A Plebeian Patient in the Industrial Revolution', in Anne Borsay and Peter Shapely (eds), *Medicine, Charity and Mutual Aid: The Consumption of Health and Welfare in Britain, c.1550–1950* (Aldershot: Ashgate, 2007), 91–110.

Hollingham, Richard, *Blood and Guts: A History of Surgery* (New York: Thomas Dunne Books, 2008).

Hurren, Elizabeth, *Dying for Victorian Medicine: English Anatomy and Its Trade in the Dead Poor, c.1834–1929* (Basingstoke: Palgrave Macmillan, 2011).

Jacob, Margaret C., and Sauter, Michael J., 'Why Did Humphry Davy and Associates Not Pursue the Pain-Alleviating Effects of Nitrous Oxide?', *Journal of the History of Medicine and Allied Sciences* 57:2 (2002), 161–76.

Jacyna, L. S., 'Images of John Hunter in the Nineteenth Century', *History of Science* 21:1 (1983), 85–108.

Jansen, Patricia, 'Breast Cancer and the Language of Risk, 1750–1950', *Social History of Medicine* 15:1 (2002), 17–43.

Jewson, Nicholas D., 'The Disappearance of the Sick Man from Medical Cosmology, 1770–1870', *Sociology* 10 (1976), 225–44.

Jewson, Nicholas D., 'Medical Knowledge and the Patronage System in 18th Century England', *Sociology* 8:3 (1974), 369–85.

Jones, Claire L, Dupree, Marguerite, Hutchison, Iain, Gardiner, Susan, and Rafferty, Anne Marie, 'Personalities, Preferences and Practicalities: Educating Nurses in Wound Sepsis in the British Hospital, 1870–1920', *Social History of Medicine* 31:3 (2018), 577–604.

Kaartinen, Marjo, *Breast Cancer in the Eighteenth Century* (London: Pickering and Chatto, 2013).

Katz, Pearl, *The Scalpel's Edge: The Culture of Surgeons* (Needham Heights, MA: Allyn & Bacon, 1999).

Kelly, Laura, *Irish Medical Education and Student Culture, c.1850–1950* (Liverpool: Liverpool University Press, 2017).

Kennaway, James, 'Celts under the Knife: Surgical Fortitude, Racial Theory and the British Army, 1800–1914', *Cultural and Social History* 17:2 (2020), 227–44.

Kennaway, James, 'Military Surgery as National Romance: The Memory of British Heroic Fortitude at Waterloo', *War & Society* 39:2 (2020), 77–92.

Kipp, Julie, *Romanticism, Maternity, and the Body Politic* (Cambridge, UK: Cambridge University Press, 2003).

Lansbury, Carol, *The Old Brown Dog: Women, Workers, and Vivisection in Edwardian England* (Madison: University of Wisconsin Press, 1985).

Latour, Bruno, *Reassembling the Social: An Introduction to Actor-Network Theory* (Oxford: Oxford University Press, 2005).

Latour, Bruno, *Science in Action: How to Follow Scientists and Engineers through Society* (Cambridge, MA: Harvard University Press, 1987).

Lawrence, Christopher, 'Anaesthesia in the Age of Reform', *History of Anaesthesia Proceedings* 20 (1997), 11–16.

Lawrence, Christopher, 'Blood and Guts: Victorian Achievements in Surgery, *Times Literary Supplement* (4 May 2018), 28–9.

Lawrence, Christopher, 'Democratic, Divine and Heroic: The History and Historiography of Surgery', in Christopher Lawrence (ed.), *Medical Theory, Surgical Practice: Studies in the History of Surgery* (London: Routledge, 1992), 1–47.

Lawrence, Christopher, 'The Edinburgh Medical School and the End of the "Old Thing" 1790–1830', *History of Universities* 1 (1988), 259–86.

Lawrence, Christopher, 'Incommunicable Knowledge: Science, Technology and the Clinical Art in Britain, 1850–1914', *Journal of Contemporary History* 20:4 (1985), 503–20.

Lawrence, Christopher, 'Medical Minds, Surgical Bodies: Corporeality and the Doctors', in Christopher Lawrence and Steven Shapin (eds), *Science Incarnate: Historical Embodiments of Natural Knowledge* (Chicago: Chicago University Press, 1998), 156–201.

Lawrence, Christopher (ed.), *Medical Theory, Surgical Practice: Studies in the History of Surgery* (London: Routledge, 1992).

Lawrence, Christopher, 'Surgery and Its Histories: Purposes and Contexts', in Thomas Schlich (ed.), *The Palgrave Handbook of the History of Surgery* (London: Palgrave Macmillan, 2018), 27–48.

Lawrence, Christopher, and Brown, Michael, 'Quintessentially Modern Heroes: Surgeons, Explorers, and Empire, c.1840–1914', *Journal of Social History* 50:1 (2016), 148–78.

Lawrence, Christopher, and Dixey, Richard, 'Practising on Principle: Joseph Lister and the Germ Theories of Disease', in Christopher Lawrence (ed.), *Medical Theory, Surgical Practice: Studies in the History of Surgery* (London: Routledge, 1992), 153–215.

Lawrence, Christopher, and Weisz, George (eds), *Greater Than the Parts: Holism in Biomedicine, 1920–1950* (Oxford: Oxford University Press, 1998).

Lawrence, Susan, *Charitable Knowledge: Hospital Pupils and Practitioners in Eighteenth-Century London* (Cambridge, UK: Cambridge University Press, 1996).

Loudon, Irvine, *Medical Care and the General Practitioner* (Oxford: Oxford University Press, 1986).

Martín-Moruno, Dolores, and Pichel, Beatriz (eds), *Emotional Bodies: The Historical Performativity of Emotions* (Urbana: University of Illinois Press, 2019).

McAlister, David, *Imagining the Dead in British Literature and Culture, 1790–1848* (London: Palgrave Macmillan, 2018).

McCalman, Ian, *Radical Underworld: Prophets, Revolutionaries and Pornographers, 1795–1840* (Cambridge, UK: Cambridge University Press, 1988).

Meyer, Jessica, *An Equal Burden: The Men of the Royal Army Medical Corps in the First World War* (Oxford: Oxford University Press, 2019).

Miles, Tim, and Sinanan, Kerry (eds), *Romanticism, Sincerity and Authenticity* (Basingstoke: Palgrave, 2010).

Milligan, Barry, 'Luke Fildes' *The Doctor*, Narrative Painting, and the Selfless Professional Ideal', *Victorian Literature and Culture* 44:3 (2016), 641–68.

Moore, Wendy, *The Mesmerist: The Society Doctor Who Held Victorian Society Spellbound* (London: Weidenfeld and Nicholson, 2017).

Moscoso, Javier, *Pain: A Cultural History* (Basingstoke: Palgrave Macmillan, 2014).

Mosucci, Ornella, *Gender and Cancer in England, 1860–1948* (London: Palgrave Macmillan, 2016).

Navickas, Katrina, *Protest and the Politics of Space and Place 1789–1848* (Manchester: Manchester University Press, 2016).

Neuendorf, Mark, *Emotions and the Making of Psychiatric Reform in Britain, c. 1770–1820* (London: Palgrave Macmillan, 2021).

Newman, Ian, *The Romantic Tavern: Literature and Conviviality in the Age of Revolution* (Cambridge, UK: Cambridge University Press, 2019).

O'Connor, Erin, *Raw Material: Producing Pathology in Victorian Culture* (Durham, NC: Duke University Press, 2000).

Ofri, Daniel, *What Doctors Feel: How Emotions Affect the Practice of Medicine* (Boston: Beacon Press, 2013).

Papper, E. M., *Romance, Poetry and Surgical Sleep: Literature Influences Medicine* (Westport, CT: Greenwood Press, 1995).

Payne, Lynda, *The Best Surgeon in England: Percivall Pott, 1713–88* (New York: Peter Lang, 2017).

Payne, Lynda, *With Words and Knives: Learning Medical Dispassion in Early Modern England* (Aldershot: Ashgate, 2007).

Pennington, T. H., 'Listerism, Its Decline and Its Persistence: The Introduction of Aseptic Surgical Techniques in Three British Teaching Hospitals, 1890–99', *Medical History* 39:1 (1995), 35–60.

Pernick, Martin S., *A Calculus of Suffering: Pain, Professionalism and Anaesthesia in Nineteenth-Century America* (New York: Columbia University Press, 1985).

Pladek, Brittany, '"A Variety of Tastes: *The Lancet* in the Early Nineteenth-Century Periodical Press', *Bulletin of the History of Medicine* 85:4 (2011), 560–86.

Poole, Robert, '"To the Last Drop of my Blood": Melodrama and Politics in Late Georgian England', in Peter Yeandle, Katherine Newey, and Jeffrey Richards (eds), *Politics, Performance and Popular Culture: Theatre and Society in Nineteenth-Century Britain* (Manchester: Manchester University Press, 2016), 21–43.

Porter, Roy, 'Accidents in the Eighteenth Century', in Roger Cooter and Bill Luckin (eds), *Accidents in History: Injuries, Fatalities and Social Relations* (Amsterdam: Rodopi, 1997), 90–106.

Porter, Roy, *Bodies Politic: Death, Disease and the Doctors in Britain, 1650–1900* (London: Reaktion, 2001).

Porter, Roy, 'The Gift Relation: Philanthropy and Provincial Hospitals in Eighteenth-Century England', in Roy Porter and Lindsay Granshaw (eds), *The Hospital in History* (London: Routledge, 1989), 149–78.

Porter, Roy, 'Laymen, Doctors and Medical Knowledge in the Eighteenth Century: The Evidence of the *Gentleman's Magazine*', in Roy Porter (ed.), *Patients and Practitioners: Lay Perceptions of Medicine in Pre-Industrial Society* (Cambridge, UK: Cambridge University Press, 1985), 283–314.

Porter, Roy, 'The Patient's View: Doing Medical History from Below', *Theory and Society* 14:2 (1985), 175–98.

Prentice, Rachel, *Bodies in Formation: An Ethnography of Anatomy and Surgery Education* (Durham, NC: Duke University Press, 2013).

Prentice, Rachel, 'Drilling Surgeons: The Social Lessons of Embodied Surgical Learning', *Science, Technology and Human Values* 32:5 (2007), 534–53.

Reddy, William, *The Navigation of Feeling: A Framework for the History of the Emotions* (Cambridge, UK: Cambridge University Press, 2001).

Richardson, Alan, *British Romanticism and the Science of the Mind* (Cambridge, UK: Cambridge University Press, 2001).

Richardson, Ruth, *Death, Dissection and the Destitute* (London: Routledge and Kegan Paul, 1987).

Rosenwein, Barbara H., *Emotional Communities in the Early Middle Ages* (Ithaca, NY: Cornell University Press, 2006).

Rosenwein, Barbara H., *Generations of Feeling: A History of Emotions, 600–1700* (Cambridge, UK: Cambridge University Press, 2015).

Ruston, Sharon, *Shelley and Vitality* (Basingstoke: Palgrave Macmillan, 2005).

Sabor, Peter, and Trodie, Lars E. (eds), *Frances Burney: Journals and Letters* (London: Penguin, 2001).

Sanders, Mike, 'The Platform and the Stage: The Primary Aesthetics of Chartism', in Peter Yeandle, Katherine Newey, and Jeffrey Richards (eds), *Politics, Performance and Popular Culture: Theatre and Society in Nineteenth-Century Britain* (Manchester: Manchester University Press, 2016), 44–58.

Scarry, Elaine, *The Body in Pain: The Making and the Unmaking of the World* (Oxford: Oxford University Press, 1985).

Schlich, Thomas, 'The Days of Brilliancy Are Past': Skill, Styles and the Changing Rule of Surgical Performance', *Medical History* 59:3 (2015), 379–403.

Schlich, Thomas, 'The History of Anaesthesia and the Patient – Reduced to a Body?', *Lancet* 390:10099 (9–15 September 2017), 1020–1.

Schlich, Thomas, 'No Time for Statistics: Joseph Lister's Antisepsis and Types of Knowledge in Nineteenth-Century British Surgery', *Bulletin of the History of Medicine* 94:3 (2020), 394–422.

Schlich, Thomas, '"One and the Same the World Over": The International Culture of Surgical Exchange in an Age of Globalization, 1870–1914', *Journal of the History of Medicine and Allied Sciences* 71:3 (2016), 247–70.

Schlich, Thomas, *The Origins of Transplant Surgery: Surgery and Laboratory Science, 1880–1930* (Rochester, NY: University of Rochester Press, 2010).

Schlich, Thomas (ed.), *The Palgrave Handbook of the History of Surgery* (London: Palgrave Macmillan, 2018).

Schlich, Thomas, 'The Technological Fix and the Modern Body: Surgery as a Paradigmatic Case', in Ivan Crozier (ed.), *The Cultural History of the Human Body in the Modern Age* (London: Bloomsbury, 2010), 71–92.

Scott, Anne L., 'Physical Purity Feminism and State Medicine in Late Nineteenth-Century England', *Women's History Review* 8:4 (1999), 625–53.

Shaw, Philip, 'Longing for Home: Robert Hamilton, Nostalgia and the Emotional Life of the Eighteenth-Century Soldier', *Journal for Eighteenth-Century Studies* 39:1 (2016), 25–40.

Shaw, Philip, *Suffering and Sentiment in Romantic Military Art* (Aldershot: Ashgate, 2013).

Shepherd, John, 'The Civil Hospitals in the Crimea (1855–1856)', *Proceedings of the Royal Society of Medicine* 59:3 (1966), 199–204.

Skuse, Alana, *Constructions of Cancer in Early Modern England* (London: Palgrave Macmillan, 2015).

Smith, Mark, and Boddice, Rob, *Emotions, Sense, Experience* (Cambridge, UK: Cambridge University Press, 2020).

Smith, Olivia, *The Politics of Language, 1791–1819* (Oxford: Oxford University Press, 1984).

Snell, K. D. M., 'Belonging and Community: Understanding of "Home" and "Friends" among the English Poor', *Economic History Review* 65:1 (2012), 1–25.

Snow, Stephanie, *Blessed Days of Anaesthesia: How Anaesthetics Changed the World* (Oxford: Oxford University Press, 2008).

Snow, Stephanie, *Operations without Pain: The Practice and Science of Anaesthesia in Victorian Britain* (Basingstoke: Palgrave Macmillan, 2006).

Stanley, Peter, *For Fear of Pain: British Surgery, 1790–1850* (Amsterdam: Rodopi, 2003).

Steinke, Hubert, *Irritating Experiments: Haller's Concept and the European Controversy on Irritability and Sensibility, 1750–90* (Amsterdam: Rodopi, 2005).

Temkin, Owsei, 'The Role of Surgery in the Rise of Modern Medical Thought', *Bulletin of the History of Medicine* 25:3 (1951), 248–59.

Thompson, E. P., *The Making of the English Working Class* (New York: Pantheon Books, 1964).

Trilling, Lionel, *Sincerity and Authenticity* (London: Oxford University Press, 1972).

Tröhler, Ulrich, 'Statistics and the British Controversy about the Effects of Joseph Lister's System of Antisepsis for Surgery, 1867–1890', *Journal of the Royal Society of Medicine* 108:7 (2015), 280–7.

Waddington, Ivan, *The Medical Profession in the Industrial Revolution* (Dublin: Gill and Macmillan, 1984).

Waddington, Keir, 'Mayhem and Medical Students: Image, Conduct, and Control in the Victorian and Edwardian London Teaching Hospital', *Social History of Medicine* 15:1 (2002), 45–64.

Wahrman, Dror, *The Making of the Modern Self: Identity and Culture in Eighteenth-Century England* (New Haven: Yale University Press, 2004).

Wall, Rosemary, *Bacteria in Britain, 1880–1939* (London: Pickering and Chatto, 2013).

Wangensteen, Owen D., and Wangensteen, Sarah D., *The Rise of Surgery: From Empiric Craft to Scientific Discipline* (Minneapolis: University of Minnesota Press, 1978).

Warner, John Harley, 'The Aesthetic Grounding of Modern Medicine', *Bulletin of the History of Medicine* 88:1 (2014), 1–47.

Warner, John Harley, 'The Idea of Science in English Medicine: The "Decline of Science" and the Rhetoric of Reform, 1815–45', in Roger French and Andrew Wear (eds), *British Medicine in an Age of Reform* (London: Routledge, 1992), 136–64.

Wild, Wayne, *Medicine by Post: The Changing Voice of Illness in Eighteenth-Century British Consultation Letters and Literature* (Amsterdam: Rodopi, 2006).

Williams, Guy, *The Age of Agony: The Art of Healing, c.1700–1800* (Chicago: Academy Chicago Publishers, 1986 [1975]).

Williams, Guy, *The Age of Miracles: Medicine and Surgery in the Nineteenth Century* (Chicago: Academy Chicago Publishers, 1987 [1981]).

Winter, Alison, *Mesmerised: Powers of Mind in Victorian Britain* (Chicago: Chicago University Press, 1998).

Winter, Alison, 'Mesmerism and Popular Culture in Early Victorian England', *History of Science* 32:3 (1994), 317–43.

White, Paul, 'Introduction: The Emotional Economy of Science', *Isis* 100:4 (2009), 792–7.

Worboys, Michael, *Spreading Germs: Disease Theories and Medical Practice in Britain, 1865–1900* (Cambridge, UK: Cambridge University Press, 2000).

Yeandle, Peter, Newey, Katherine, and Richards, Jeffrey (eds), *Politics, Performance and Popular Culture: Theatre and Society in Nineteenth-Century Britain* (Manchester: Manchester University Press, 2016).

Youngston, A. J., *The Scientific Revolution in Victorian Medicine* (London: Croom Helm, 1979).

Index

of surgeons, 56, 67, 68, 75, 78, 80–1, 86–7,
94, 109, 180–1, 259, 260, 261, 263, 280
apothecaries, 118, 166; *see also* Society of
Apothecaries
Apothecaries Act, The, 156
Arnold, Edwin, 273
Ashwell, Samuel, 217
Association for the Advancement of Medicine
by Research, 265
Atkinson, James, 133–4

bacteriology. *See* germ theory
Baillie, Matthew, 24, 26
Barbers' Company, 19
Baume, Pierre Henri Joseph, 207
Bell, Benjamin, 32
Bell, Charles, 12, 20, 22, 36, 40, 59, 84, 86,
94, 157, 158, 175, 279, 282, 283
and detachment, 85–6
and masculinity, 88
and pain, 215–16
and vivisection, 187
emotional disposition of, 77–8, 81–2, 87, 260
natural theology of, 159
paintings of, 97
Bell, George, 72
Bell, John, 12, 34, 55, 79, 80, 173, 193
and embodied sensation, 109
and Romantic surgery, 8, 28, 32–3, 39–40,
76, 198, 262
and self-composure, 50
and surgical anatomy, 20, 28, 36, 37, 198
legacy of, 40–1
relations with patients, 91, 93–4
Bentham, Jeremy, 189, 204, 210
and anatomical dissection, 200–1
and emotion, 201, 202
and happiness, 201
dissection of, 201, 205–6
on pain, 191–2, 216
Bildung, 75, 186
biography, 15, 16, 31, 53, 77, 161, 162, 185–8,
237, 249, 262, 263, 268, 277, 281, 282
Birmingham General Hospital, 178
Bishop, John, 211
blood-letting. *See* therapeutics: blood-letting
Board, Ernest, 52
bodies, 28, 63, 74, 79, 99, 100, 115, 140, 145,
170, 190, 191, 195, 202, 205, 212, 229,
235, 241, 250, 251, 286; *see also* dead
bodies; embodiment
quiescent, 189, 213, 232–3
bones, 37, 144, 207
broken, 125, 129, 137, 138
compound fracture of, 128, 136, 137, 145,
173, 245

excision of, 51, 60, 61, 142
setting of, 82, 158
Brande, William Thomas, 224
Braxton Hicks, John, 253
British Medical Association, 155, 213, 239;
see also Provincial Medical and Surgical
Association
Brodie, Benjamin, 24, 71, 74, 90, 124, 223
and anatomical dissection, 204
and emotional self-restraint, 86–8
relations with patients, 94
Brown, John, 41–2, 87, 277
Burke, William, 207–8, 211
Burney, Frances, 84, 98, 110, 112
butchery. *See* surgeons: caricature of

Callaway, Thomas, 146, 158
Cameron, Hector Charles, 277
Cameron, Hector Clare, 255, 277
Camperdown, Battle of, 194
cancer, 119, 140
breast, 16, 41, 65–7, 69, 82, 91, 95–7,
99–105, 108, 111–2, 116–25, 127, 130,
131, 135
causes of, 98–9, 105–6, 118
facial, 60–1, 127–8, 142
historiography of, 97–8, 111
penile, 50
testicular, 101
Cargil, Lionel Vernon, 261
caricature. *See* surgeons: caricature of
casebooks, 15, 16, 91, 95–106, 107, 111, 115,
124, 127, 128, 130, 133, 136, 219, 226
cataract, 34, 234
Chalmers, Thomas, 235
charity, medical, 132, 134, 154, 176, 177, 218
chemistry, 10, 94, 215, 224, 240, 246, 250
Chesleden, William, 20, 24, 181, 259
Cheyne, William Watson, 237, 251, 252,
262, 271
Chiene, John, 252
children
as objects of sentiment, 9, 51, 68, 106–7,
116–17, 150, 177, 179, 208, 268–70
illness of, as cause of anxiety, 102–3
Clarke, James Fernandez, 161, 162
class, 15, 21, 111, 114, 158, 160, 162, 181,
189–90, 197, 208
Cline, Henry, 91, 93, 158–9, 186–7, 280
clinical medicine, 66, 68, 71, 105, 113–15,
123, 127, 131, 132, 156, 216–17, 252,
265; *see also* Paris: clinical revolution in
clothing, surgical, 85, 89
Cobbe, Frances Power, 266–8
Cobbett, William, 152, 209, 210
Coleridge, Samuel Taylor, 10, 139, 168

Webb Street School of Anatomy and
  Medicine, 157
Wellcome, Henry, 52
Westaby, Stephen, 285
Westminster Hospital, 39, 50, 142, 158, 226
Whelpdale, Andrew, 20–1, 23, 30, 55
widowhood, 103–4, 116–17, 200, 208
Williams, Thomas, 211
Wilson, George, 1–3, 6, 110, 126–7
Wintle, Frederick Thomas, 225
Wolseley, Garnet, Sir, 273

women's movement, 266–7
workhouse, 106, 132, 191, 196, 200, 203
wounds, 29, 83, 126, 128, 137, 140, 219, 232,
  243
  care of, 27, 133, 136, 158, 175, 240–1,
    245–50, 251, 255–7, 259
  surgical, 29, 80, 81, 109
  war, 85, 97, 194, 275

Yeo, Isaac Burney, 265
York County Hospital, 133–4

Printed in the United States
by Baker & Taylor Publisher Services